JOHN A. PUPILLO, M.D.

AN ATLAS OF
CARDIAC ARRHYTHMIAS

Vismar Publishing Co.

To Thomas, Erik and Noelle

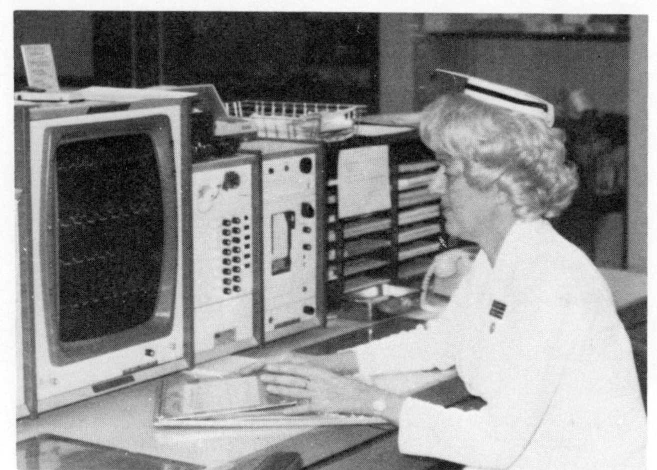

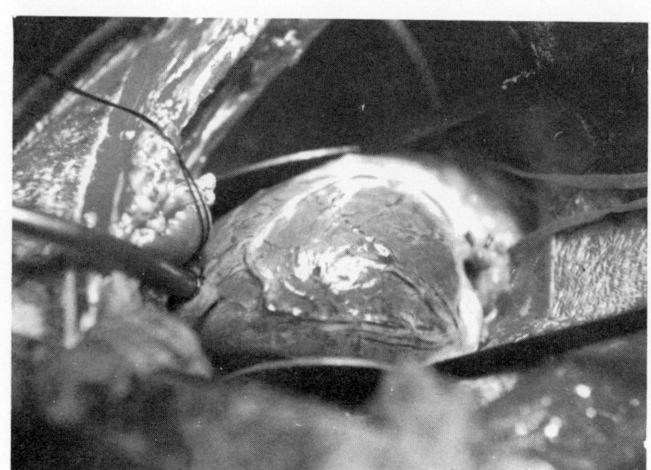

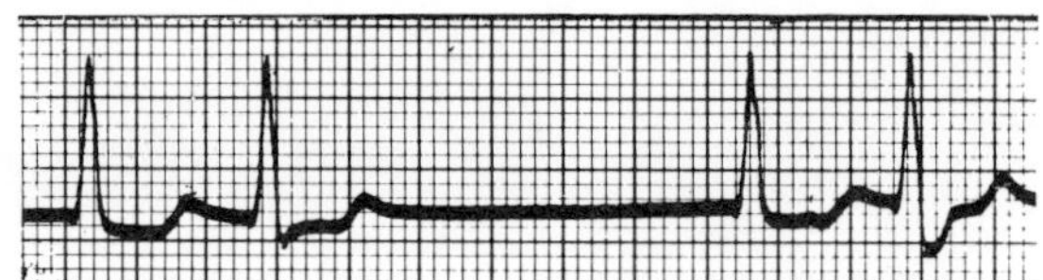

. . . to study the abnormal is the best way of understanding the normal. (William James)

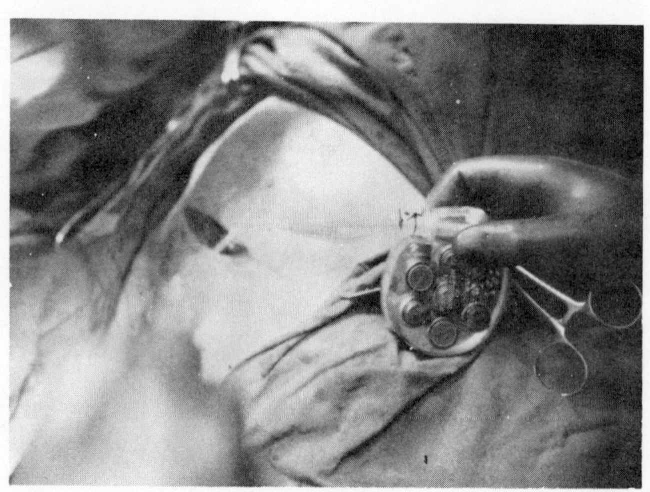

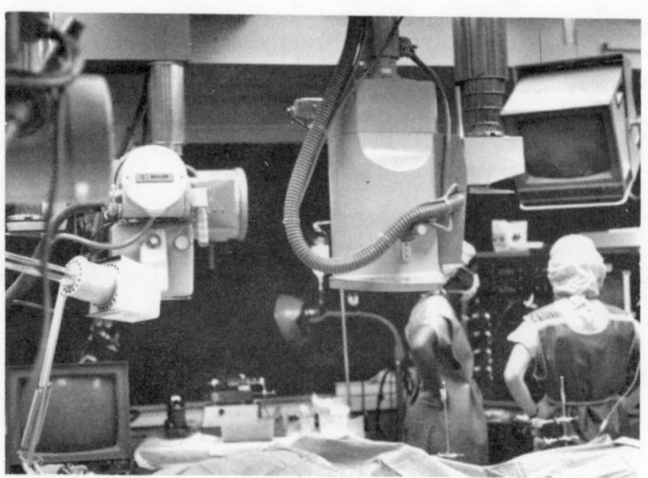

The only purpose of this Atlas is to present an illustrated classification of the most simple and most complex disturbances of the cardiac rhythm.

"The electronic cardiac era" in which we are profoundly involved has placed the cardiac arrhythmias in a position of great importance. The advent of telemetry, monitors, artificial pacemakers, cardioversion and defibrillation, and the progress of open heart surgery and resuscitation techniques require that doctors, and all those involved in the care of heart patients, be familiar with rhythms that depart from a normal sinus rhythm. The proliferation of Coronary Care Units and the better knowledge of cardiac arrhythmias permit to save many lives from "useless electrical deaths". An expert Coronary Care should not face today a sudden episode of ventricular fibrillation, since the doctor and the personnel can recognize premonitory arrhythmias, abnormal metabolic, nervous and humoral conditions which may develop, if untreated, in fatal arrhythmias. Therefore, this manual is primarly dedicated to all those who care for patients in Coronary and Intensive Care Units.

Recent is the memory of my school days when this important part of medicine was particularly difficult and confused. Enormous memory work and imagination was required, so that the student could differentiate one arrhythmia from another. Empirical methods were followed and adequate documentation was missing. Today several excellent publications are available on cardiac arrhythmias and they embrace much wider horizons. From them I have learned and to them I have referred. Convinced of the importance of visual aids in teaching, I have tried to bring a personal contribution to the field. Each arrhythmia is presented with appropriate ECG tracings, lifesize, without photographic manipulation, the way they were recorded at the bedside, in the Coronary Care Unit and in the Hemodynamic Lab. Many diagrams accompany the tracings, for a better understanding of the arrhythmias; a brief discussion about the main

*diagnostic criteria is on the opposite page. Particular evidence has been placed upon those rhythm distur-
bances which once were thought to be rare but that, with the advent of monitors, have been found to be
very common. Several pages are dedicated to parasystoles, reciprocal beats and reciprocal rhythms, aberrant ventricular conduction, "arrhythmia simulators" and the different manifestations of A-V dissociation.*

*A reference to specific mechanisms sustaining some of the arrhythmias is made only when necessary,
and when they are well known and accepted. Some arrhythmia mechanism, such as the Wenkebach
phenomenon, the Ashman phenomenon, fusion beats, etc. are treated in separate chapters, because they
are considered "key mechanisms" for the diagnosis of more complex arrhythmias. The etiology, therapy,
prognosis, and conditions associated with disturbance of the heart rhythm, have not been intentionally
considered and, therefore, the arrhythmias have been extrapolated from any clinical context.*

*Time intervals are expressed in seconds (for ex. 0.24 secs.), in milliseconds (for ex. 240 msec.) and, oc-
casionally, with entire numbers indicating hundredths of a second (for ex. 24 = 0.24 secs.). The following abbreviations have been used: ECG = electrocardiogram; PAC = premature atrial contraction; PVC
= premature ventricular contractions; PAT = paroxysmal atrial tachycardia; VT = ventricular
tachycardia; S-A = sino-atrial; A-V = atrio-ventricular; V-A = ventriculo-atrial; RBBB = right bundle branch block; LBBB = left bundle branch block; AUE = atrial unipolar electrogram; VUE =
ventricular unipolar electrogram; BE = bipolar electrogram; LV = left ventricle; BA-FA = brachial
and femoral artery.*

ACKNOWLEDGMENTS

It gives me great pleasure to acknowledge my indebtedness to those who inspired and taught me:

Dr. Henry Zimmerman	Dr. John Lister
Dr. Serge Barold	Dr. Lawrence Cohen
Dr. Philip Samet	Dr. Henry Marriott
Dr. Onkar Narula	Dr. Louis Bruno
Dr. Joseph Linhart	

TABLE OF CONTENTS

FORMATION AND CONDUCTION OF IMPULSES

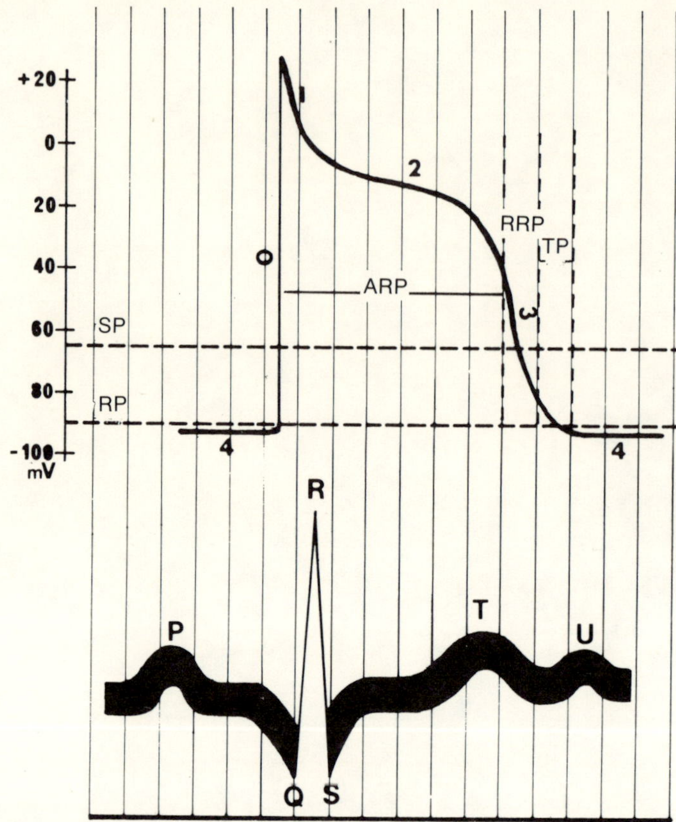

Fig. 1-A - Membrane potential of a non-automatic cell. ARP = absolute refractory period. RRP = relative refractory period. SP = supernormal period. RP = resting potential. TP = threshold potential.

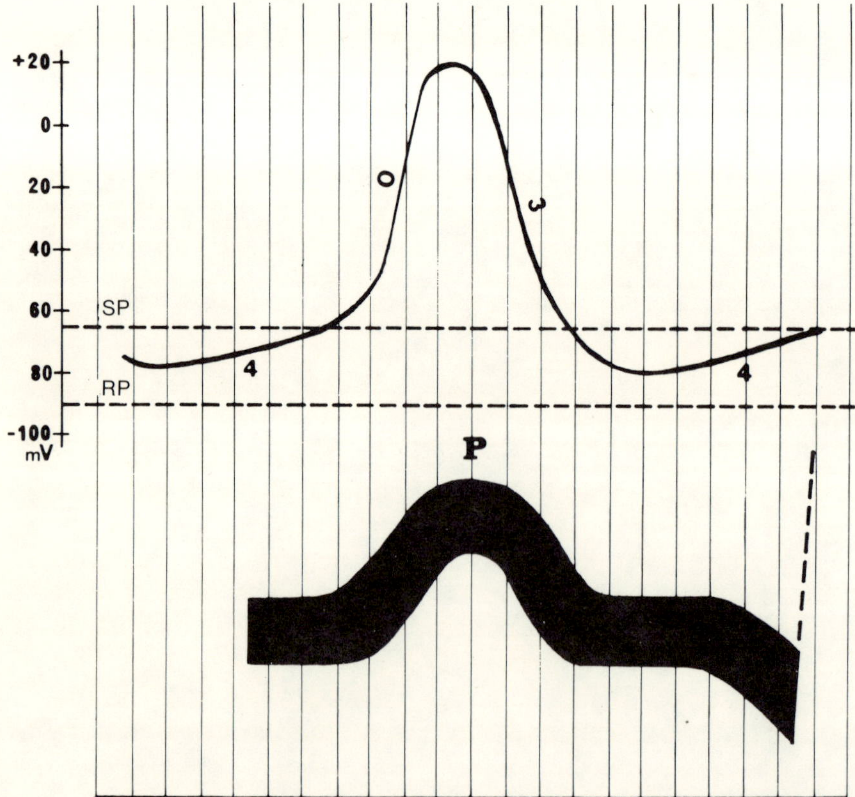

Fig. 1-B - Membrane potential of a spontaneously excitable cell (pacemaker cell). Notice the phase 4 ("diastolic depolarization"), the slower phase zero and the absence of phase 1 and 2.

FORMATION AND CONDUCTION OF IMPULSES

ELECTROPHYSIOLOGY NOTES

The myocardial fibers are excitable. They have an electric potential across the cellular membrane *(membrane potential or resting potential* = RP) which is determined by the negative intracellular and positive extracellular charges. At a resting state this is equal to -90 mV. The excitation of the myocardial fibers is obtained with passage of current (ions) through the cell membrane. It occurs if the current is sufficient enough to lower the membrane potential to a critical level called *threshold potential* (TP). The great majority of myocardial cells need a stimulus to be activated because they are not spontaneously excitable. In some special cells, however, the excitatory current flow is formed spontaneously. This property is called *"AUTOMATICITY"*. The automaticity is normally responsible for the spontaneous rhythm of the heart and for the genesis of a great number of cardiac arrhythmias.

Fig. 1-A illustrates the membrane potential of a contractile cell, which does not have the ability to form spontaneous impulses, while it is being activated. The membrane potential is characterized by five phases:

phase 4: It appears as a stable membrane potential of about -90 mV.

phase 0: The arrival of an impulse determines a rapid passage of current across the membrane. If this reaches the threshold value (TP), the cell is entirely depolarized and the potential rapidly reaches the zero mV. value, and goes up to + 20 mV., (*overshoot*).

phase 1: It is characterized by a rapid potential decline to values below zero mV.

phase 2: It is characterized by a slow repolarization plateau.

phase 3: It is characterized by a second rapid repolarization phase, till the membrane potential returns to the resting level (phase 4).

Therefore, phase 0 is the *"DEPOLARIZATION"*, while phase 1, 2 and 3 are the *"REPOLARIZATION"* phases. The depolarization results in the inscription of the QRS complex of the surface ECG, while the repolarization is included in the ST segment and the T wave.

The four phases represent the myocardial cell *"EXCITABILITY"*. Excitability is the ability to be depolarized by a stimulus. During the activation phases the cell will have: a) *an absolute refractory period* (ARP) during which a subsequent stimulus, no matter how intense, is totally ineffective; b) *a relative refractory period* (RRP) during which a subsequent stimulus may, in particular situations, again activate the cell; c) a *short supernormal excitability period* (SP) during which even a subliminal impulse may activate the cell; d) a fourth phase, also called *"diastolic phase"*, during which the cell is ready to receive a new stimulus and be depolarized.

Fig. 1-B presents the membrane potential of an automatic or pacemaker cell. It is characterized by a) a slow and spontaneous depolarization during phase 4 (*diastolic depolarization*), b) a much slower phase 0, c) an overshoot of less degree, d) a total absence of phase 1 and 2, and e) a predominant phase 3 of repolarization. The essential electrophysiological element in the *differentiation between a pacemaker and a non-pacemaker cell* resides, therefore, in phase 4. The non-automatic cells have a diastole without spontaneous depolarization, but with a constant and minimum potential. The automatic cells create, during phase 4, a spontaneous current flow across the membrane which reaches the threshold potential and thereby spontaneously depolarize.

FORMATION AND CONDUCTION OF IMPULSES

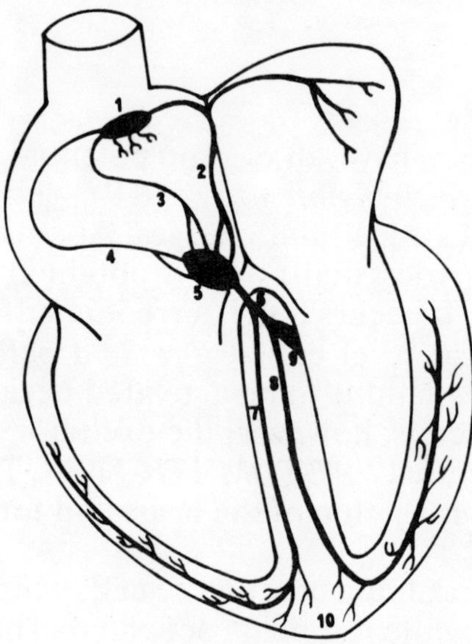

Fig. 2-A - Anatomy of specific cardiac conduction pathways. 1) S-A node 2) posterior internodal tract 3) mid-internodal tract 4) anterior internodal tract 5) A-V node 6) His bundle 7) right bundle 8) anterior fascicle of left bundle 9) posterior fascicle of left bundle 10) Purkinje fibers.

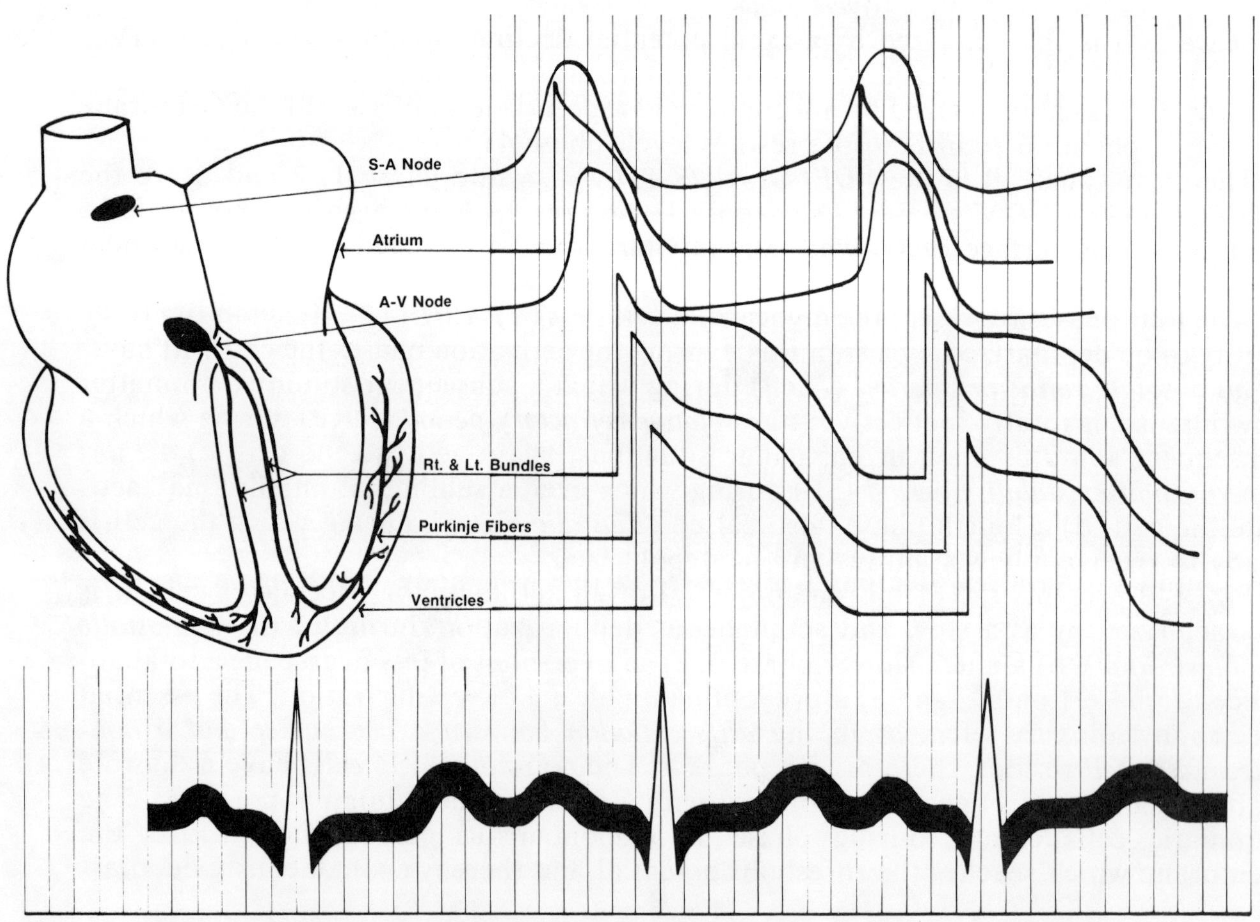

Fig. 2-B - Membrane potentials of different areas of the heart. Notice the morphology of depolarization and repolarization phases which characterize different areas of myocardial tissue.

FORMATION AND CONDUCTION OF IMPULSES

Once it is formed, the automatic pacemaker impulse is transmitted to the remaining myocardial tissue according to a well established sequence. The specific conduction pathways between the atria and the ventricles have been well defined and they are formed by:

Sino-atrial node (S-A) of Keith and Flack, located around the opening of the superior vena cava, on the right atrial epicardium (fig. 2-A n. 1).

Atrio-ventricular node (A-V) of Aschoff and Tawara situated below the orifice of the coronary sinus in the atrial septum (fig. 2-A n. 5).

His bundle, situated below the medial leaflet of the tricuspid valve (fig. 2-A n. 6).

Right bundle, made of a long, thin fascicle which runs along the ventricular septum to branch out into the Purkinje fibers of the right ventricle (fig. 2-A n. 7).

Left bundle which is formed by two fascicles, a long and thin *anterior fascicle* (fig. 2-A n. 8), and a short and thick *posterior fascicle* (fig. 2-A n. 9). Both fascicles branch out into the left ventricular Purkinje fibers.

Purkinje fibers (fig. 2-A n. 10), last and finest ramification of the specific right and left bundles which propagate within the myocardium of the two ventricles.

Recently, areas of specialized tissue have been found also within the atria; it appears that they represent specific conduction pathways for the propagation of the impulses from the S-A node to the A-V node. They are:

The anterior internodal tract of Bachman (fig. 2-A n. 4).

The mid-internodal tract of Wenckebach (fig. 2-A n. 3).

The posterior internodal tract of Thorel (fig. 2-A n. 2).

At a cellular level the impulse propagation occurs because a depolarized area of the cell works as a stimulus for the adjacent cell and so on. The repetition of this phenomenon results in the impulse *"CONDUCTION"*.

Fig. 2-B is the representation of the different membrane potentials recorded in different cardiac cells. From the morphology of the membrane potentials, it may be understood why the impulse propagation velocity is rapid in the atria, decreases markedly in the A-V node, resulting in an isoelectric line of the surface ECG (P-R interval), and becomes faster in more distal areas of the A-V node.

LADDER DIAGRAM

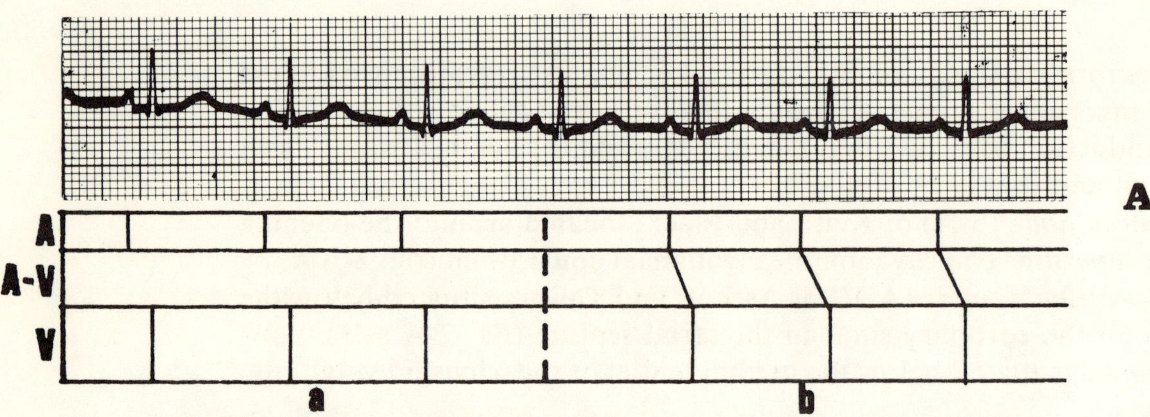

Fig. 3-A - Ladder diagram. A = atrial depolarization; A-V = conduction in the A-V junction; V = ventricular depolarization. The vertical lines in section "a" of the diagram represent the P waves and the QRS complexes. The diagonal line in "b" represents the A-V conduction.

Fig. 3-B - Ladder diagram. Section A can be enlarged to emphasize the atrial activation.

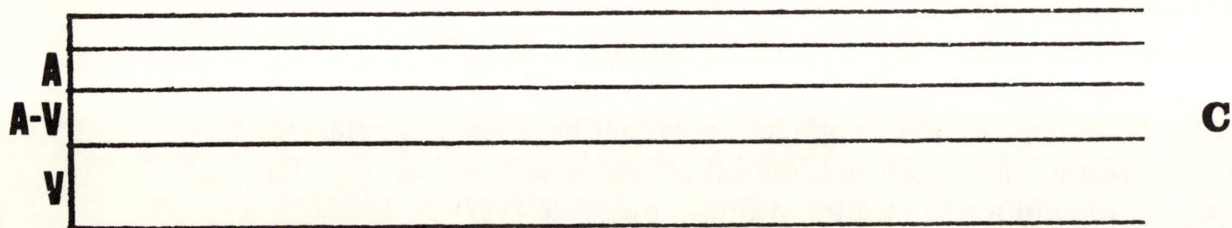

Fig. 3-C - Ladder diagram. An additional space may be added above "A" when the stimulus conduction between the S-A node and the adjacent atrial tissue must be emphasized.

Fig. 3-D - Ladder diagram. A space added below "V" can be used to show a parasystolic focus, an artificial pacemaker, etc.

LADDER DIAGRAMS

The ladder diagrams, also known as "Lewis lines", were first used by Sir Thomas Lewis in explaining the most complex arrhythmias. They will be used to elucidate difficult rhythms and to enhance the understanding of the underlying mechanisms.

Fig. 3-A shows the most commonly used ladder diagram. Each one of the spaces A, A-V and V are enclosed by four horizontal lines, which represent the atria, the A-V junction and the ventricles. The transmission of the impulse through the atria and ventricles will be represented by a vertical line just below the ECG tracing being examined. Line A must coincide with the P wave and line V will be drawn exactly below the QRS complex (fig. 3-A).

While the atrial and ventricular depolarizations write their own message clearly on the surface ECG, what happens in the A-V conduction tissue is understood only indirectly. As a general rule, therefore, when using this diagram, the first phenomenon to be diagrammed will be the P waves and then the QRS's (fig. 3-A a). When the atrial and ventricular activations are clearly depicted on the diagram, the connection of the A and V lines will elucidate what is happening in the A-V junction (fig. 3-A b). The direction in which the impulse travels will become evident when connecting the atrial and the ventricular activation lines. When it is necessary to underline what happens in a particular cardiac chamber, e.g. in the atria, the diagram will be represented as in fig. 3-B.

Additional horizontal lines can be added when focusing on the impulse conduction between the S-A node and the atrium (fig. 3-C), between a parasystolic focus and the adjacent myocardial tissue, or when representing the mechanism of an artificial pacemaker (fig. 3-D).

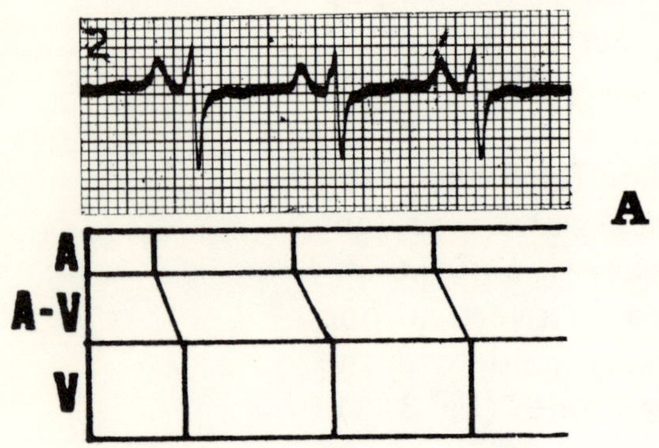

Fig. 4-A - Normal sinus rhythm.

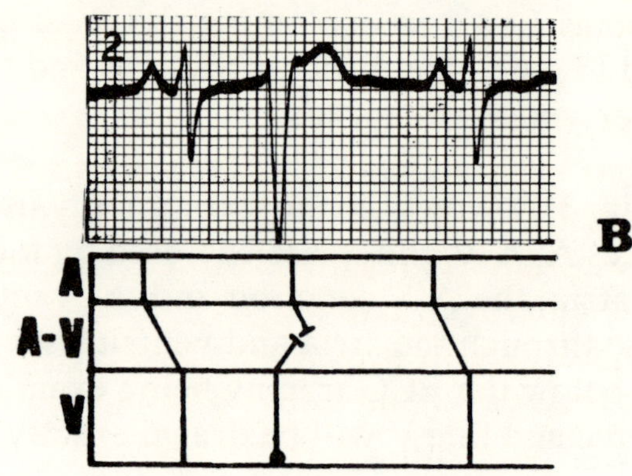

Fig. 4-B - Ventricular extrasystole.

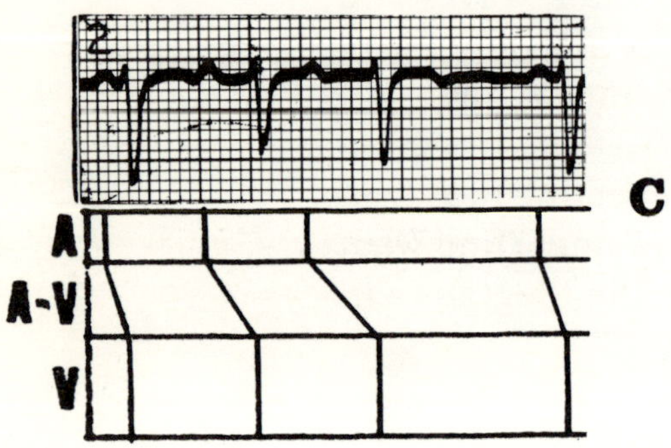

Fig. 4-C - Atrial extrasystoles.

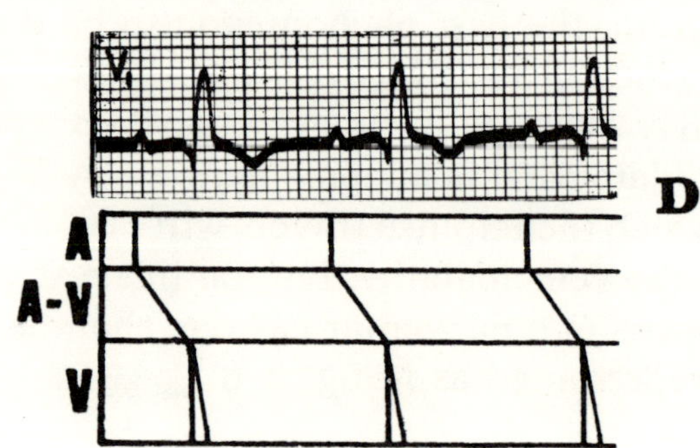

Fig. 4-D - Right bundle branch block.

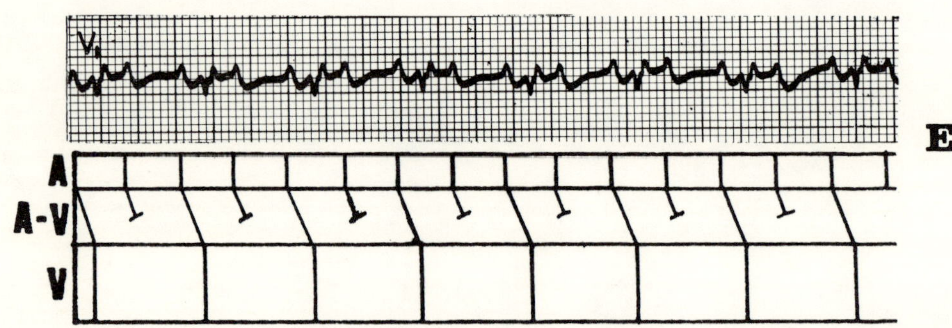

Fig. 4-E - Atrial tachycardia with 2:1 A-V block.

LADDER DIAGRAMS

A dot will be used to point out the site of ectopic impulse formation; a dash at a right angle to the main line will indicate a block in the propagation of the impulse, and a diagonal line will represent the A-V conduction. Bundle branch blocks and aberrant ventricular conduction will be represented by two slightly diverging lines.

Tracings of Fig. 4-A through 4-E and the corresponding ladder diagrams show: (A) normal sinus rhythm, (B) a normal sinus rhythm interrupted by a ventricular extrasystole, (C) a normal sinus rhythm and two atrial extrasystoles with progressive prolongation of the P-R interval, (D) a sinus rhythm with complete right bundle branch block, (E) and an atrial tachycardia with 2:1 A-V block.

MEASUREMENT OF THE HEART RATE

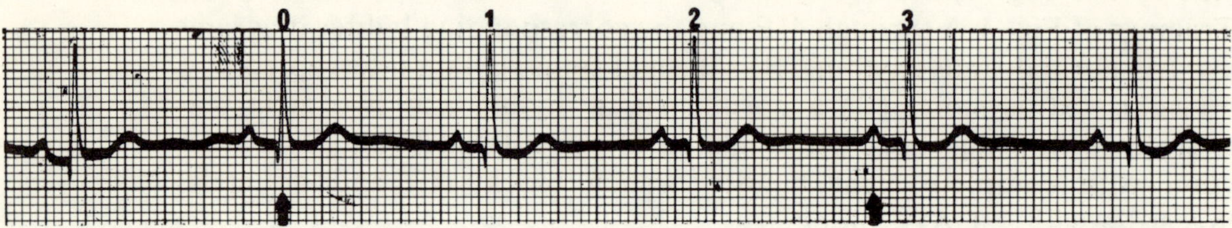

Fig. 5-A - Measurement of the heart rate. 2.8 R-R intervals are inscribed in three seconds (interval between the two arrows). Therefore, the rate will be 2.8 X 20 = 56/min.

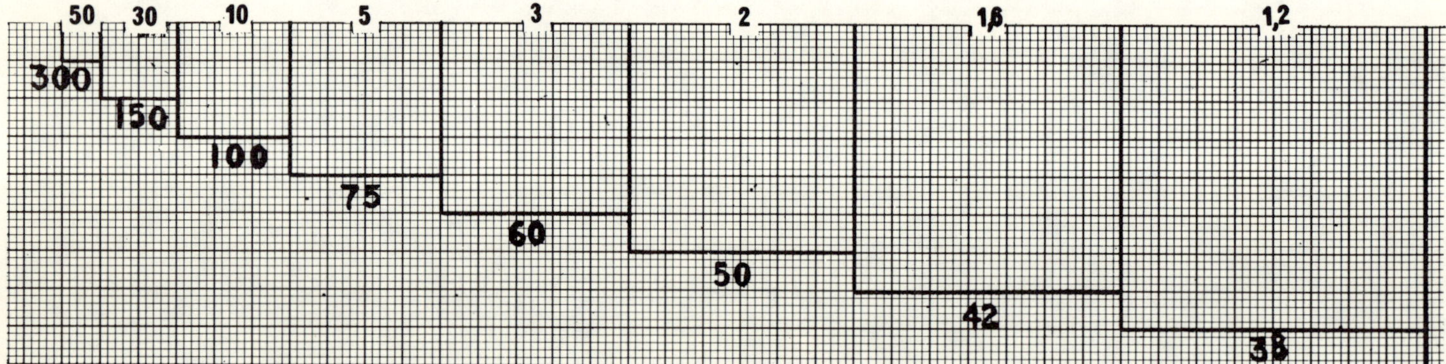

Fig. 5-B - Measurement of the heart rate. The bottom numbers indicate the rate values in relation to the 200 msec. squares. The top numbers indicate the additional rate values for each 40 msec. squares.

MEASUREMENT OF THE HEART RATE

The heart rate can be measured exactly by dividing the R-R interval (in seconds) into 60. (For example, if the R-R interval is equal to 0.70, the heart rate will be:

$$\frac{60}{0.70} = 85/min.$$

Figs. 5-A and 5-B present two quick ways of determining the heart rate by a simple glance at the ECG tracing.

In fig. 5-A, the heart rate can be measured as follows:

a)   first count the number of R-R intervals which appear during three seconds (fifteen big squares of 200 msec.). In fig. 5-A there are 2.8 R-R intervals.

b)   multiply the number of R-R intervals by 20 to obtain the heart rate/minute (2.8 x 20 = 56/min.).

Another easy and rapid method is presented in fig. 5-B. This enables one to immediately establish if the heart rate is above 100/min. or below 60/min. It is only necessary to determine how many big squares (the 200 msec. squares) are included within one R-R interval. If there are less than three, the heart rate is more than 100/min.; if there are more than five, the heart rate is below 60/min. Furthermore, fig. 5-B shows different values of heart rates in relation to the big and small squares of the standard ECG paper, e.g. if the R-R interval is equal to one large square, the rate will be 300/min.; if equal to four large squares the rate will be 75/min., and so on.

On the top of the tracing are indicated the values of rate increase and decrease in relation to each small square (40 msec.), e.g., if the R-R interval is equal to five large squares plus a small one (1240 msec.), it can be immediately stated that the heart rate is below 60/min. For the exact determination proceed as follows:

a)   the rates of 60 and 50 (difference = 10) are separated by a large square which is made up of five small squares. Each of the small squares will be

$$\frac{10}{5} = 2$$

and the heart rate will therefore be 60-2 = 58/min.

A second example:

b)   between 150 and 100 the difference is 50. Each small square is therefore equal to

$$\frac{50}{5} = 10 \text{ and so on.}$$

Once this method becomes familiar, it is quite easy to measure the heart rate with remarkable speed and accuracy.

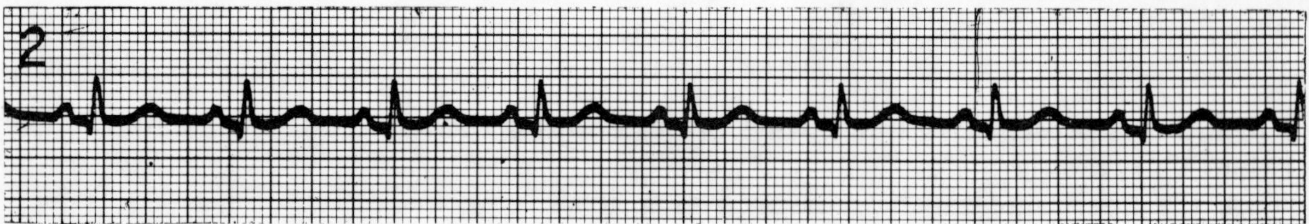

Fig. 6-A - Normal sinus rhythm.

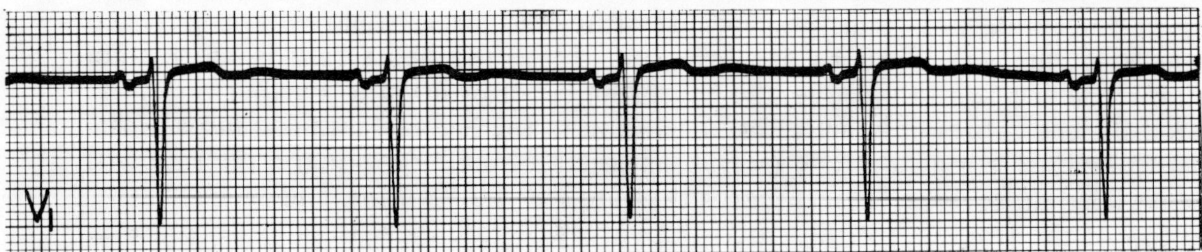

Fig. 6-B - Sinus bradycardia - The heart rate is below 60/min.

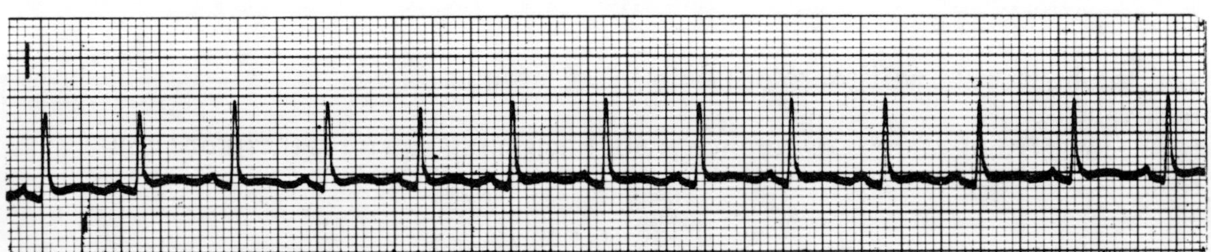

Fig. 6-C - Sinus tachycardia - The heart rate is above 100/min.

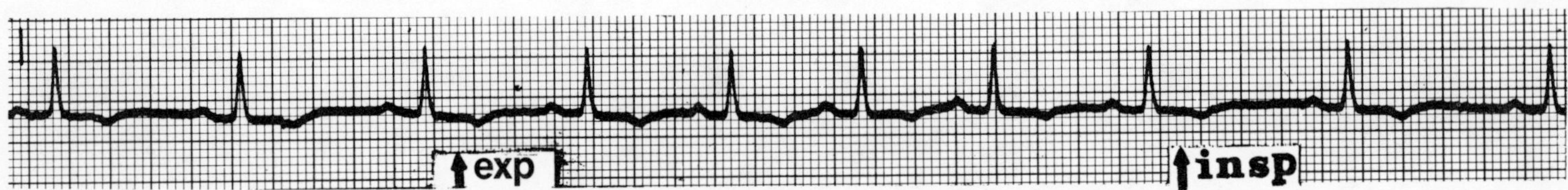

Fig. 6-D - Sinus arrhythmia - There is a relationship with the respiratory phases. A cyclic increase and decrease of the heart rate is present in relation to expiration and inspiration.

NORMAL SINUS RHYTHM

Fig. 6-A presents a normal sinus rhythm. The rate is 85/min. and the QRS complexes show a normal morphology and are all preceded by a P wave. The P-R interval is normal (between 120-200 msec.).

SINUS BRADYCARDIA

A sinus bradycardia is shown in fig. 6-B. The only difference from a normal sinus rhythm is the rate which, in this case, is equal to 48/min. The minimal rate limit for a normal sinus rhythm has been conventionally set at 60/min.

SINUS TACHYCARDIA

When the rate of formation of impulses in the S-A node is above 100/min., the resulting rhythm is called sinus tachycardia (fig. 6-C).

SINUS ARRHYTHMIA

When the sinus rhythm presents cyclic rate variations in phase with respiration, it is called respiratory sinus arrhythmia (fig. 6-D).

ARRHYTHMIAS DUE TO ABNORMAL IMPULSE FORMATION

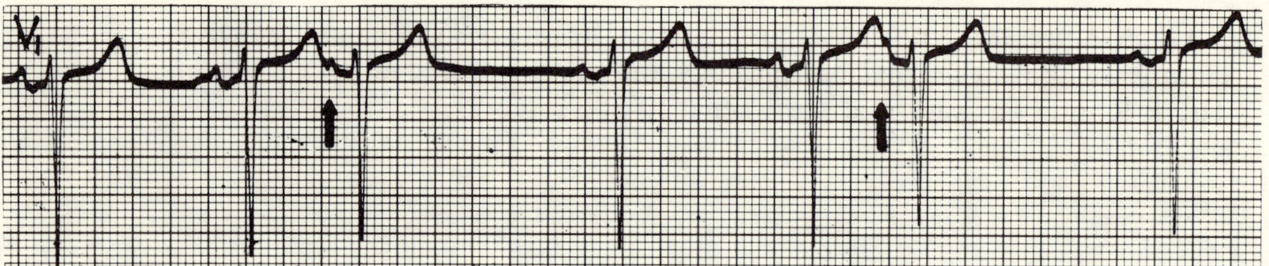

Fig. 7-A PAC's - P¹ waves are easily recognized and the extrasystolic QRS complexes are similar to those of sinus beats.

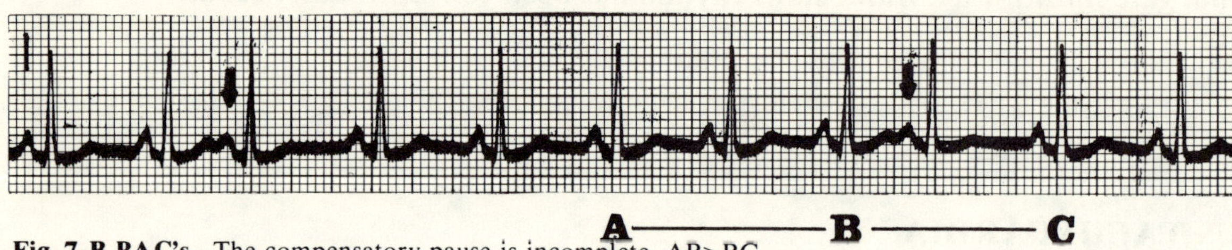

Fig. 7-B PAC's - The compensatory pause is incomplete. AB>BC.

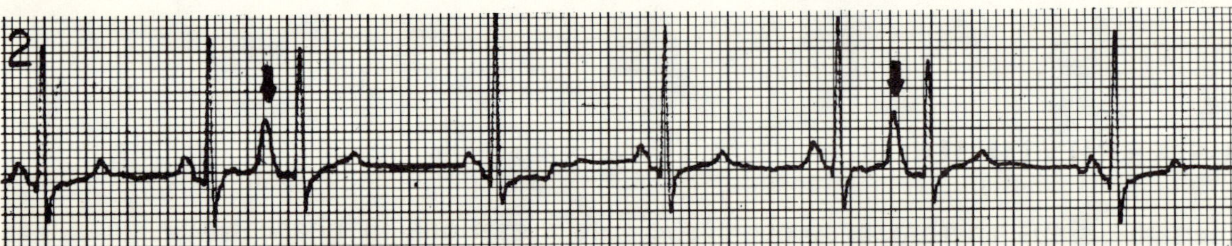

Fig. 7-C PAC's - Arrows indicate the P¹ waves concealed within the preceding tall and peaked T waves.

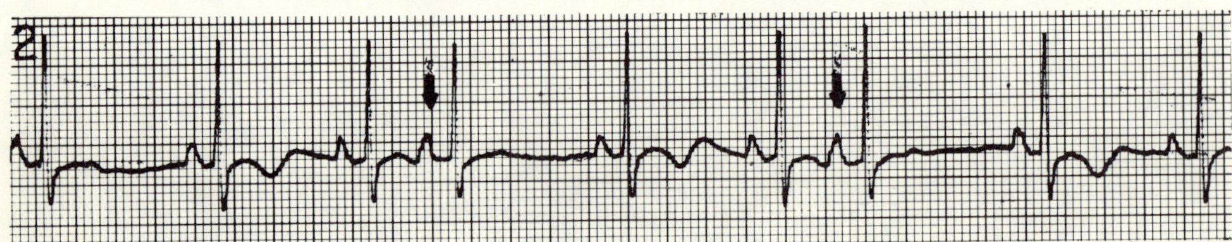

Fig. 7-D PAC's - P¹ waves alter the morphology of the preceding T waves which appear biphasic.

ARRHYTHMIAS DUE TO ABNORMAL IMPULSE FORMATION

A - ISOLATED OR INTERMITTENT

ATRIAL EXTRASYSTOLES (PAC = Premature atrial contraction)

In the classic form of atrial extrasystole the basic cardiac rhythm is prematurely interrupted by a QRS complex with a normal morphology and preceded by a premature P wave (P^1 wave). The letter "P^1" indicates an atrial depolarization of other than sinus origin (e.g., from an atrial ectopic focus or from a retrograde impulse).

Fig. 7-A and 7-B show two cases of sinus rhythm punctuated by atrial premature beats. P^1 waves are easily recognized and they appear on the descending limb of the preceding T waves (arrows). The P^1-R intervals and the QRS complexes are similar to those of sinus beats. The compensatory pause following the PAC's is incomplete (AB>BC), (fig. 7-B). The compensatory pause will be discussed in detail when illustrating the ventricular extrasystoles (page 19).

VARIANTS:

Three factors can disguise the presence of atrial extrasystoles and interfere with their recognition:
a) *"Cherchez le P^1"*.
In the majority of cases, the P^1 wave is so premature within the cardiac cycles of sinus origin that it falls within the preceding T wave. This fact produces a T wave markedly different from other T waves and usually taller, peaked or biphasic. A quick comparison between this and other T waves is generally sufficient to spot a premature P^1 wave.

The two arrows in fig. 7-C point to two obviously unusual T waves which precede two premature but normal looking QRS's. They indicate two atrial premature beats (PAC's) whose P^1 waves are fused with the preceding T waves and result in high amplitude T waves.

In fig. 7-D, the P^1 waves are again buried within the preceding T waves and result, this time, in biphasic P^1 waves. Note that the morphology and amplitude of these waves result from the algebraic summation of T and P^1 amplitudes.

ARRHYTHMIAS DUE TO ABNORMAL IMPULSE FORMATION

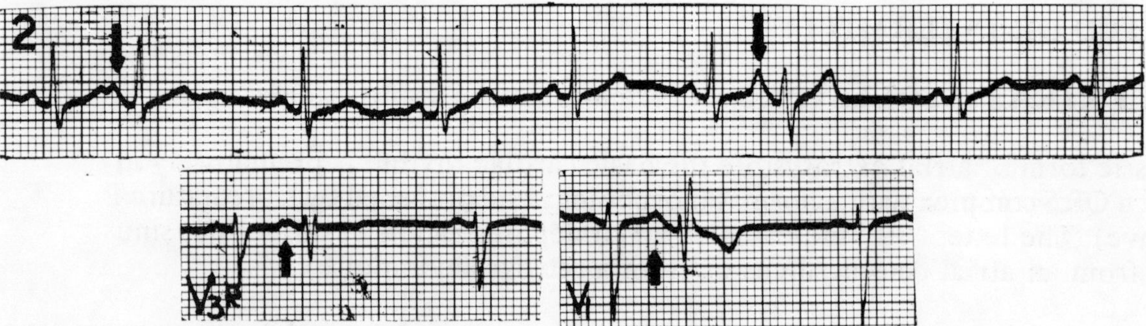

Fig. 8-A - PAC with aberrant conduction. P¹ waves are indicated by the arrows. The aberrant conduction is of a right bundle branch block type.

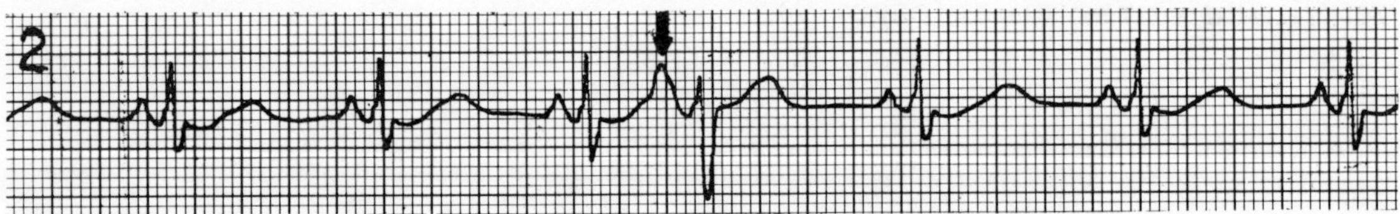

Fig. 8-B - PAC with aberrant ventricular conduction.

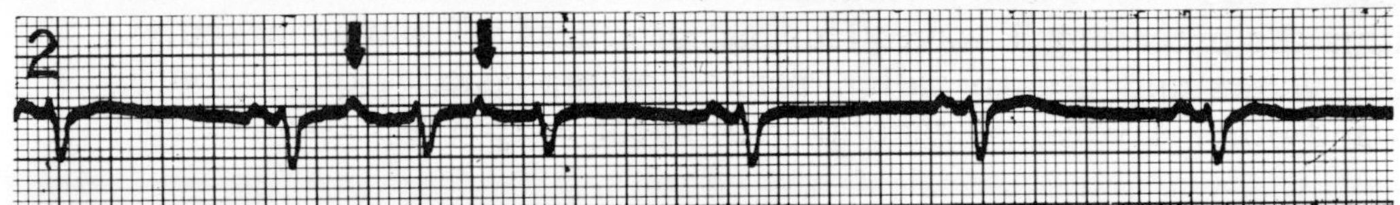

Fig. 8-C - PAC's with prolongation of the P¹-R interval.

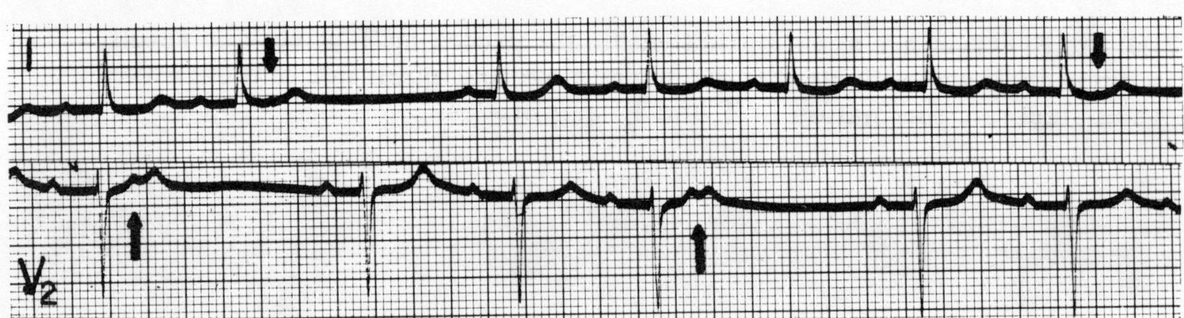

Fig. 8-D - Blocked PAC's. The arrows indicate the blocked premature P¹ waves. They are not followed by a QRS complex.

ATRIAL EXTRASYSTOLES (PAC's)

VARIANTS:

b) Aberrant ventricular conduction.

This is a situation which very often simulates the presence of ventricular extrasystoles. *Aberrant conduction or ventricular aberration* indicates an intraventricular conduction disturbance of a supraventricular impulse. Unlike a continuous or intermittent bundle branch block, aberrant ventricular conduction does not indicate a pathology of the A-V conduction system. It is an electrophysiologic phenomenon induced by sudden variations of cardiac rate.

The upper tracing (L2) of fig. 8-A shows two atrial extrasystoles. While the QRS morphology of the first PAC is equal to that of sinus beats, the second PAC shows a delay in the terminal forces and a deviation of the electrical axis to the left. The atrial premature beats recorded in V3R and V1 show an rSR^1 type of complex, which indicates a conduction delay within the right bundle.

A similar situation is presented in fig. 8-B. Electrophysiologically, the right bundle has the longest repolarization time of the entire A-V conduction system. Therefore, in the majority of cases, very premature impulses coming from the atria, or from anywhere above the His bundle, may show an aberrant ventricular conduction of the right bundle branch block type, incomplete or complete. The knowledge of this possibility and the identification of a P^1 wave may help in differentiating PAC's with aberrant ventricular conduction from ventricular extrasystoles.

Atrial extrasystoles may have a shorter, normal or prolonged P^1-R interval. The length of the P^1-R interval depends on the prematurity of the extrasystole, the state of repolarization of the A-V junction and the origin of the ectopic focus.

Fig. 8-C has two PAC's following two sinus beats. Both extrasystoles show a clearly prolonged P^1-R interval. (Note, however, that when the P^1 wave is overimposed on the preceding T wave, it is sometimes difficult to determine the exact length of the P^1-R interval). The atrial extrasystoles are quite premature and are conducted to the ventricles with delay. They find the A-V conduction tissue partly refractory and, therefore, with a decreased conduction velocity.

c) Blocked atrial extrasystoles.

They are very common but not easily recognized, especially when the premature P^1 wave is not conspicuous and clearly visible in the lead being recorded (fig. 8-D). A careful examination of the tracing usually enables one to identify the P^1 waves buried with the ST segment of the preceding beat (arrows).

The extrasystoles are so premature that they are blocked within the totally refractory A-V conduction tissue. The compensatory pause is not complete. The presence of blocked PAC's must be kept in mind when facing sudden asystolic pauses. Again *"Cherchez le P^1"* and compare the T wave of the beat preceding the extrasystole with other T waves.

ARRHYTHMIAS DUE TO ABNORMAL IMPULSE FORMATION

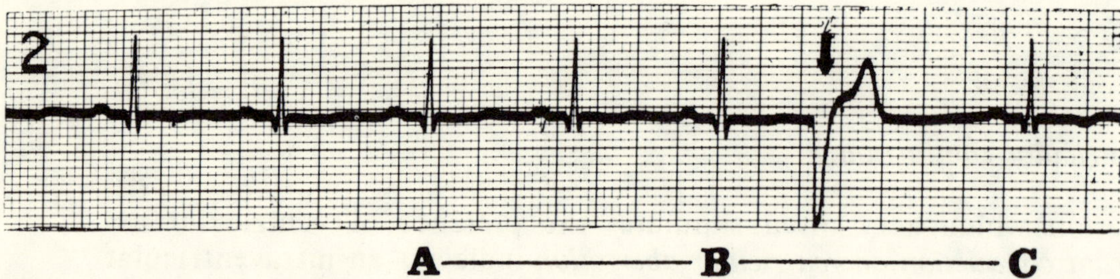

Fig. 9-A - Ventricular extrasystoles. The morphology of the PVC's is bizarre and different from that of other QRS's. The compensatory pause is complete.

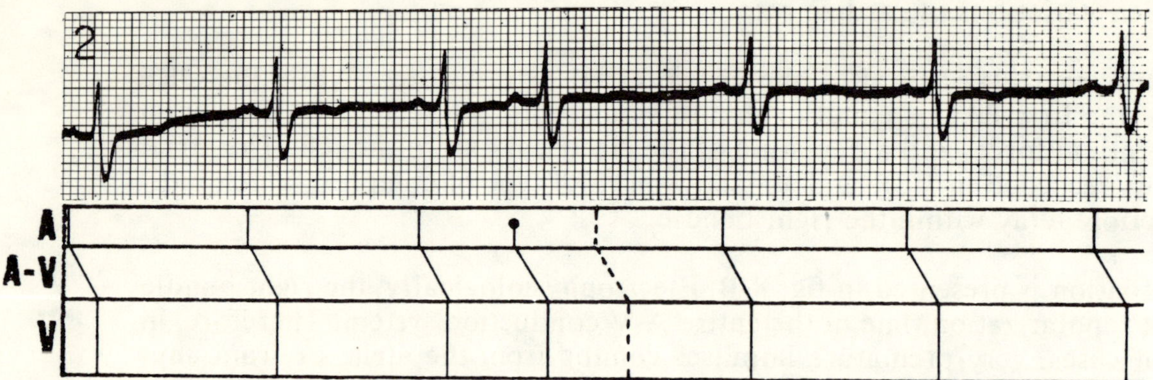

Fig. 9-B - Atrial extrasystoles. The S-A node is prematurely depolarized by the PAC. Dashes indicate the moment in which a sinus beat would appear if the S-A node is not suppressed by the ectopic stimulus. The compensatory pause is not complete.

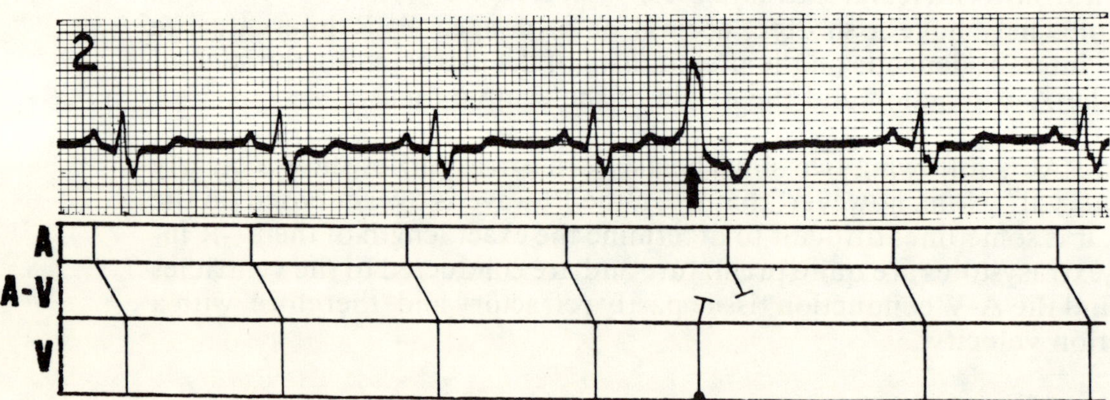

Fig. 9-C - Ventricular extrasystole. The PVC penetrates the A-V junction but does not reach the S-A node. The following sinus impulse propagates normally into the atria and is blocked in the A-V junction. The compensatory pause is complete.

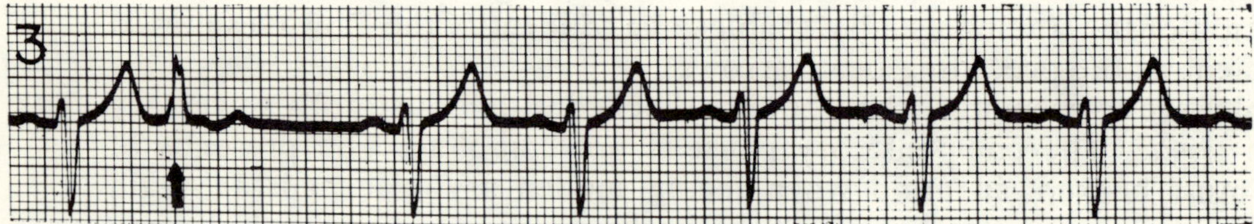

Fig. 9-D - Ventricular extrasystole. The compensatory pause is complete.

ARRHYTHMIAS DUE TO ABNORMAL IMPULSE FORMATION

VENTRICULAR EXTRASYSTOLES (PVC = Premature Ventricular Contraction)

In the contest of a tranquil sinus rhythm, the classical form of ventricular extrasystole (PVC) sticks out suddenly as a "bizarre, wide and abnormal QRS complex" (fig. 9-A). The impulse originates in a ventricular ectopic focus and it propagates by following a specific conduction tissue. The vectorial representation of the QRS is anomalous and resembles that of a QRS complex with a right or left bundle branch block. The QRS is wide, bizarre, premature and not preceded by a P wave. Unlike atrial extrasystoles (fig. 9-B) PVC's are usually followed by a *complete compensatory pause* (AB = BC).

THE COMPENSATORY PAUSE

As a general rule, a premature beat coming from an ectopic atrial or ventricular focus may reach the sino-atrial node and depolarize it prematurely, before it delivers its own impulse, (which normally controls the heart rhythm and propagates according to specific conduction pathways). If this happens, the sino-atrial node is depolarized and it restarts a new impulse-formation cycle. This determines a pause which terminates with the propagation of the following sinus impulse. The pause is called *compensatory pause or complementary pause* and it is calculated by measuring the interval of time between the two QRS complexes which include the extrasystole and by comparing it to two successive regular R-R intervals.

The different length of the compensatory pause following atrial or ventricular extrasystoles, is due to what happens in the sino-atrial node during the propagation of the extrasystolic impulse. In the majority of cases, *the sino-atrial node is penetrated and depolarized prematurely by atrial extrasystoles and not by ventricular extrasystoles* (fig. 9-B). The latter usually die during their retrograde trip in the A-V junction following the aberrant ventricular depolarization. The next sinus impulse, undisturbed by the ventricular extrasystole, is blocked in the refractory A-V junction (fig. 9-C and 9-D).

Therefore, the *compensatory pause determined by atrial extrasystoles* is usually shorter than two normal cardiac cycles and it is called *incomplete* (fig. 9-B). *A ventricular extrasystole*, instead, *determines* a pause equal to two sinus cycles which is called *complete compensatory pause* (figs. 9-A, 9-C and 9-D). However, note that the type of compensatory pause is only an indication and not a differential criteria between atrial and ventricular extrasystoles. The pause only indicates whether the sinus node is or is not being depolarized by the premature beat. Occasionally it is possible to find a ventricular extrasystole with an incomplete compensatory pause and an atrial extrasystole with a complete compensatory pause.

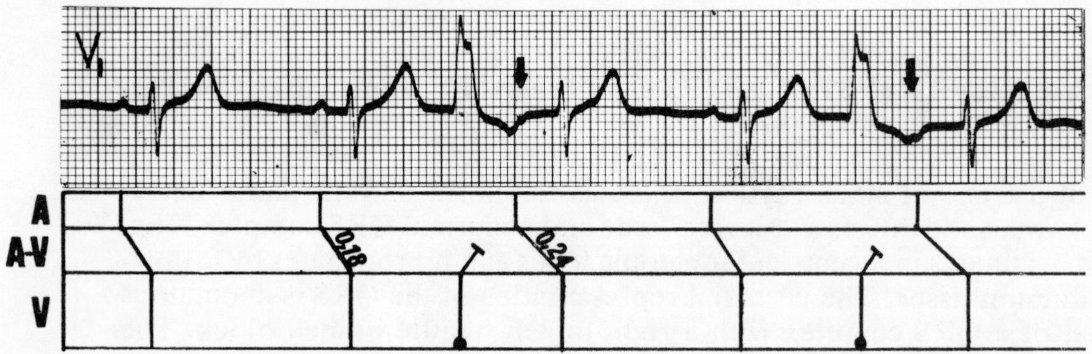

Fig. 10-A - Interpolated PVC's. The sinus rhythm is not altered. The arrows indicate sinus P waves, with prolonged P-R intervals, for the retrograde, "concealed" conduction of the PVC in the A-V junction.

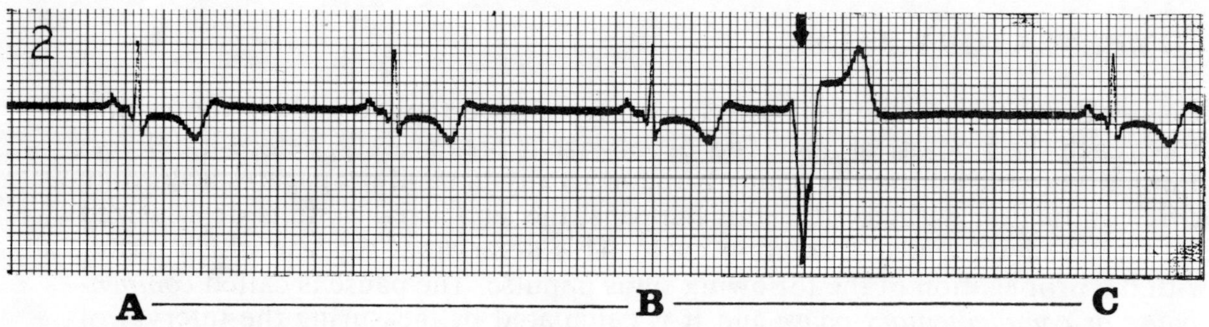

Fig. 10-B - Ventricular extrasystole with incomplete compensatory pause. The PVC penetrates in a retrograde fashion into the atria and depolarizes the S-A node. The compensatory pause is not complete.

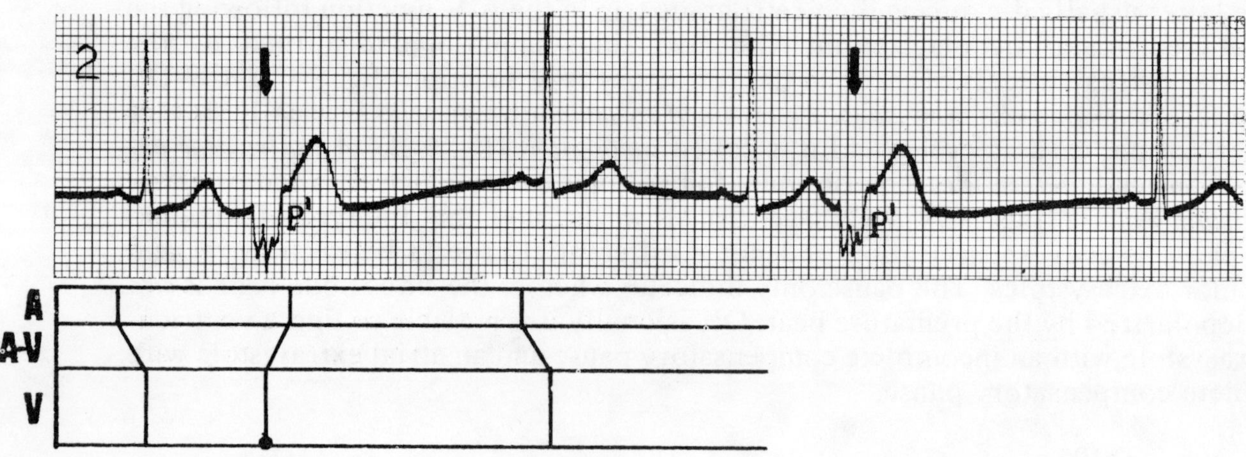

Fig. 10-C - PVC's with retrograde conduction to the atria (P¹). The compensatory pause is not complete.

VARIANTS:

a) INTERPOLATED VENTRICULAR EXTRASYSTOLES

Occasionally a ventricular extrasystole may be "sandwiched" between two normal ventricular complexes. These extrasystoles are called *interpolated* and are usually found within the contest of bradycardic rhythms.

Fig. 10-A shows two interpolated ventricular extrasystoles with an incomplete compensatory pause. The sinus rhythm is not altered by the extrasystoles. A closer observation of the tracing reveals that the P-R interval of the sinus beats following the PVC is prolonged when compared to other P-R intervals. This occurs quite often and indicates a *concealed retrograde ventriculo-atrial conduction of the PVC.* In a retrograde fashion, the extrasystole has penetrated the A-V junction and has rendered it partially refractory so that the A-V conduction of the following sinus beat is prolonged. Therefore, the presence of a *concealed V-A conduction* is revealed by the length of the P-R interval of the sinus beat following the extrasystoles.

b) VENTRICULAR EXTRASYSTOLES WITH RETROGRADE CONDUCTION TO THE ATRIA

It is also quite common to find PVC's which penetrate the A-V junction and depolarize the atria in a retrograde fashion (figs. 10-B and 10-C). The compensatory pause following this type of extrasystoles is always incomplete (AB>BC) because of the PVC's suppress the sinus node.

The P^1 waves are not easily recognized and frequently they are buried in the extrasystolic ST segment (fig. 10-B). They are negative waves when compared to sinus P waves, and premature when compared to basic P-P intervals (fig. 10-C). When P^1 waves are evident the R-P^1 interval, and by that the retrograde V-A conduction time, may be determined. This is measured from the beginning of the QRS to the beginning of the P^1 wave and it usually measures between 0.16-0.20 seconds. When it is prolonged it indicates a *retrograde ventriculo-atrial block.*

ARRHYTHMIAS DUE TO ABNORMAL IMPULSE FORMATION

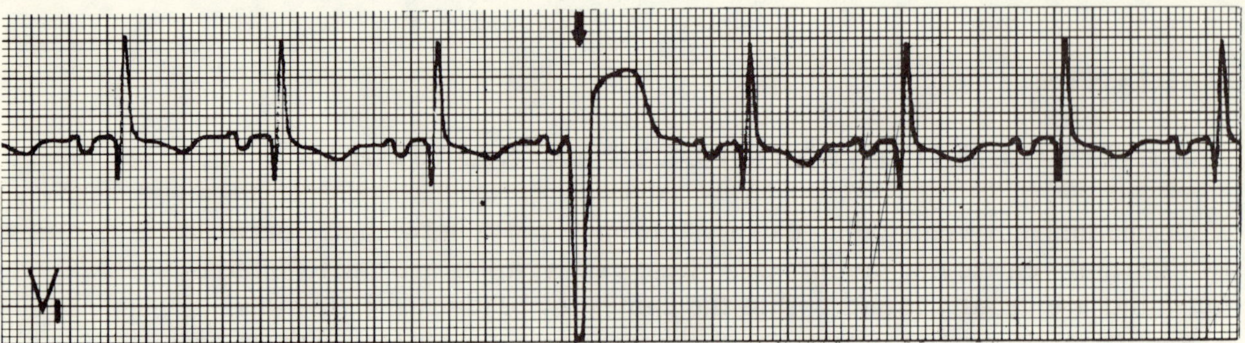

Fig. 11-A - Endiastolic ventricular extrasystoles. The PVC follows the sinus P wave and does not modify significantly the cardiac rhythm.

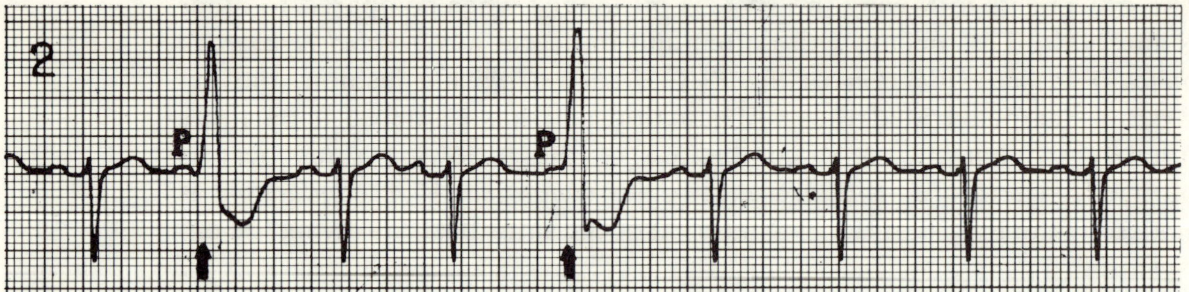

Fig. 11-B - Endiastolic ventricular extrasystoles. Notice the different relation between sinus P waves and PVC's.

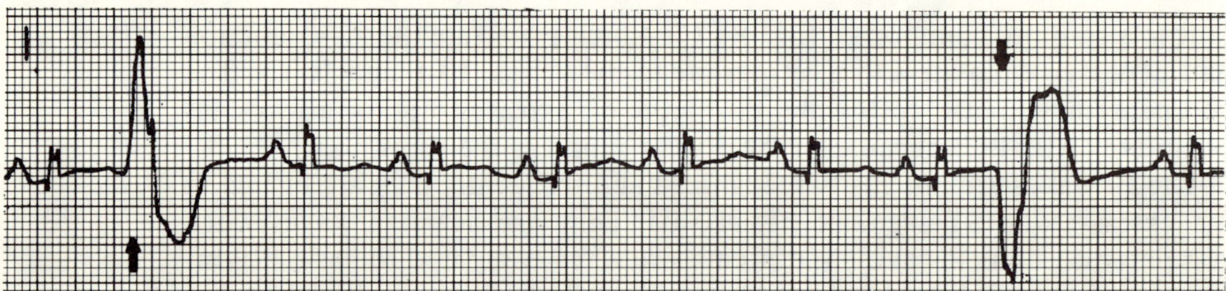

Fig. 11-C - Multifocal or multiform ventricular extrasystoles. The morphology of the PVC's, recorded in the same lead, is different.

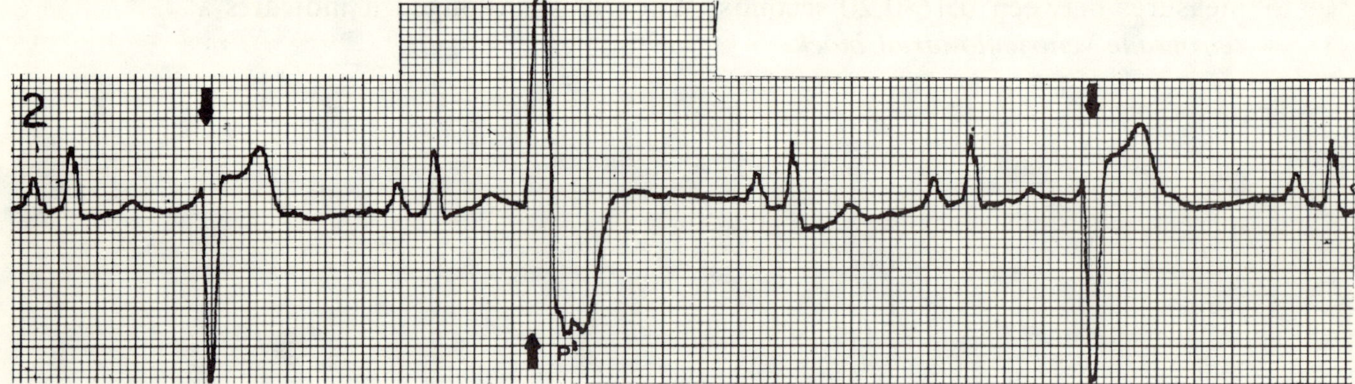

Fig. 11-D - Multifocal or multiform PVC's. Extrasystoles with a different QRS morphology are recorded in the same lead.

c) ENDIASTOLIC VENTRICULAR EXTRASYSTOLES (PVC with a P)

This is a type of extrasystole which, although hemodynamically benign, seems to herald more dangerous arrhythmias and it may be associated with ventricular parasystoles and sudden degenerations into ventricular tachycardias (fig. 11-A).

The extrasystoles have a *long and variable coupling interval,* which is that interval of time that separates them from the preceding beat, and they usually appear immediately after a sinus P wave (see page 24). Hemodynamically they behave almost like sinus beats because, falling at the end of diastole, they allow for an almost complete ventricular diastolic filling period. Since they follow the atrial contraction, they maintain an almost normal atrio-ventricular synchronism.

However, the P-PVC ratio may be quite variable and it is not unusual to find an extrasystole inscribed right on top of a P wave (fig. 11-B). This type of extrasystole may sometimes be confused with the intermittent W-P-W syndrome (see page 162).

d) MULTIFOCAL OR MULTIFORM EXTRASYSTOLES:

When extrasystoles, recorded in the same lead, show different morphologies they are called *multifocal extrasystoles.* They are considered as coming from different ventricular foci (figs. 11-C and 11-D).

Others call them *multiform extrasystoles* because they may have a unifocal origin and propagate into the ventricles through different pathways and therefore result in different type of aberration.

ARRHYTHMIAS DUE TO ABNORMAL IMPULSE FORMATION

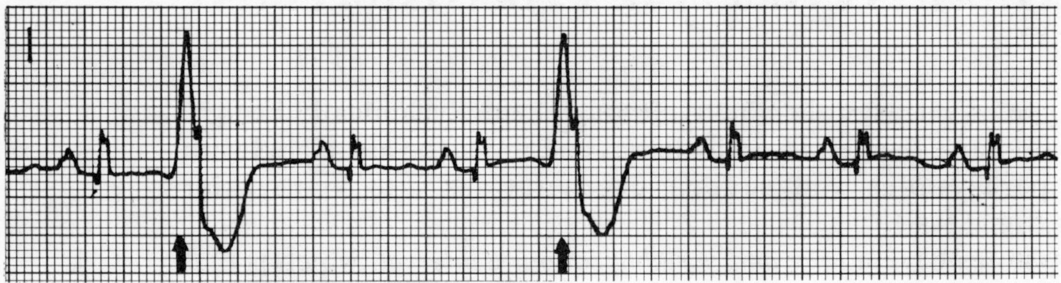

Fig. 12-A - PVC's with fixed coupling intervals.

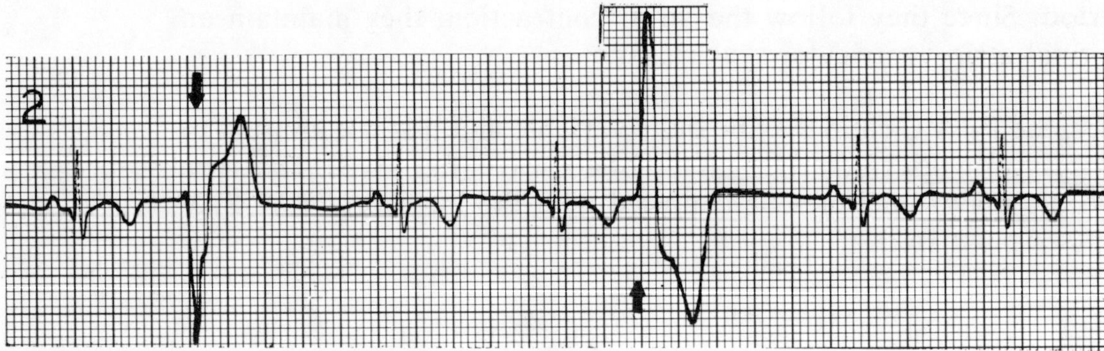

Fig. 12-B - PVC's with variable coupling interval.

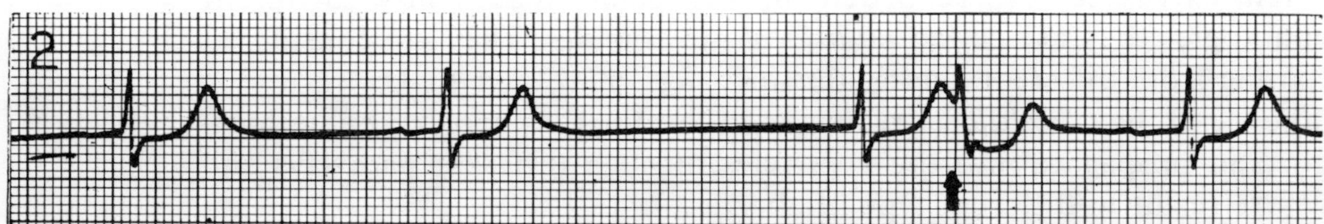

Fig. 12-C - PVC's with early coupling interval ("R on T phenomenon").

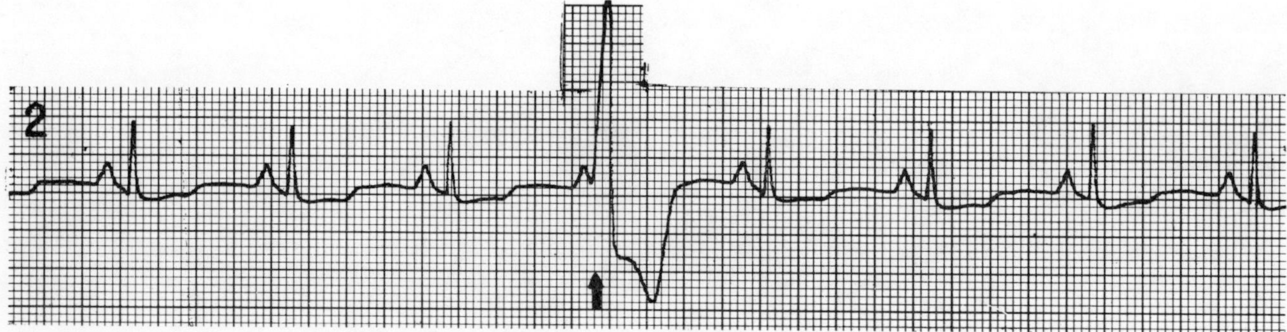

Fig. 12-D - PVC's with late coupling interval (endiastolic PVC).

VENTRICULAR EXTRASYSTOLES

THE COUPLING INTERVAL

Although the production mechanism of ventricular extrasystoles is not exactly known, it is a common opinion that a cause and effect relationship exists between the extrasystoles and the preceding sinus beats. PVC's may or may not show a constant interval of time with the preceding beat. This is called *coupling interval*. The coupling interval is measured from the beginning of the extrasystolic QRS to the beginning of the preceding QRS. Therefore, ventricular extrasystoles may have different types of coupling intervals:

a) *fixed:* when the temporal relation of the extrasystole with the preceding beat is constant (fig. 12-A).

b) *variable:* when the interval is not constant and the difference between two coupling intervals is more than 0.10 seconds (fig. 12-B).

c) *early:* the ventricular extrasystole is inscribed on the descending branch of the preceding T wave and determines the so-called *"R on T phenomenon"* (fig. 12-C).

d) *late:* this is typical of endiastolic ventricular extrasystoles (fig. 12-D).

ARRHYTHMIAS DUE TO ABNORMAL IMPULSE FORMATION

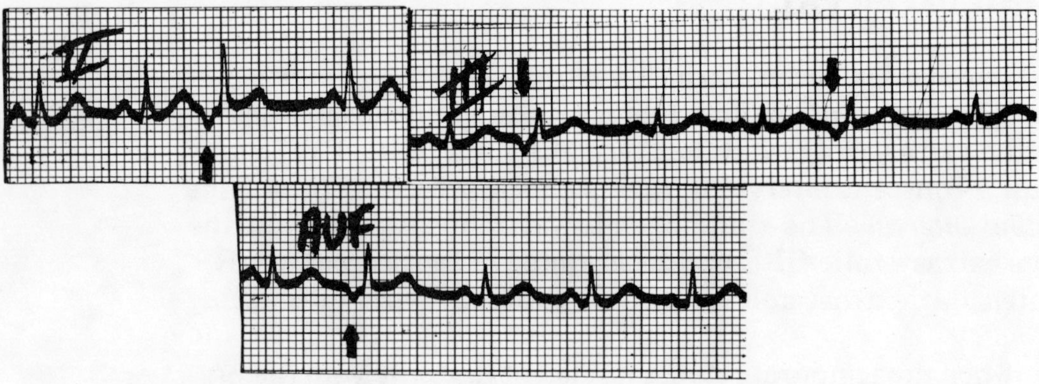

Fig. 13-A - "High" junctional extrasystoles. P¹ waves are negatives in L2, L3 and aVF and the
P¹-R interval is less than 0.12 secs.

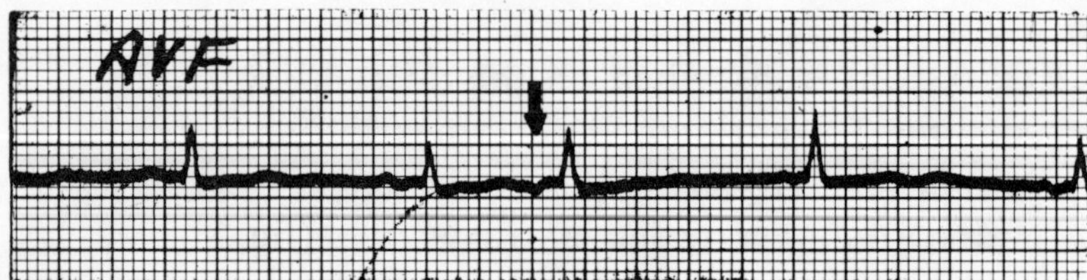

Fig. 13-B - "High" junctional extrasystoles.

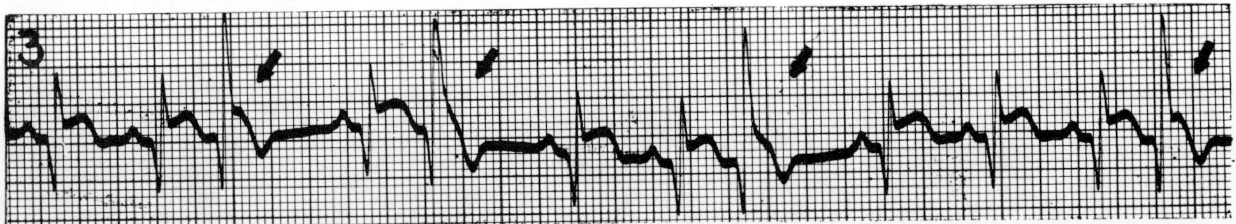

Fig. 13-C - "Mid"-junctional extrasystoles. P¹ waves are not present and the QRS complexes are similar to
those of sinus beat and show the injury current of an acute myocardial infarction.

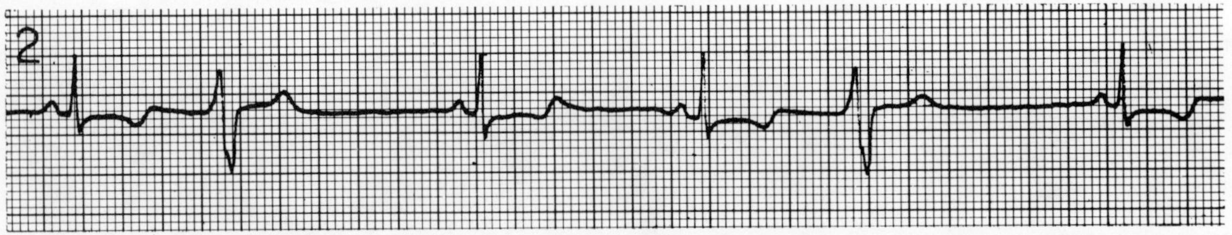

Fig. 13-D - "Mid"-junctional extrasystoles with ventricular aberration.

JUNCTIONAL EXTRASYSTOLES (A-V NODAL)

They are usually of the *high junctional or mid-junctional types* (see page 36).

In the *high junctional type,* the atria are depolarized in a retrograde fashion and the P[1] waves, which are negative in L2, L3 and in aVF, appear before the QRS's (fig. 13-A and 13-B).

The P[1]-QRS interval is short and less than 0.12 seconds. The QRS may be normal or may show a ventricular aberration. The compensatory pause is not complete.

In the *mid-junctional* type, P[1] waves are absent because the atrial and the ventricular depolarizations occur almost simultaneously. The P[1] waves are absorbed by the QRS complexes (fig. 13-C).

Fig. 13-D shows two mid-junctional extrasystoles with ventricular aberration. It is very difficult to distinguish this type of extrasystole from PVC's. The absence of recognizable P[1] waves, the presence of an incomplete compensatory pause, and the aberrant ventricular conduction of the right bundle branch block type are highly suggestive of an origin of these beats above or within the His bundle.

ARRHYTHMIAS DUE TO ABNORMAL IMPULSE FORMATION

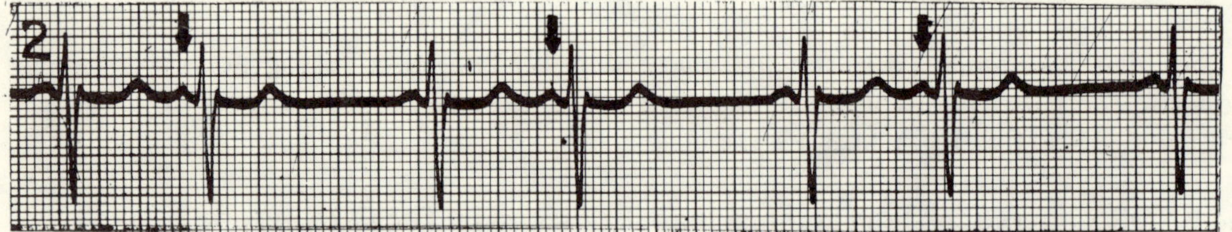

Fig. 14-A - Atrial bigeminy. Arrows indicate the ectopic P^1 wave which follows each sinus beat.

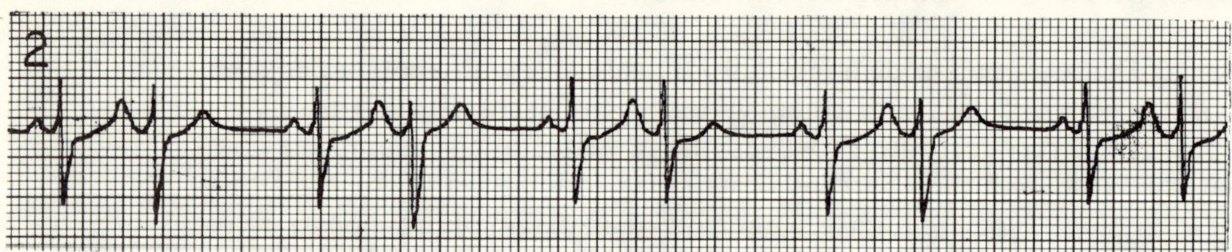

Fig. 14-B - Atrial bigeminy. The "couplet" is formed by a sinus beat and a PAC. The P^1 waves are buried in the preceding T waves.

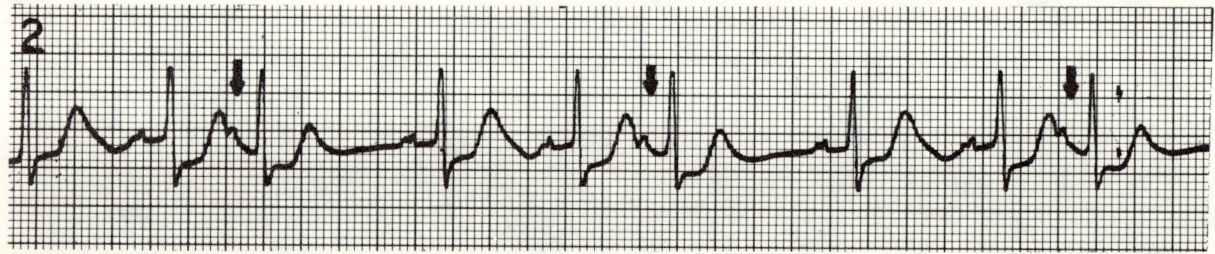

Fig. 14-C - Atrial trigeminy. The third beat of each "triplet" is a PAC.

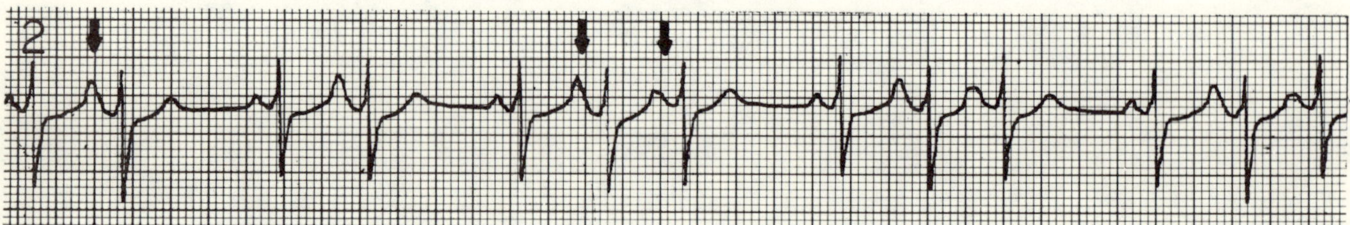

Fig. 14-D - Atrial bigeminy and trigeminy. They may be present in the same tracing. The arrows indicate the atrial extrasystoles.

ATRIAL BIGEMINY AND TRIGEMINY

These are intermittent extrasystolic rhythms, also called ALLO-RYTHMIAS.

In *atrial bigeminy,* an atrial extrasystole alternates with a sinus beat (figs. 14-A and 14-B).

The *atrial trigeminy* may have, instead, two forms. The most common is where the atrial premature beat follows the sinus beat (fig. 14-C), while the less common is when a sinus beat is followed by two atrial extrasystoles (fig. 14-D).
The compensatory pause of the extrasystoles determines "the grouping" of sinus and extrasystolic beats in "couplets and triplets". Usually, it is the group beating which is first noticed on a superficial examination of the electrocardiogram.

All the variations encountered for sporadic atrial extrasystoles are also valid for atrial bigeminy and trigeminy. Therefore, it is possible to find atrial bigeminy where P^1 waves are easily recognizable (fig. 14-A), or where P^1 waves are inscribed in the preceding T waves (fig. 14-B). Atrial bigeminy or trigeminy may have PAC's with ventricular aberration or blocked within the A-V junction.

Atrial bigeminy and trigeminy may also be present in the same tracing (fig. 14-D).

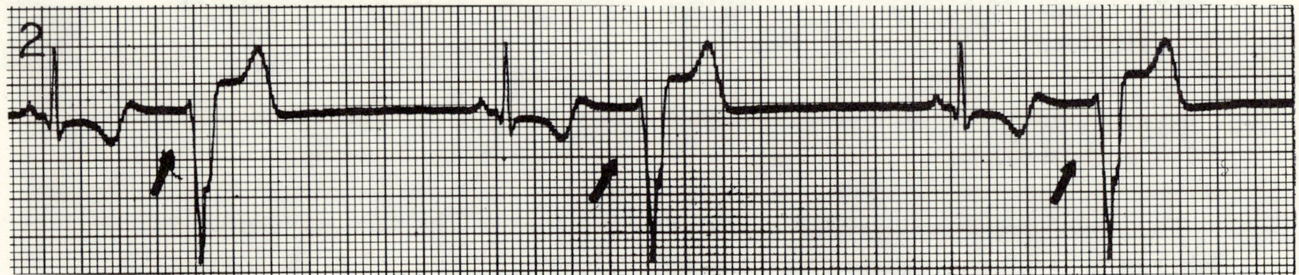

Fig. 15-A - Ventricular bigeminy. A ventricular extrasystole follows each sinus beat.

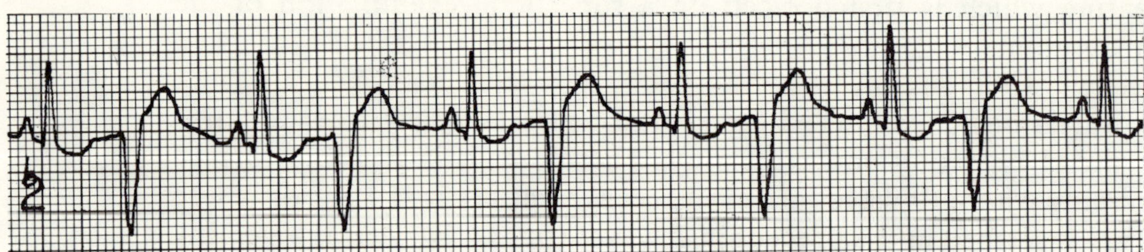

Fig. 15-B - Ventricular bigeminy.

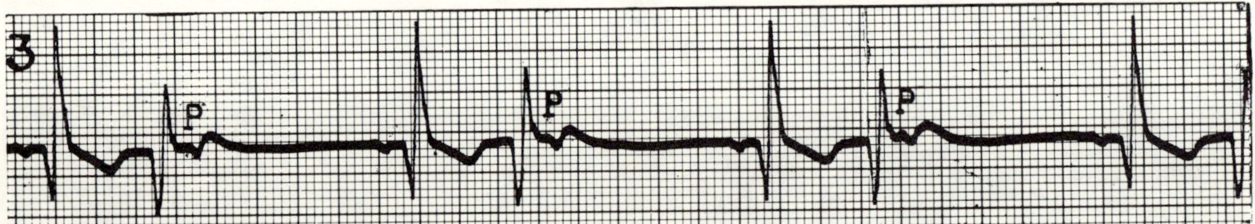

Fig. 15-C - "Mid"-junctional bigeminy. A sinus P wave follows the extrasystolic QRS.

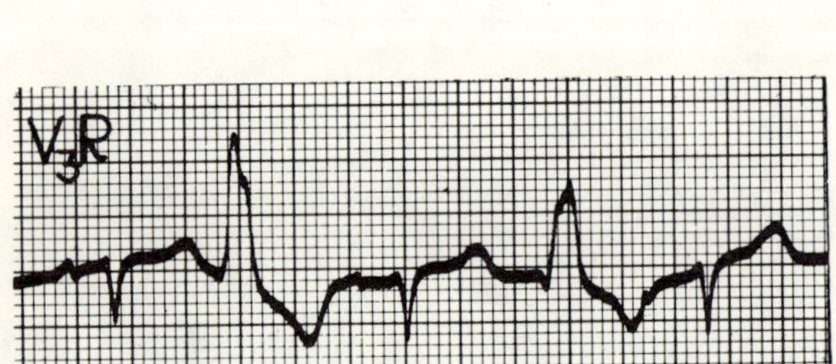

Fig. 15-D - Interpolated ventricular bigeminy.

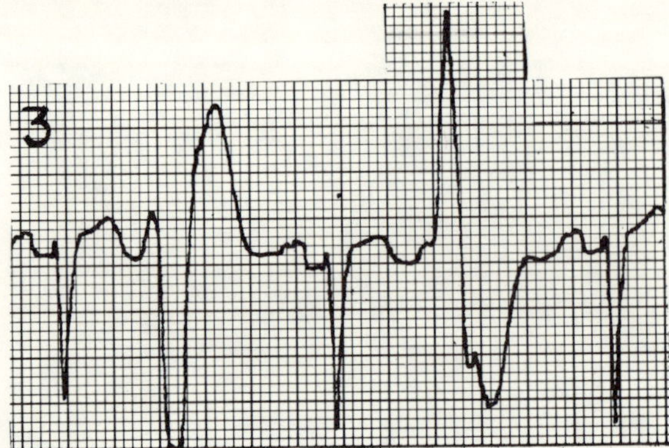

Fig. 15-E - Multifocal or multiform ventricular bigeminy.

VENTRICULAR BIGEMINY

In ventricular bigeminy, a ventricular extrasystole follows a normal sinus complex.

Fig. 15-A shows a ventricular bigeminy resulting in a bradycardic rhythm accentuated by long compensatory pauses. The coupling intervals of the extrasystoles are fixed.

In the ventricular bigeminy of fig. 15-B, the extrasystoles have fixed coupling intervals with the preceding sinus beats and the resulting ventricular rate is 150 beats/min. Hemodynamically, however, each extrasystole may not be able to generate enough systolic volume and a peripheral arterial pulse; it often happens that the radial pulse rate may be lower than the apical rate.

The *low-junctional bigeminy* of fig. 15-C shows evident P[1] waves following each extrasystolic QRS which has a morphology similar to that of sinus beats.

An *interpolated ventricular bigeminy* is presented in fig. 15-D. The configuration of the extrasystoles is slightly different and the second PVC is followed by a sinus beat with a longer P-R interval. This indicates a retrograde penetration of the second PVC higher into the A-V junction which, therefore, is made partially refractory (see page 27).

It is not unusual to find a *multiform or multifocal ventricular bigeminy* as the one illustrated in fig. 15-A.

ARRHYTHMIAS DUE TO ABNORMAL IMPULSE FORMATION

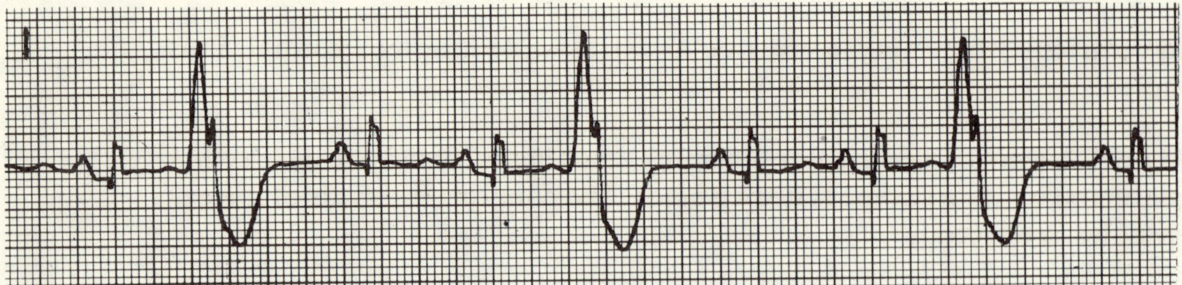

Fig. 16-A - Ventricular trigeminy. The "triplet" is formed by two sinus beats and a PVC.

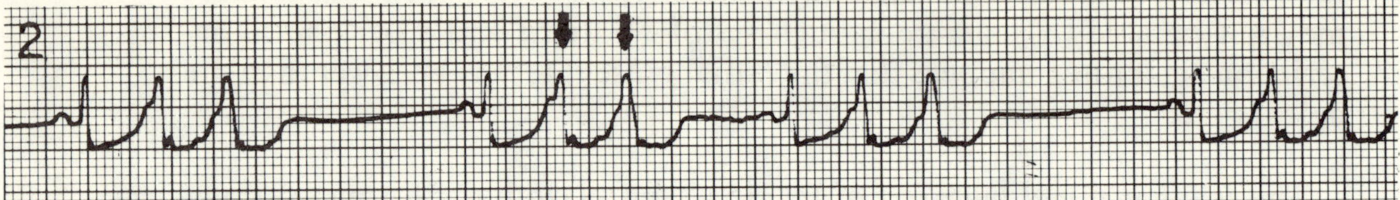

Fig. 16-B - Ventricular trigeminy. The "triplet" is formed by a sinus beat and two PVC's.

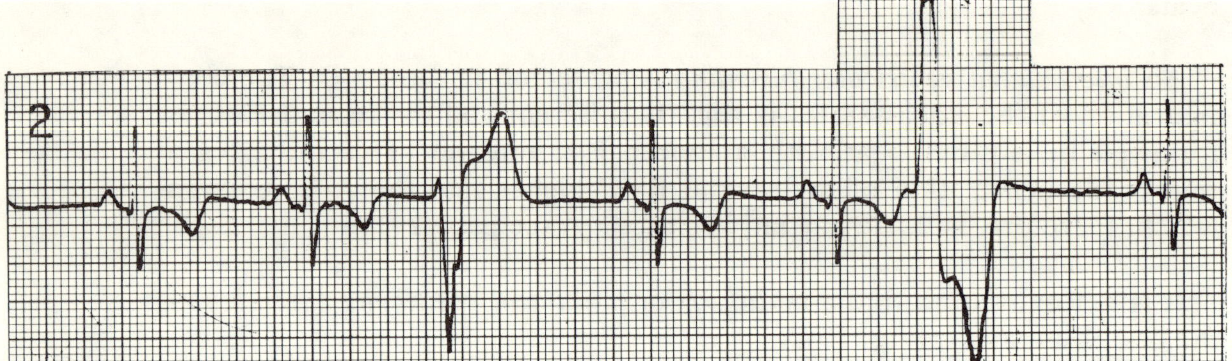

Fig. 16-C - Multifocal or multiform ventricular trigeminy.

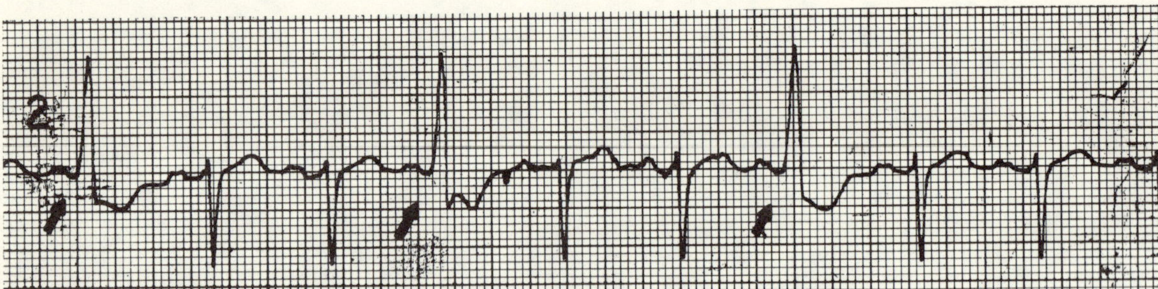

Fig. 16-D - Endiastolic ventricular trigemin

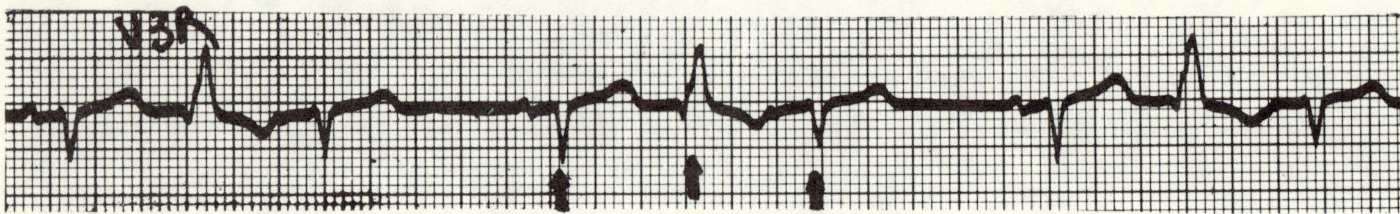

Fig. 16-E - Interpolated ventricular trigeminy.

VENTRICULAR TRIGEMINY

It has two forms:
a) a ventricular extrasystole follows two sinus beats (fig. 16-A).
b) two ventricular extrasystoles follow a sinus beat (fig. 16-B).

Of the two forms, the second is more rare and dangerous because it easily degenerates in a repetitive arrhythmia and may initiate episodes of ventricular tachycardia.

Variants of the classical forms of trigeminy are:
a) *multifocal or multiform ventricular trigeminy.* The PVC's show variable coupling intervals and different morphologies (fig. 16-C).
b) *endiastolic ventricular trigeminy.* The ventricular extrasystoles are preceded by sinus P waves and have variable coupling intervals (fig. 16-D).
c) *interpolated ventricular trigeminy.* The triplet (see arrows) is formed by the PVC sandwiched between two sinus beats (fig. 16-E).

ARRHYTHMIAS DUE TO ABNORMAL IMPULSE FORMATION

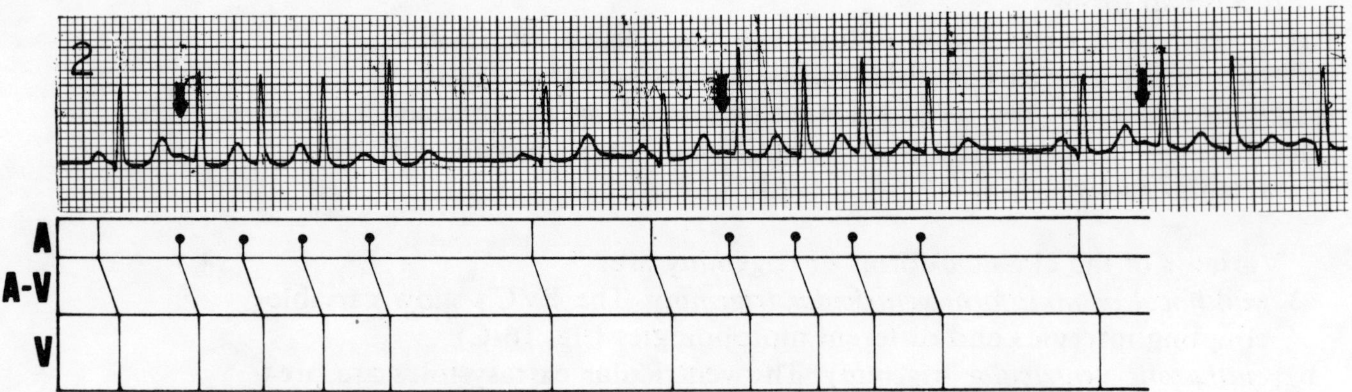

Fig. 17-A - Paroxysmal atrial tachycardia. The arrows indicate the atrial extrasystoles which initiate the salvos of PAT.

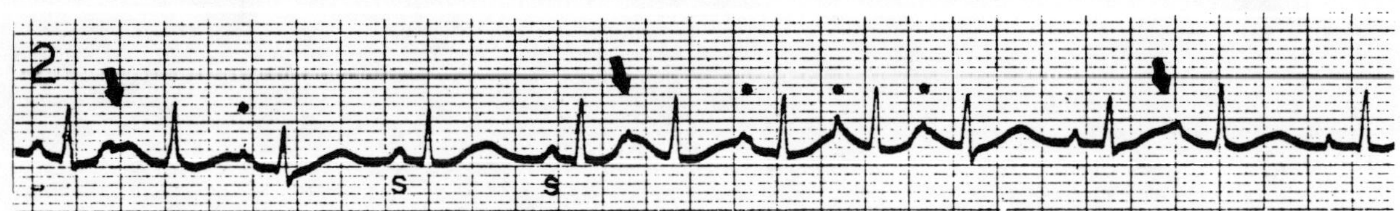

Fig. 17-B - Multifocal atrial tachycardia. The ventricular rate is irregular and P^1 waves originate from different atrial foci (arrows and dots) and are mixed with sinus beats (S).

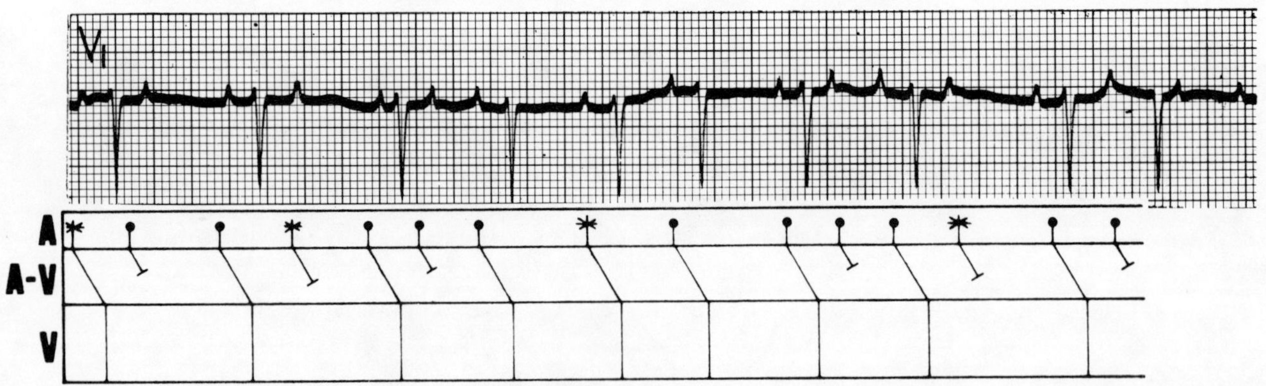

Fig. 17-C - Chaotic atrial tachycardia. The dots and asterisks in the diagram indicate different atrial ectopic foci. Several P^1 waves are blocked in the A-V junction. The ventricular rate is irregular.

ARRHYTHMIAS DUE TO ABNORMAL IMPULSE FORMATION

B - SUSTAINED RHYTHMS

SUPRAVENTRICULAR TACHYCARDIAS (SVT)

The term SVT indicates all tachyarrhythmias with foci situated above the His bundle. Therefore, the tachycardic ventricular rhythms secondary to atrial flutter or fibrillation, may also be part of this group. However, since they are well defined and recognized entities, they will be considered separately. What remains are the paroxysmal atrial and junctional (A-V nodal) tachycardias. Since it is often difficult to distinguish and separate these two forms of tachyarrhythmias, and since their etiology, treatment and prognosis are practically the same, they are often considered together and grouped under the not so compromising title of "Supraventricular Tachycardias" (SVT).

PAROXYSMAL ATRIAL TACHYCARDIA (PAT)

It is commonly believed that atrial tachycardia is an easy bedside diagnosis. The truth of the matter is that even the electrocardiographic recognition of this arrhythmia is often difficult, because a) it is practically undistinguishable from a junctional tachycardia (A-V nodal), b) it may perfectly simulate a ventricular tachycardia, especially in patients with a bundle branch block or with aberrant ventricular conduction and c) may be so irregular as to be mistaken for an atrial fibrillation. The diagnostic insufficiency of the 12 leads surface ECG is such that this type of arrhythmia often requires the help of particular maneuvers and diagnostic techniques (see pages 122 and 215).

In the classic form, a PAT appears as a more or less prolonged episode of tachycardia, with rates fluctuating between 120 and 250 beats/min., and with normal QRS complexes preceded by a P^1 wave and with a P^1-R interval usually shorter than 0.12 secs.
Fig. 17-A shows three episodes of PAT. As is usually the case, the paroxysms are initiated by atrial premature beats (arrows) and they start and cease abruptly. The cessation of the PAT is followed by an incomplete compensatory pause before the sinus node regains control of the heart rate for one or more beats.

A PAT may be *unifocal* (fig. 17-A) or *multifocal* (figs. 17-B and 17-C). In the latter circumstance, especially if P^1 waves are not clearly visible and occasionally blocked within the A-V junction, the ventricular rhythm may be so irregular as to simulate the ventricular response of an atrial fibrillation. This type of PAT is also known as *chaotic atrial tachycardia.*

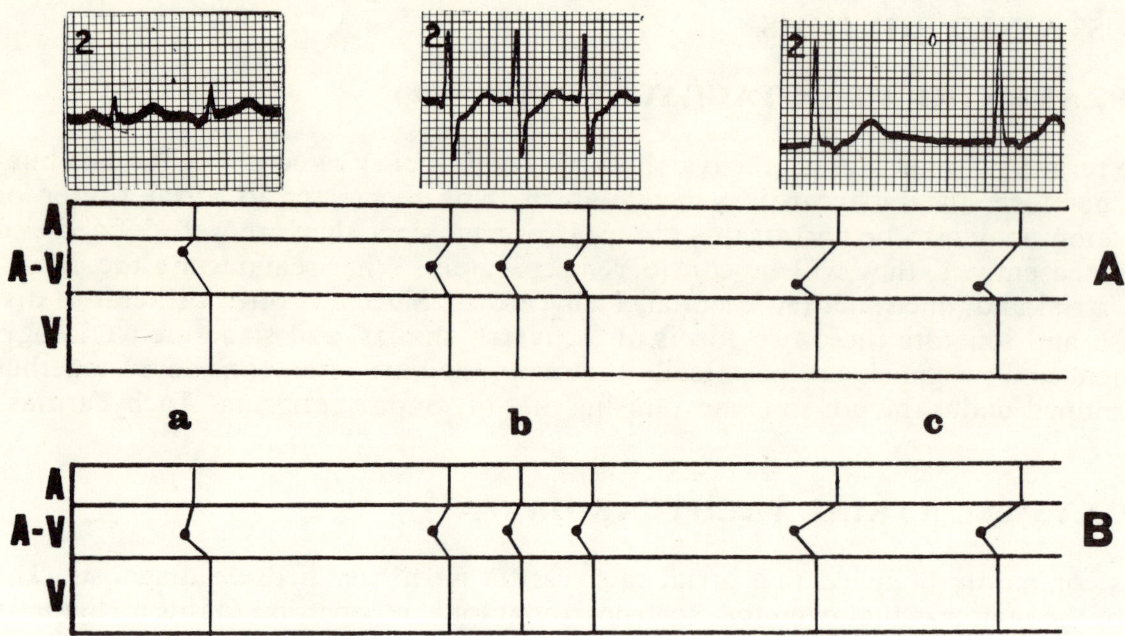

Fig. 18-A - **Junctional rhythms and tachycardias.** The diagram illustrates the different relationship between the P¹ waves and the QRS complexes. This is due to the junctional pacemaker position (diagram A) and to the anterograde and retrograde impulse conduction velocity (diagram B).

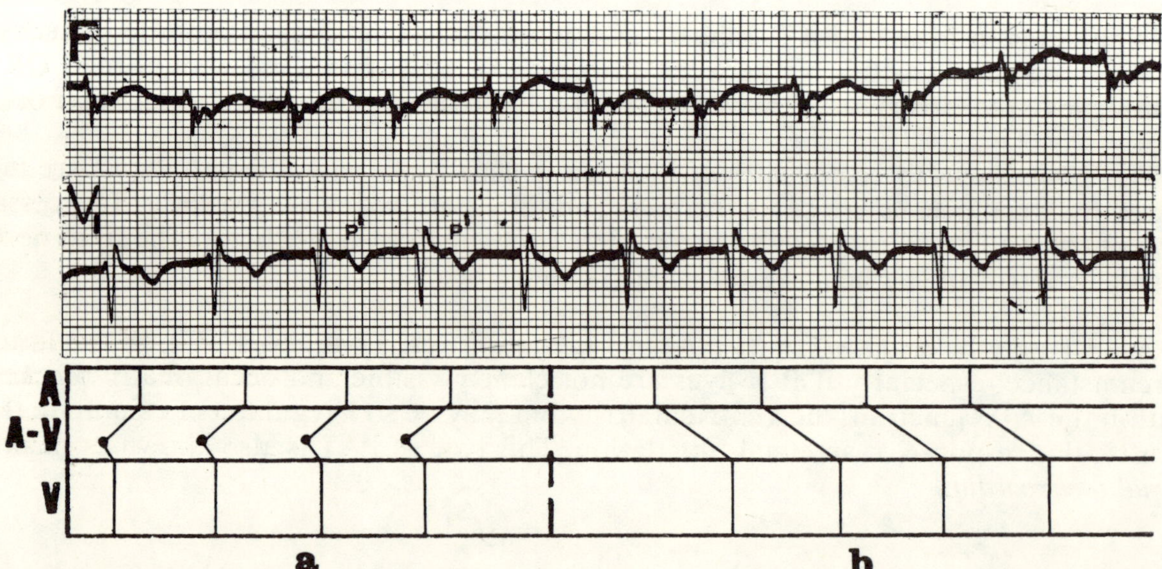

Fig. 18-B - **Junctional rhythms and tachycardias.** The pacemaker may be junctional, with a delay in the conduction to the atria (a), or atrial with a conduction delay to the ventricles (b).

SUPRAVENTRICULAR TACHYCARDIA

JUNCTIONAL RHYTHM AND JUNCTIONAL TACHCARDIA (A-V nodal)

In this type of arrhythmias the impulses originate in the A-V junction (where cells with pacemaker activity are present) and simultaneously propagate to the ventricles, through normal conduction pathways, and to the atria, in a retrograde fashion. The QRS complex is usually normal, unless aberrant ventricular conduction is present, and P[1] waves may precede (P[1]-R<0.12 sec.), be buried within, or follow the QRS's.

It is a common belief that the P[1] waves - QRS's relation is determined by the point of origin of the impulse within the A-V junction. Therefore, when the secondary pacemaker is situated in high areas of the A-V node, the rhythm has been called "high nodal" and P[1] waves precede the QRS's; if located in central A-V nodal areas, the rhythm will be a "mid-nodal rhythm" and P[1] waves will not appear on the ECG because atria and ventricles are depolarized simultaneously. If P[1] waves follow the QRS's, the rhythm is called "low nodal" and the secondary pacemaker will be situated in the lower parts of the A-V node. This is diagrammed in A of fig. 18-A where three junctional rhythms are presented (a,b,c).

However, histologists and physiologists have not been able to find pacemaker cells in the A-V node, while they have found them in the transitional areas between the A-V node and the His bundle, and within the His bundle itself. Therefore, the term "nodal" has been slowly substituted by *junctional* which is anatomically more generic and less committing (the term *A-V junction* indicates the specific A-V conduction tissue from the A-V node to the His-Purkinje system).

The other important factor in determining the position of the P[1] wave in relation to the QRS, is the retrograde and anterograde conduction velocity of the impulse which originates in the A-V junction and, simultaneously or almost, travels toward the atria and ventricles.

In diagram B of fig. 18-A, the pacemaker site and the anterograde conduction velocity to the ventricles is maintained constant, while the retrograde conduction to the atria is made variable. Therefore, the atrial activation (P[1]) may appear before (a), simultaneously (b) or after the ventricular activation (c). The same results, but in an opposite sequence, would be obtained if the conduction velocity toward the atria is constant while that to the ventricles is changing. Therefore, the relationship P[1]-QRS and QRS-P[1] is nothing else than the difference between the anterograde and retrograde conduction times. Although it indicates a less important aspect of the P[1]-QRS relationship, the terminology "high, mid and low junctional rhythms or tachycardias" is more descriptive and it becomes handy when facing rhythms such as those presented in fig. 18-A. For example, a "low junctional rhythm" is a less complicated definition than "mid junctional rhythm with delay of retrograde conduction," etc.

The typical rate of an A-V junctional subsidiary pacemaker usually fluctuates between 40-60 beats/min. When it appears with a rate as in fig. 18-A-c, it is a *"passive rhythm"* coming into being for the absence of the primary sinus pacemaker *(junctional escape rhythm)* (see page 112). However, when the rate is above 60/min. (fig. 18-A-b) the rhythm is indicated as a *junctional tachycardia* and it will be an "active rhythm," which takes command above the normal sinus rhythm because of an increased excitability of a subsidiary junctional pacemaker.

Occasionally, a diagnostic dilemma may result from the fact that the P[1]-R intervals of a PAT may be prolonged and above 0.12 sec.

Fig. 18-B shows a tachycardia whose origin may have two explanations:

a) "low" junctional, with P[1] waves following the QRS's.

b) atrial, with marked prolongation of P[1]-R interval.

In such a case the exact diagnosis is almost impossible and the only differential element is the vectorial configuration of the P[1] wave.

ARRHYTHMIAS DUE TO ABNORMAL IMPULSE FORMATION

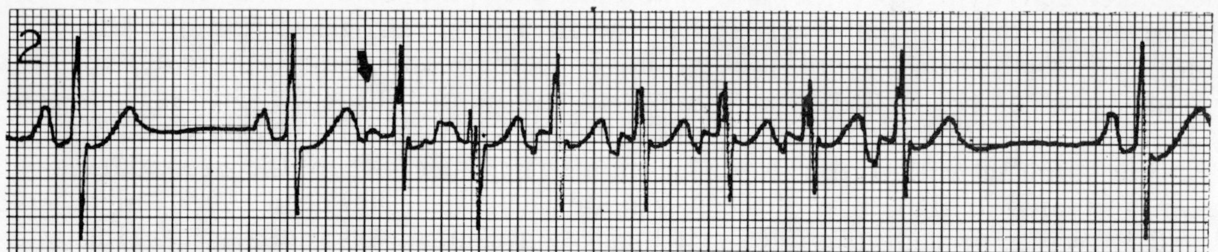

Fig. 19-A - Paroxysmal atrial tachycardia. The arrow indicates the PAC which initiates the paroxysm of tachycardia with a rate of 140/min. The QRS complexes are slightly aberrant and preceded by obvious P¹ waves.

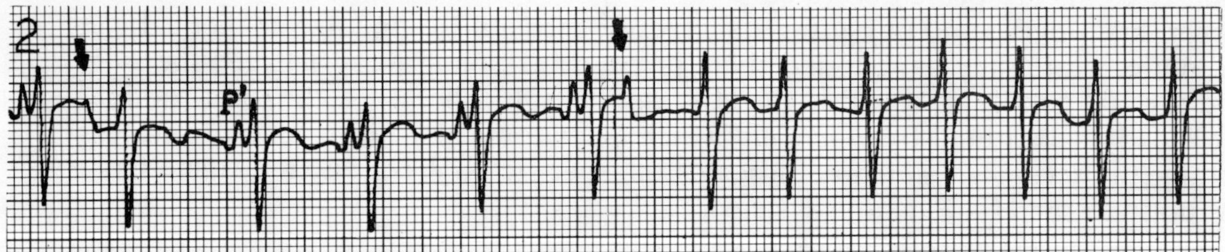

Fig. 19-B - Junctional tachycardia. The first arrow indicates a PAC conducted with delay to the ventricles; the second arrow indicates a blocked PAC which is followed by a "mid"-junctional tachycardia.

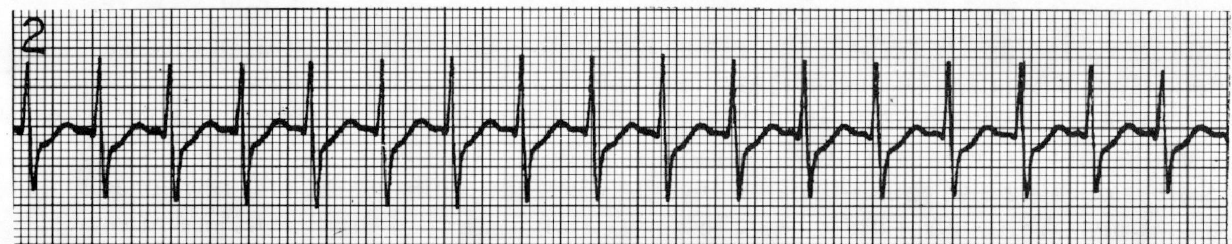

Fig. 19-C - Junctional tachycardia. P¹ waves are not evident. The QRS complexes show a normal morphology and a regular rate (180/min.). The ventricular and atrial activation are simultaneous and the rhythm is defined as a "mid"-junctional tachycardia.

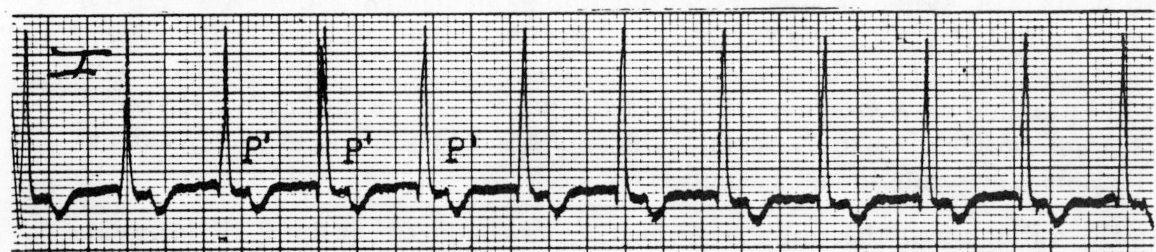

Fig. 19-D - Supraventricular tachycardia. A "low" junctional tachycardia or an atrial tachycardia with prolongation of the P¹-R interval? This rhythm may create doubts and controversies.

Fig. 19-A shows a salvo of seven beats of a paroxysmal atrial tachycardia. Each QRS complex shows a slight aberration in the ventricular conduction and P¹ waves are present before each QRS. The paroxysm is initiated by a PAC and it ends abruptly, causing the appearance of a sinus beat.

Fig. 19-B shows a predominant rhythm of a probable atrial or *high junctional* origin, as is suggested by the configuration of the P¹ wave and by the P¹-R intervals. Two atrial extrasystoles are present (arrows). The first is conducted, although with some delay, to the ventricles, while the second is blocked in the A-V junction and is followed by a tachycardic rhythm (rate = 150/min.). P¹ waves are not recognized and, if present, must be buried within the QRS's, suggesting a simultaneous activation of the atria and ventricles. Therefore, the last part of the rhythm is a *mid-junctional tachycardia*.

Fig. 19-C shows again a *mid-junctional tachycardia* with a rate of 180/min.

In fig. 19-D the QRS complexes, which show a normal morphology and a rate of 120/min., are followed by easily recognizable P¹ waves. Therefore, the rhythm must be a *junctional tachycardia;* the P¹ waves indicate a retrograde atrial activation. An alternative explanation is that the arrhythmia originates from an atrial focus with a P¹-R interval which is markedly prolonged (0.40 sec.) and it is an *atrial tachycardia* with a first degree A-V block.

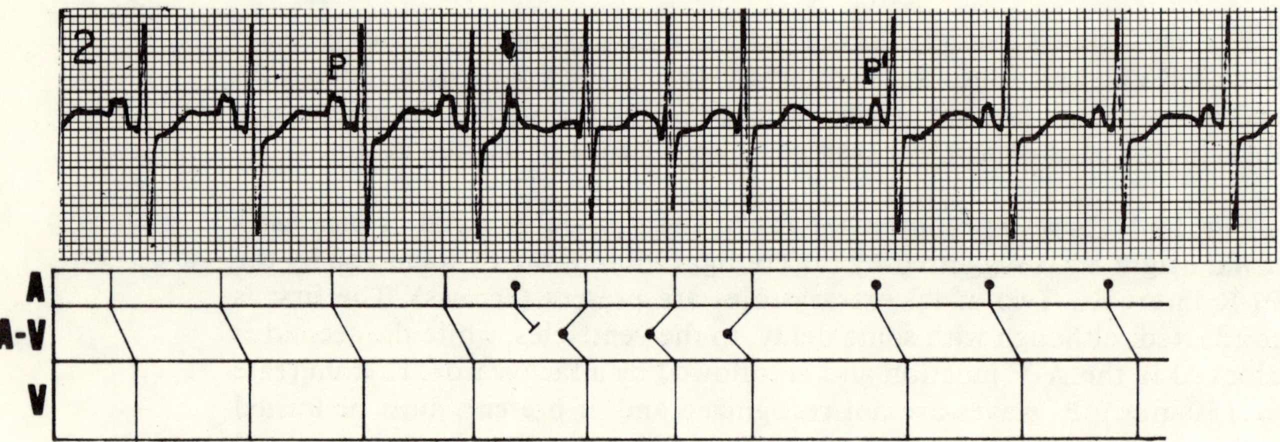

Fig. 20-A - Supraventricular tachycardia. A PAC (arrow) interrupts the sinus rhythm and is blocked in the A-V junction. This is followed by a brief salvo of three mid-junctional beats and by a new atrial pacemaker (as it is suggested by the different P^1 wave configurations and the shorter P^1-R intervals).

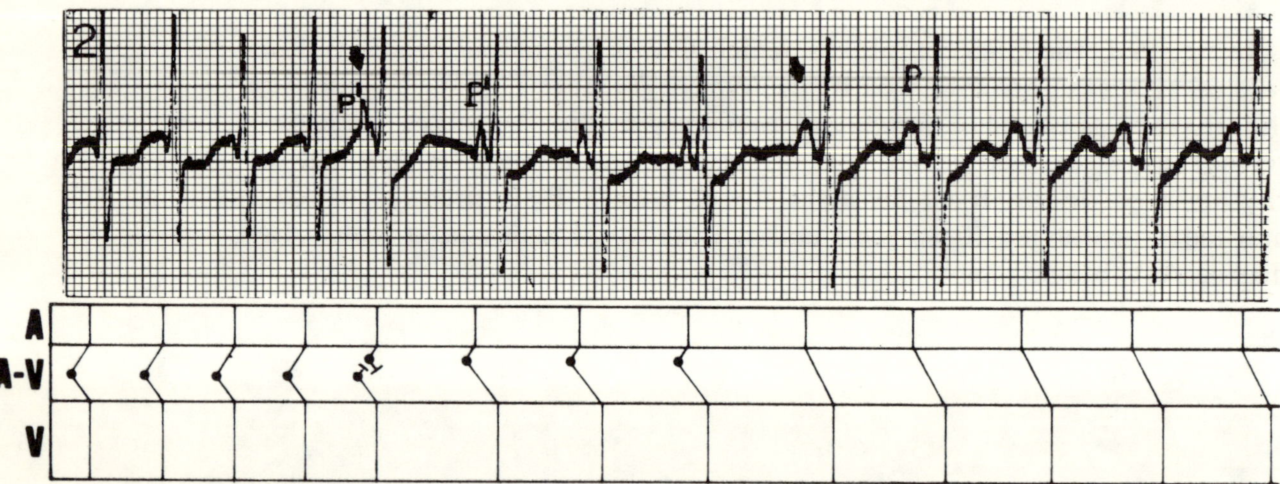

Fig. 20-B - Supraventricular tachycardia. An interesting arrhythmia which goes from a "mid"-junctional tachycardia (180/min.) to a "high" junctional rhythm (110/min.) and, finally, into a more stable sinus rhythm (100/min.).

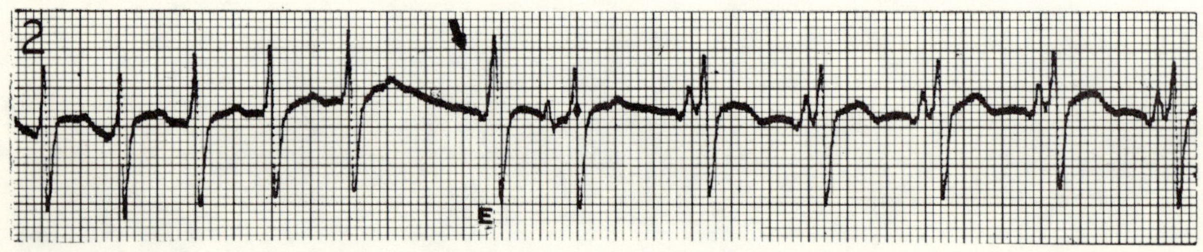

Fig. 20-C - Supraventricular tachycardia. The paroxysm is followed by a junctional escape beat (E) and by an atrial (or a high junctional) pacemaker.

SUPRAVENTRICULAR TACHYCARDIA

Fig. 20-A starts with a sinus rhythm that is interrupted, after the fourth beat, by a blocked atrial extrasystole. This permits a brief burst of a *mid-junctional tachycardia* with simultaneous activation of the atria and ventricles (rate = 150/min.). The tachycardia, which only lasts for three beats and ceases suddenly is followed by an ectopic and more stable atrial focus. (Notice the different morphology of sinus P waves and P[1] waves and the different length of P-R and P[1]-R intervals.)

Fig. 20-B starts with the final sequence of a *mid-junctional tachycardia*. When the fifth impulse is being formed, a new ectopic impulse appears (P[1]) from a different high junctional or atrial focus. (See the diagram.) The simultaneous firing of the two pacemakers blocks the retrograde propagation of the mid-junctional impulse, and the rhythm is controlled, for the next three beats by the high junctional focus before the sinus node has a chance to reappear.

When ceasing abruptly, a paroxysm of a supraventricular tachycardia may be followed by an asystolic pause. This usually terminates with an *escape beat* (E) (such as in fig. 20-C), before a new pacemaker takes control of the cardiac rhythm (see page 112).

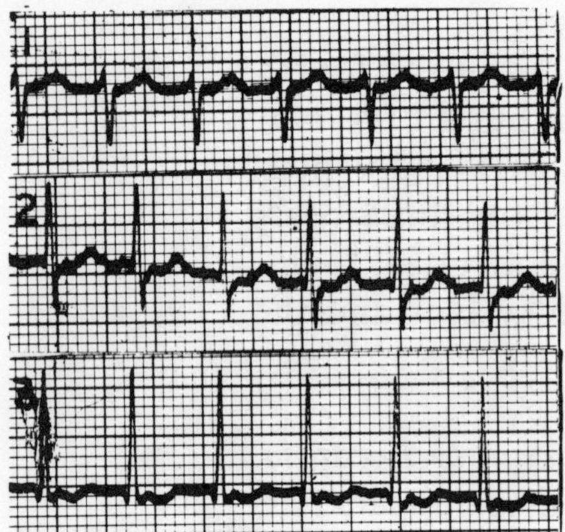

Fig. 21-A - Supraventricular tachycardia with normal ventricular conduction.

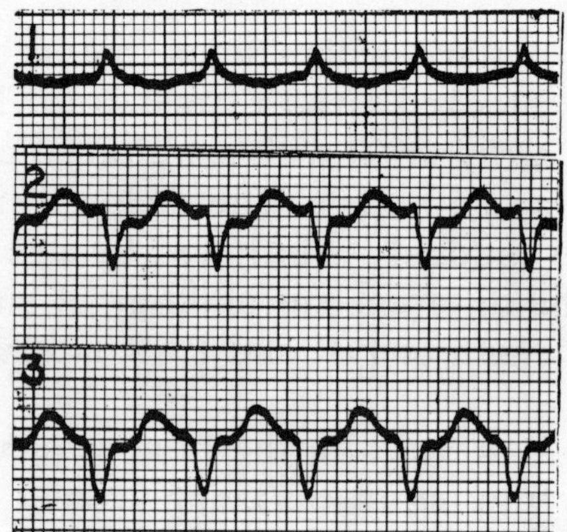

Fig. 21-B - Supraventricular tachycardia with aberrant ventricular conduction.

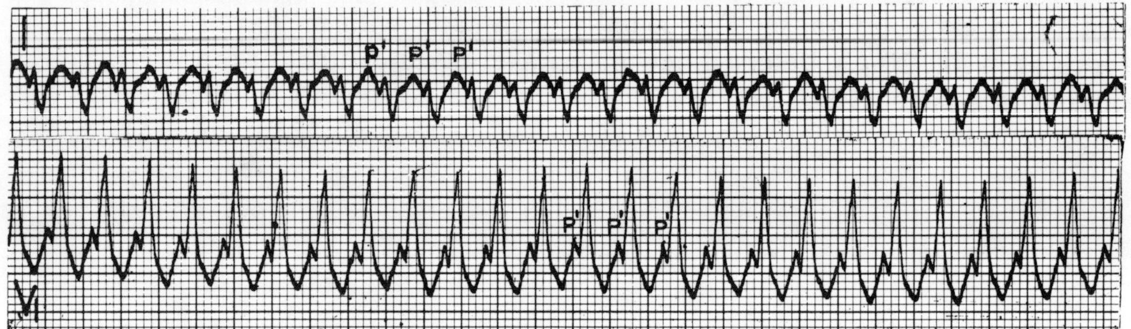

Fig. 21-C - Supraventricular tachycardia with aberrant ventricular conduction. The aberrant conduction is of a right bundle branch block type. P[1] waves are present before each QRS.

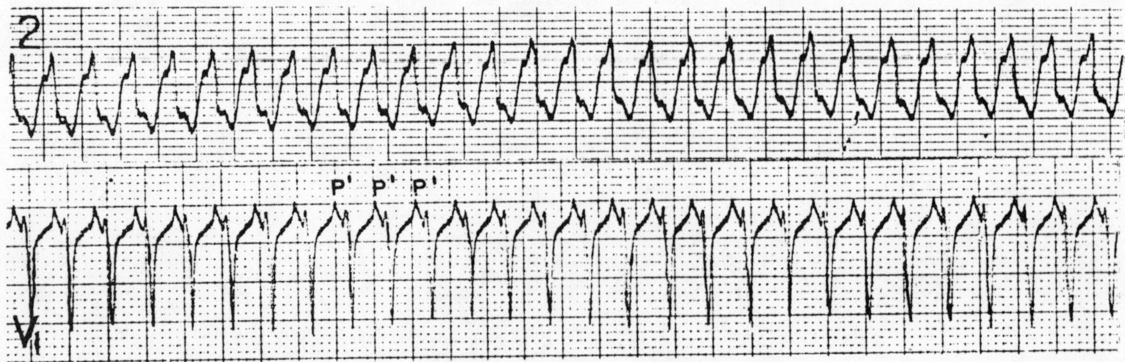

Fig. 21-D - Supraventricular tachycardia with aberrant ventricular conduction. P[1] waves precede each QRS and the aberration is of left bundle branch block type.

SUPRAVENTRICULAR TACHYCARDIA

Fig. 21-A and 21-B present a situation that is often encountered in the presence of a supraventricular tachycardia and may be easily misdiagnosed. The SVT of fig. 21-A has a rate of 175/min. and shows QRS complexes with a normal configuration. The SVT of fig. 21-B, although slower, has an aberrant ventricular conduction. The importance of recognizing an *aberrant ventricular conduction*, during supraventricular tachycardias, is usually underestimated. Ventricular aberration is more common than one would think. Supraventricular tachycardias (SVT) may simulate to perfection their more ominous cousins: ventricular tachycardias (VT). It has already been seen that PAC's may have morphologies totally similar to PVC's. This is due to the aberrant conduction of the PAC (see page 16) which presents a configuration of the right bundle branch block type. The same may happen for repetitive beats and supreventricular tachycardias.

Tracings of fig. 21-C dramatically illustrate how easily one type of tachycardia may be mistaken for another. At first glance the tracing suggests a ventricular tachycardia. The rate is rapid (270/min.) and the QRS complexes are bizarre and of an ectopic type. With careful examination, however, it may be noted that a P[1] wave precedes each QRS and that the ventricular aberration is a RBBB type. It was also noted that the ventricular activation of this patient would come back to normal at slower sinus rates. Therefore, the rhythm is a *supraventricular tachycardia with aberrant ventricular conduction.*

Two factors may make it arduous for a differential diagnosis between a ventricular tachycardia and a supraventricular tachycardia with aberration:
a) VT impulses may conduct 1:1 in a retrograde fashion to the atria and P[1] waves may follow each QRS (see pages 72 and 78).
b) occasionally the ventricular aberration may be of a LBBB type. This is usually a sign of latent pathology of the left bundle, which is revealed by fast cardiac rates.
Tracings of fig. 21-D present a tachycardia with a rate of 280/min. and with a ventricular aberration of LBBB type. Again, P[1] waves are easily recognized preceding each QRS and indicate a supraventricular origin of the tachycardia.

Therefore, in the presence of a tachycardia with aberrant complexes:
1) first, think of the aberration of an SVT; it is very common.
2) "cherchez le P[1]".
3) obtain, if possible, a previous tracing of the patient. If PAC's or PVC's have been previously documented, their morphology may help in localizing the focus of the tachycardia.
4) if the aberration is of the RBBB type, chances are that the arrhythmia is a SVT.

ARRHYTHMIAS DUE TO ABNORMAL IMPULSE FORMATION

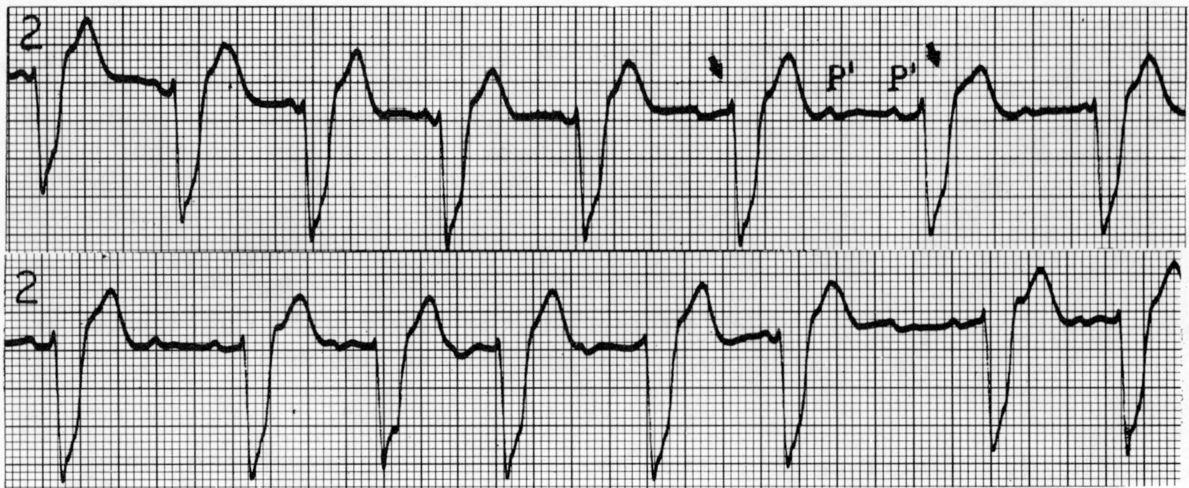

Fig. 22-A - Atrial tachycardia with a variable A-V block. The A-V block is basically of a 2:1 type and the longer pauses are due to a 3:1 A-V block. During the asystolic pauses P¹ waves appear evident and the atrial rate may be determined (190/min.).

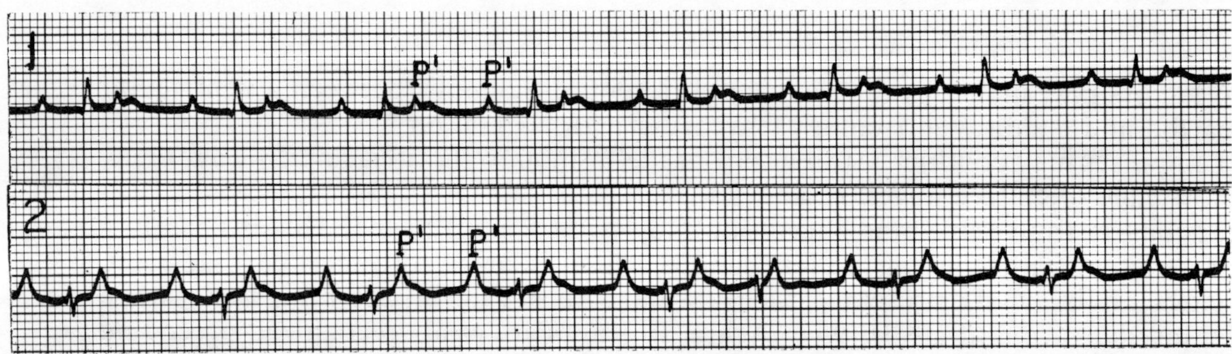

Fig. 22-B - Atrial tachycardia with a 2:1 A-V block. The P¹ wave which reaches the ventricles has a prolonged P¹-R interval and the atrial rate is 150/min.

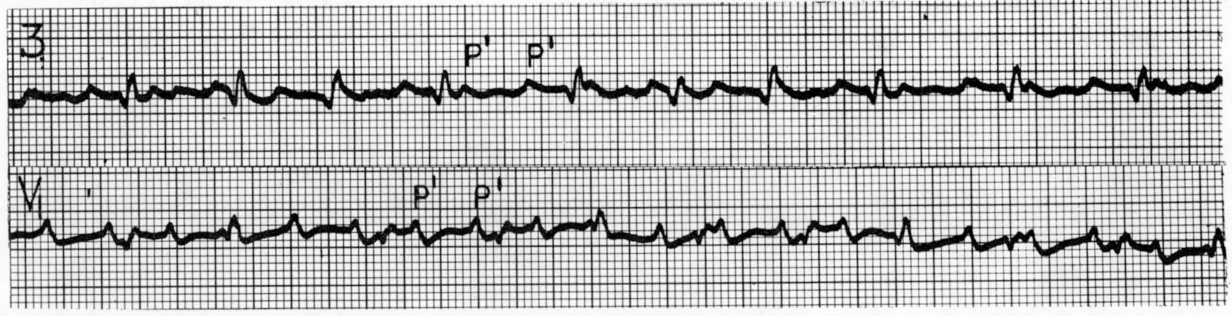

Fig. 22-C - Atrial tachycardia with a variable A-V block. The A-V block is of a variable type for the presence of a Wenckebach phenomenon into the A-V junction.

SUPRAVENTRICULAR TACHYCARDIA

It is not uncommon to find SVT's with different degrees of A-V block. The most common type is the 2:1 A-V block. This type of block is in relation to the rate of the atrial waves and the functional state of the A-V junction.

Fig. 22-A presents a rhythm with QRS complexes of the left bundle branch block type (LBBB) and which are closely preceded by atrial waves (P¹-R = 0.10 sec.). The rhythm mechanism is revealed by the sixth QRS of the upper tracing (preceded by a more distant atrial wave) and by the seventh QRS, preceded by a pause which clearly shows two P¹ waves and enables the measurement of the atrial rate (190/min.). Therefore, the arrhythmia is a *supraventricular tachycardia with a 2:1 A-V block* and moments of a *3:1 A-V block*. The lower tracing reveals other moments of variable A-V block with easilyn identifiable p¹ waves. One of the P¹ waves is always buried in the ST segment of the conducted beat. The atrial impulses are conducted with a LBBB abberation.

Fig. 22-B shows a *supraventricular tachycardia* with an atrial rate of 150/min. (as it can be derived by the P¹-P¹ interval) and a *stable 2:1 A-V block*. The P¹ wave which conducts to the ventricle, has a P¹-R interval of 0.22 secs.

A *supraventricular tachycardia with a variable A-V block* is presented in fig. 22-C. The A-V block varies because of a Wenckebach mechanism in action in the conduction of the atrial impulses through the A-V junction (see page 172).

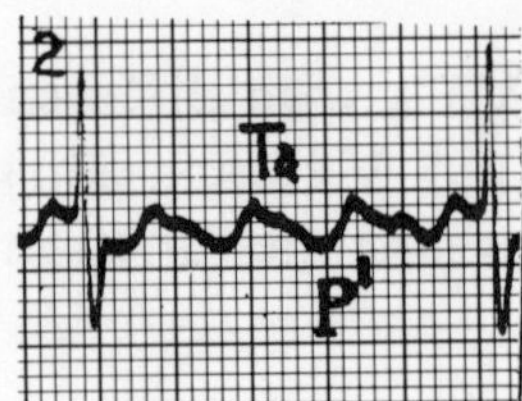

Fig. 23-A - Atrial flutter. F waves.

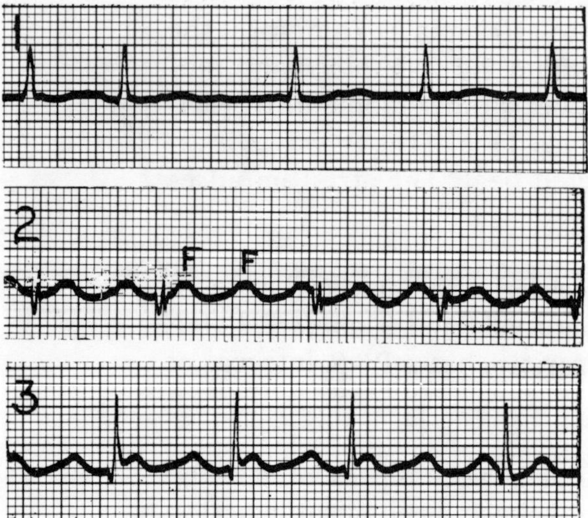

Fig. 23-B - Atrial flutter. Classical "saw-tooth" appearance of atrial complexes (F waves).

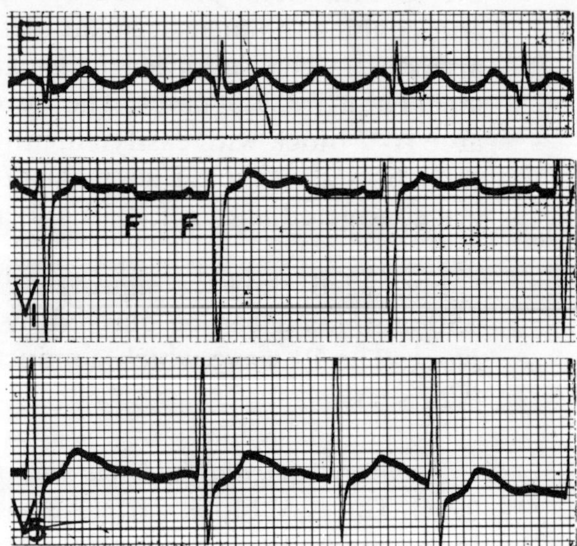

Fig. 23-C - Atrial flutter. F waves are recognized in some leads but not in others.

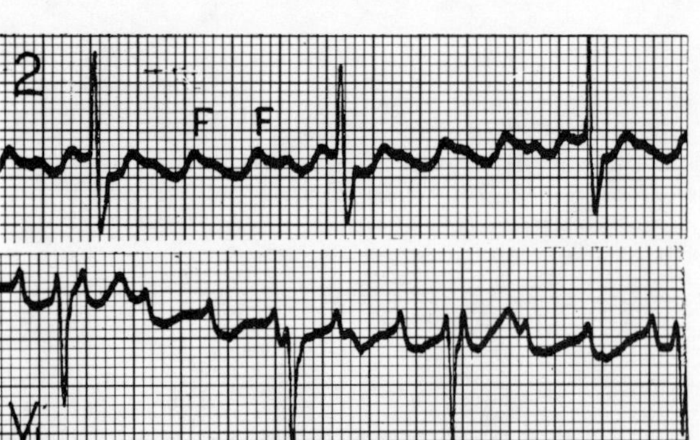

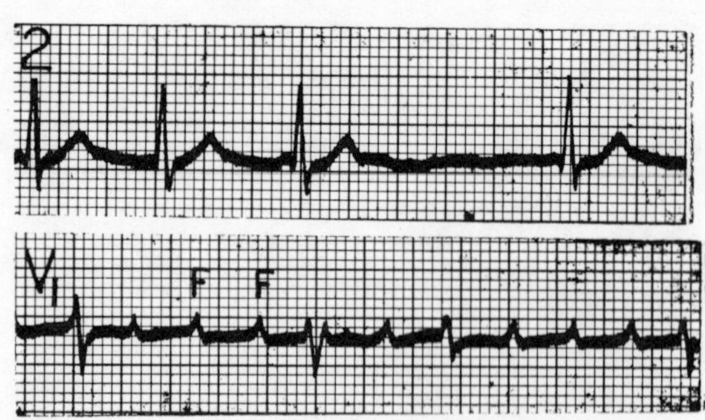

Fig. 23-D - Atrial flutter. F waves are well recognized in L2 and V1.

Fig. 23-E - Atrial flutter. F waves are present only in the precordial leads.

ATRIAL FLUTTER

Atrial flutter is a "limbo" within atrial tachyarrhythmias. In fact, there are not yet well established criteria for the recognition and definition of this arrhythmia. Attempts have been made to separate an atrial flutter from both a supraventricular tachycardia and an atrial fibrillation on the following criteria:

a) *the morphology of atrial complexes:* the presence on the surface ECG of an undulating baseline with a "saw-tooth appearance", would be due to rapid atrial depolarization waves of an atrial flutter (F waves).

b) *the rate of atrial waves:* conventionally established between a maximum of 350/min. and minimum of 250/min.

c) *the A-V conduction ratio.*

A. - MORPHOLOGY OF ATRIAL COMPLEXES

The F waves, which show a rapid ascending and a more gradual descending slopes, represent atrial P¹ waves fused with a prominent preceding Ta wave (atrial repolarization wave). F waves are indicative of atrial flutter (fig. 23-A).

F waves are usually present in L2, L3, and aVF; they may be sometimes recognized in L1, V5, and V6 and they usually are small, peaked and positive waves in the right precordial leads (figs. 23-B and 23-C).

Fig. 23-D presents an atrial flutter with F waves clearly visible in L2 and V1, while fig. 23-E shows how the recording of only L2 may be sometimes misleading. While in L2 the baseline is almost isolectric, F waves are clearly recorded in the V1 lead.

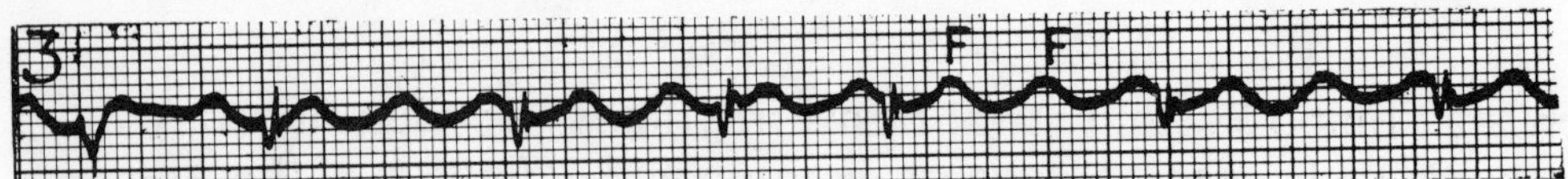

Fig. 24-A - Atrial flutter. F waves with a rate of 200/min.

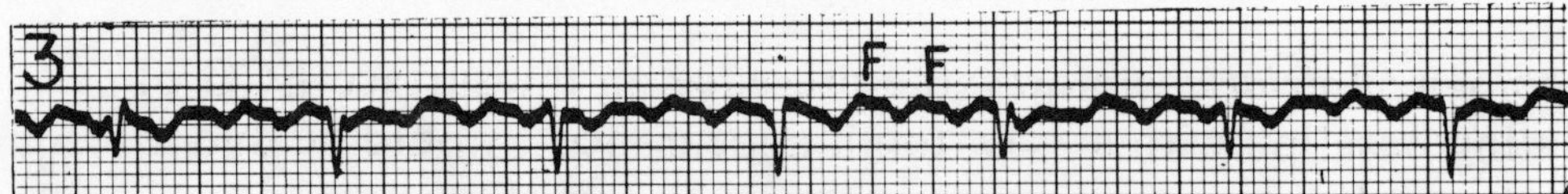

Fig. 24-B - Atrial flutter. Classical F waves with a rate of 220/min.

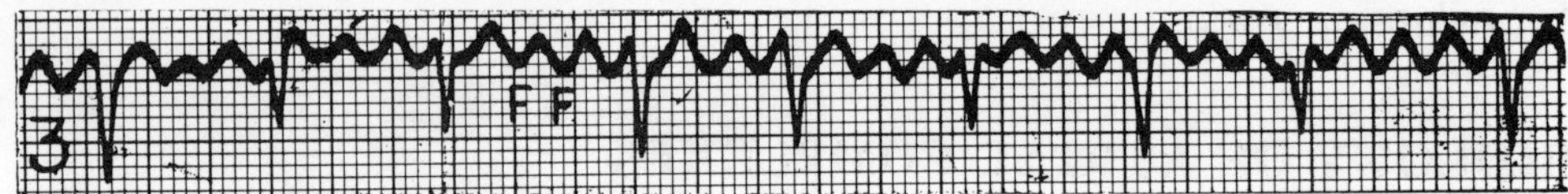

Fig. 24-C - Atrial flutter. The atrial rate is 380/min. This rhythm is also called "flutter-fibrillation."

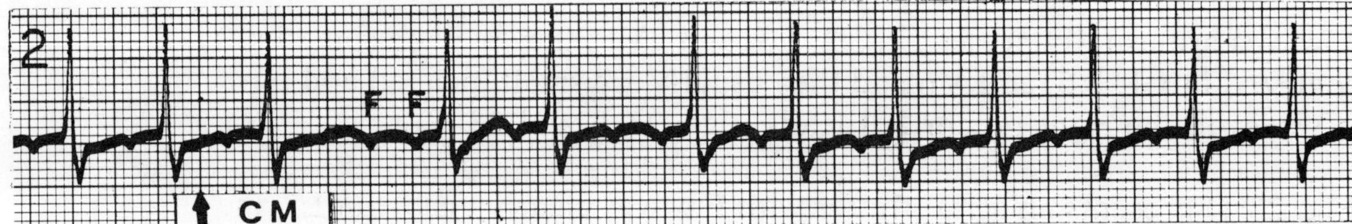

Fig. 25-A - Atrial flutter. The A-V ratio is of a 2:1 type. F waves appear evident during the increased A-V block obtained with a carotid sinus massage (CM).

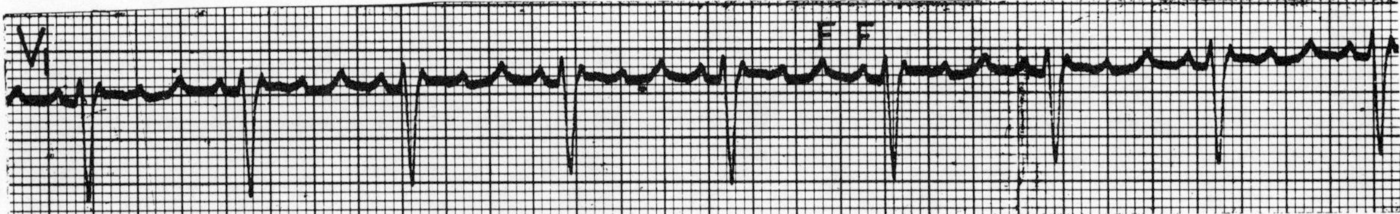

Fig. 25-B - Atrial flutter. Stable 4:1 A-V ratio.

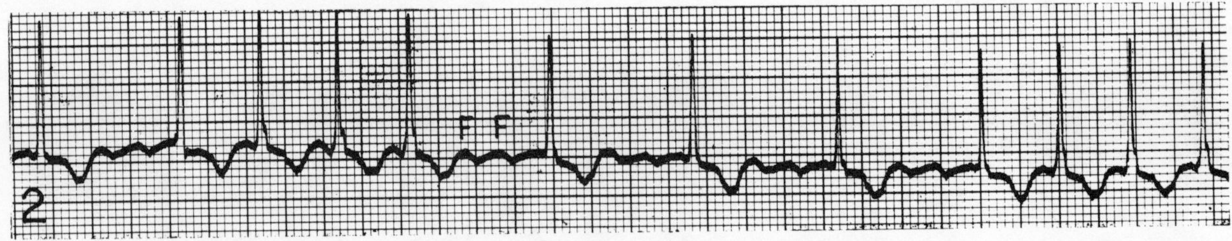

Fig. 25-C - Atrial flutter. The A-V ratio changes between a 2:1 and a 4:1 type.

B. - RATE OF ATRIAL WAVES

The lower and upper limits of atrial rates of an atrial flutter have been conventionally established between 250 and 350 impulses/min. Since these limits are not rigid it is not uncommon to find ECG tracings with the classical saw-tooth waves (F waves) in L2, L3 and aVF, and with atrial rate below 200 beats/min. or above 400 beats/min.

Figs. 24-A, 24-B, and 24-C show three cases of atrial flutter with different atrial rates. F waves are clearly evident in all three tracings and the atrial rates are respectively 220/min. (fig. 24-A), 330/min. (fig. 24-B) and 380 beats/min. (fig. 24-C).

In fig. 24-A the atrial rate is within the limits of an atrial tachycardia, but the diagnosis of *atrial flutter* is made on the typical saw-tooth appearance of F waves.

In fig. 24-C, instead, the atrial rate is very high (380/min.) and the F waves are slightly irregular. This rhythm is at the threshold of an atrial fibrillation and is also called *flutter-fibrillation*.

C. - A-V CONDUCTION RATIO

The most common ratio between the atrial and ventricular rate of an atrial flutter is the 2:1 type. Therefore, only every other F wave crosses the A-V junction and reaches the ventricles originating a QRS complex.

This type of A-V conduction is also commonly called *2:1 A-V block*. The term block, in this circumstance, does not indicate a pathology of the A-V conduction tissue, but is the expression of a physiological refractoriness of the A-V junction to the continuous bombardment and concealed penetration of numerous atrial impulses. The A-V block is a protective mechanism. It protects the ventricles from the fast atrial rates by allowing only half of the atrial impulses to filter through the A-V junction and to reach the ventricles.

With an A-V conduction ratio of 2:1, every other F wave may be buried in a QRS complex and the mechanism of the arrhythmia may not appear clear. Vagal maneuvers, such as the carotid massage (CM), may easily unveil the real rhythm disturbance (fig. 25-A).

Other types of A-V ratios may also be found. The 4:1 A-V ratio is common enough (fig. 25-B). A-V ratios of 1:1, 5:1, 6:1, 7:1, and 8:1 are less common but are occasionally found. A-V ratios of 3:1 and higher usually suggest something more than a simple physiological refractoriness and are probably caused by drugs which delay A-V conduction velocity or by an organic A-V block.

A-V ratios of 4:1 and 2:1 may be present in the same tracing (fig. 25-C). Sudden changes in the A-V block may lead to an irregular ventricular rate and, therefore, may simulate the ventricular response of an atrial fibrillation.

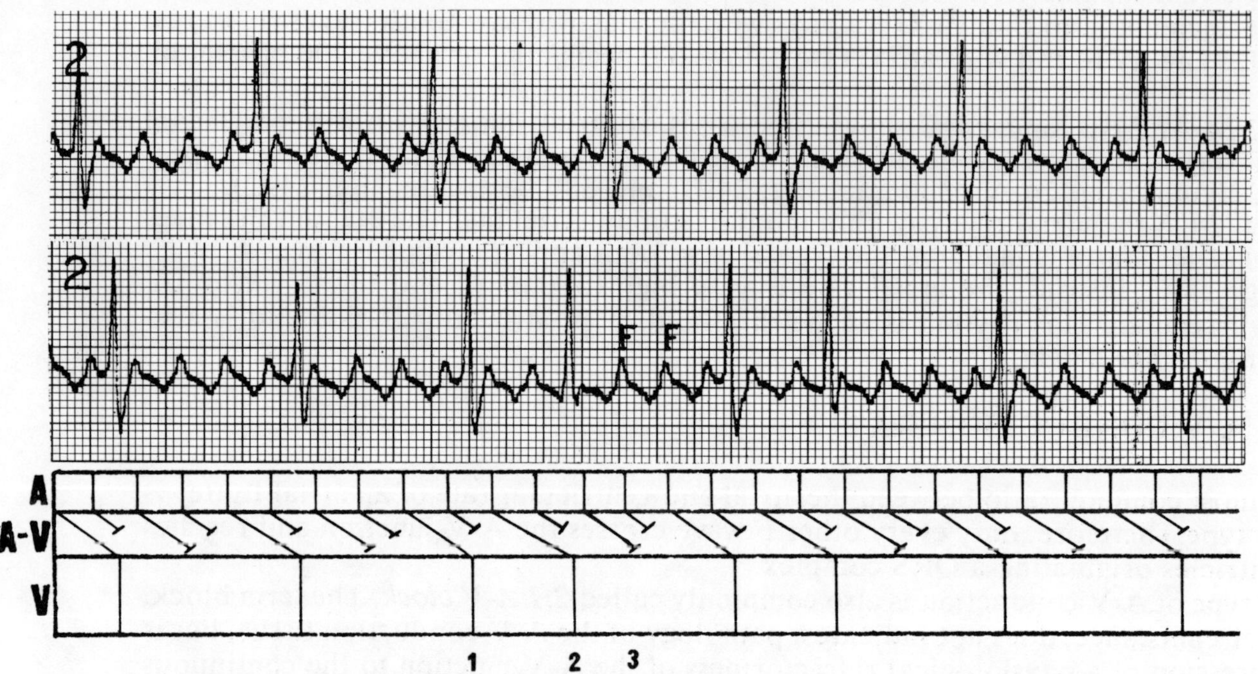

Fig. 26-A - Atrial flutter with variable A-V block. The diagram illustrates the A-V Wenckebach phenomenon which determines the variable A-V block from a 4:1 to a 2:1 type.

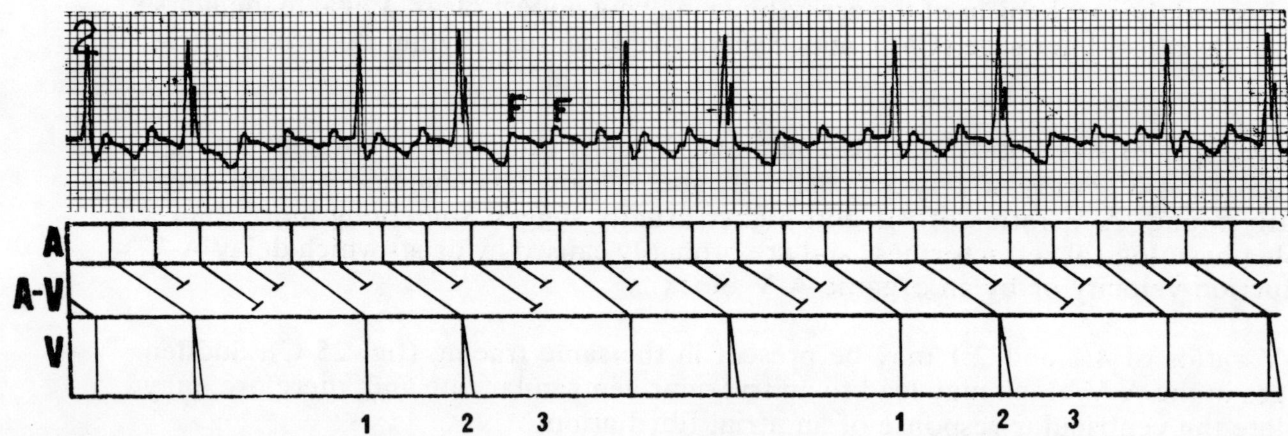

Fig. 26-B - Atrial flutter with a variable A-V block and bigeminal rhythm. The QRS conducted to the ventricles, with a prolongation of the F-R interval, shows a slight ventricular aberration.

A-V RATIO

When an A-V ratio changes from 2, 3, 4 to 1 in the same tracing and produces an irregular ventricular rate, one must always think of the presence of a *Wenckebach phenomenon* in the A-V conduction of atrial impulses (see page 70).

The atrial flutter of fig. 26-A, with a rate of 270 beats/min. and a 4:1 A-V block, shows irregularly spaced R-R intervals (second tracing) and shorter cardiac cycles which alternate with longer ones. The diagram illustrates how *concealed atrial impulses penetrate continuously both in the proximal and distal portions of the A-V junction*.

During a 4:1 A-V block only one of the four F waves is conducted to the ventricles. Of the other three, one is blocked in the high portion of the A-V junction, the following penetrates slightly further, but it is still blocked, and the third is again blocked in higher areas of the A-V junction. Therefore, while a constant 2:1 block is present in the high portions of the A-V junction, a simultaneous 4:1 block is working distally.

The penetration of every other F wave in lower areas of the A-V junction is demonstrated by the occasional transformation of the A-V block from a 4:1 into a 2:1 type. In fact, during the alternating 4:1 and 2:1 A-V block the *concealed Wenckebach sequence* is as follows:

a) one F wave reaches the ventricles (fig. 26-A no. 1) while the following is blocked in proximal areas of the A-V junction.

b) the following F wave is again conducted to the ventricles, but with a prolongation of the F-R interval (fig. 26-A no. 2).

c) the next F wave is again blocked proximally in the A-V junction and the following one, although penetrating more distally, is again blocked (fig. 26-A no. 3), closing the Wenckebach sequence.

Therefore, while a constant 2:1 A-V block is present proximally in the A-V junction, a *Wenckebach phenomenon* operates distally with periods of 3:2.

Fig. 26-B presents, again, an atrial flutter, with an A-V conduction which alternates from 4:1 to 2:1, and a production of a bigeminal rhythm. In this case the QRS complex, which closes the shorter cardiac cycle shows a ventricular aberration. The *3:2 Wenckebach* is formed by:

1) the beat conducted normally to the ventricle;

2) the beat aberrantly conducted to the ventricle with a prolongation of the F-R interval;

3) the beat blocked in the distal areas of the A-V junction.

While the Wenckebach operates distally, a 2:1 A-V block is simultaneously present in the higher areas of the A-V junction.

ARRHYTHMIAS DUE TO ABNORMAL IMPULSE FORMATION

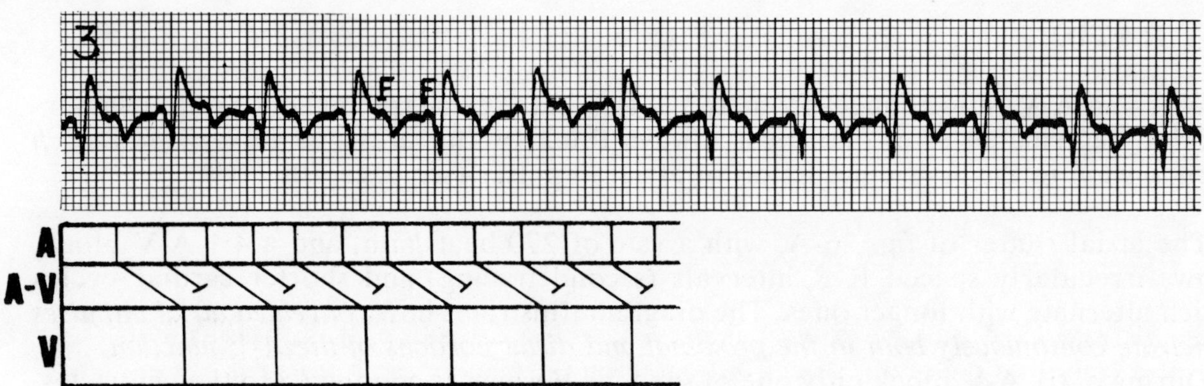

Fig. 27-A - Atrial flutter. The A-V block is of a 2:1 type. The first of the two F waves is conducted to the ventricles while the second is blocked in the A-V junction.

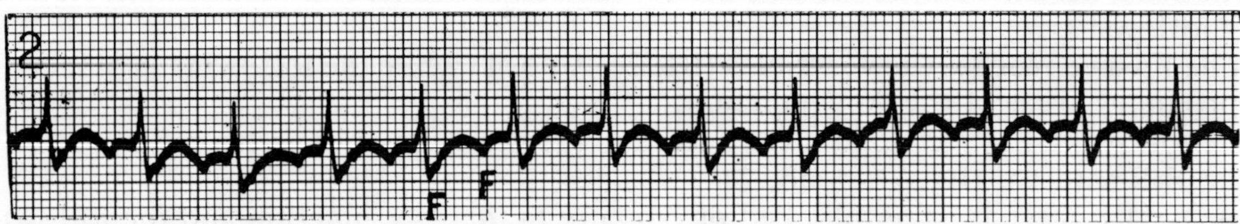

Fig. 27-B - Atrial flutter with 2:1 A-V block.

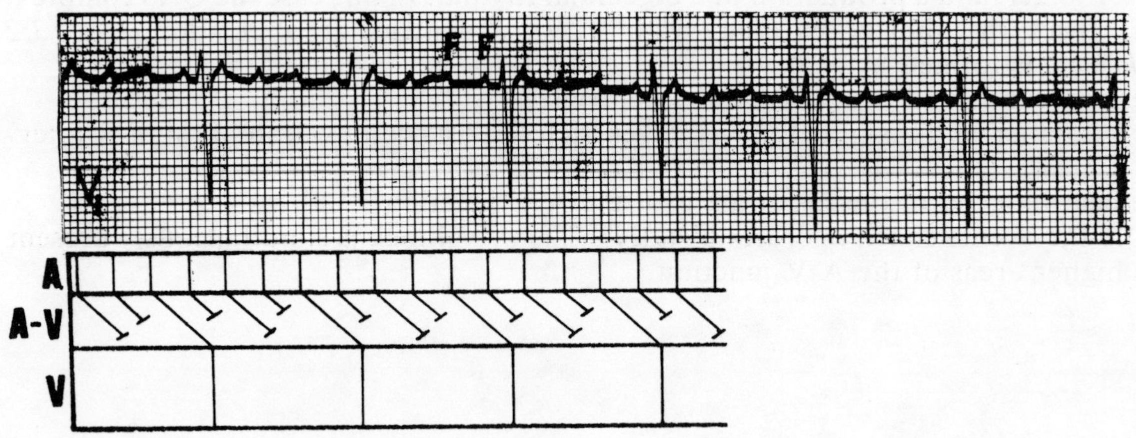

Fig. 27-C - Atrial flutter with 4:1 A-V block.

During an atrial flutter it is usually difficult to exactly measure the F-R interval because it is not always clear where the F wave starts and, therefore, where to begin the measurement. However, it is commonly believed that the F-R interval is constantly prolonged because the atrial impulses bombard and penetrate the A-V junction at different levels, maintaining it in a partial refractory state. Usually the length of F-R intervals fluctuate between 0.26 and 0.45 secs.

In fig. 27-A, an atrial flutter is present with a 2:1 block. It is obvious that the second of the two F waves indicated on the tracing can not possibly conduct to the ventricles because it falls too close to the QRS. Therefore, the F wave, with an F-R interval of 0.32 secs., is the one which conducts to the ventricles.

In fig. 27-B, although both F waves show quite prolonged F-R intervals, the first F wave is the one that conducts to the ventricles, with an F-R interval of 0.38 secs.

In fig. 27-C, an atrial flutter with a 4:1 A-V block is presented. The F wave immediately preceding the QRS is blocked because of the very short F-R interval and because the A-V junction is in a state of partial refractoriness for the concealed penetration of preceding F waves. Therefore, it is conceivable that the F wave which conducts to the ventricles is the one with an F-R interval of 0.30 sec.

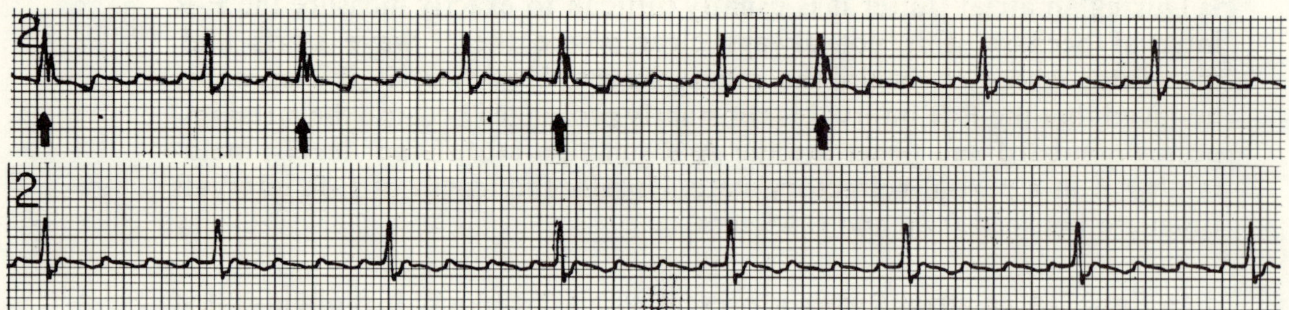

Fig. 28-A - Atrial flutter with a variable A-V block. The arrows indicate the beats with aberrant ventricular conduction.

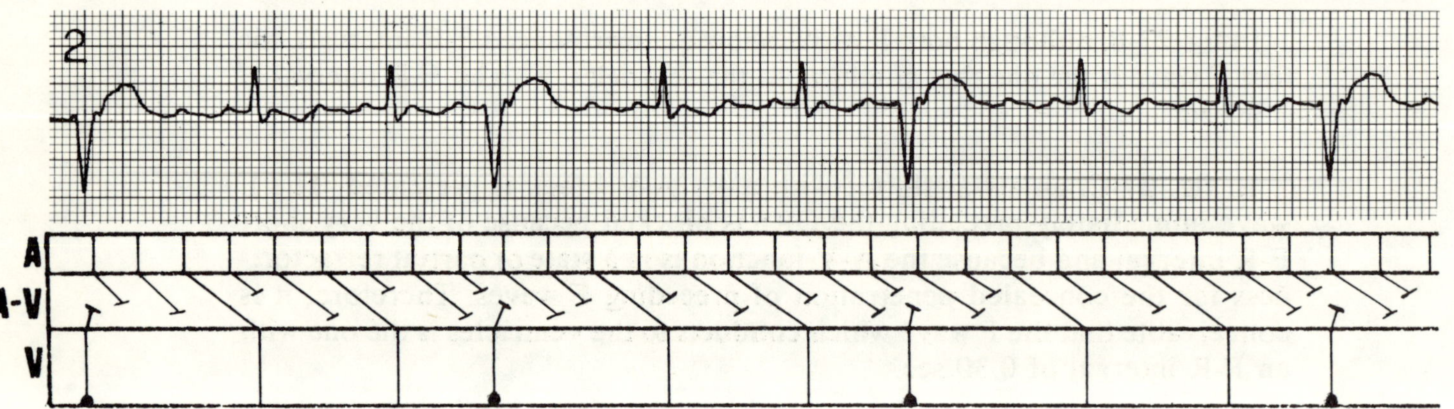

Fig. 28-B - Atrial flutter. The retrograde conduction of the ventricular extrasystoles increases the refractoriness of the A-V junction.

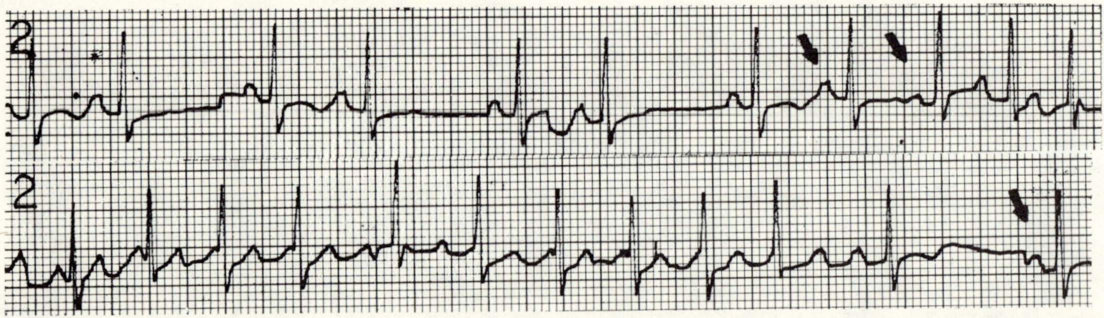

Fig. 28-C - Atrial flutter. The paroxysmal flutter (lower tracing) is anticipated by several PAC's with a bigeminal pattern (upper tracing).

Fig. 28-A presents an example of an atrial flutter with A-V ratio varying from 4:1 to 2:1 and an aberrant ventricular conduction of the beats closing the shortest cardiac cycles. The first, third, fifth, and seventh QRS show an aberrant ventricular conduction and determine a bigeminal rhythm because of the alternating 4:1 and 2:1 A-V block. The aberrant conduction disappears when the ventricular rhythm becomes regular for the stabilization of the A-V block in a 4:1 type (lower tracing).

A *ventricular trigeminy* is present in the atrial flutter of fig. 28-B. Two normal looking QRS's are followed by a PVC with a fixed coupling interval and a complete compensatory pause. This indicates a partial retrograde penetration of the PVC into the A-V junction while the atrial rate remains undisturbed. Therefore, while the atrial flutter has a basic 3:1 A-V block, the cardiac cycle which includes the PVC has a 6:1 A-V ratio; this is for the *retrograde penetration* of the PVC's which prolongs the refractoriness of the A-V junction.

The tracing of fig. 28-C starts with an *atrial bigeminy* which degenerates into a brief paroxysmal atrial flutter with a variable 3:1 and 2:1 A-V block. Two atrial premature beats mark the beginning of the paroxysm (upper tracing) and a sinus beat reappears promptly after the cessation of the arrhythmia (lower tracing).

ARRHYTHMIAS DUE TO ABNORMAL IMPULSE FORMATION

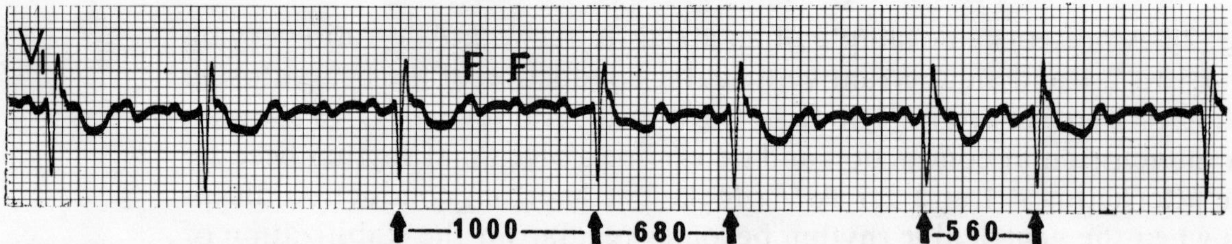

Fig. 29-A - Atrial flutter with a variable A-V ratio. The ventricular rate is irregular.

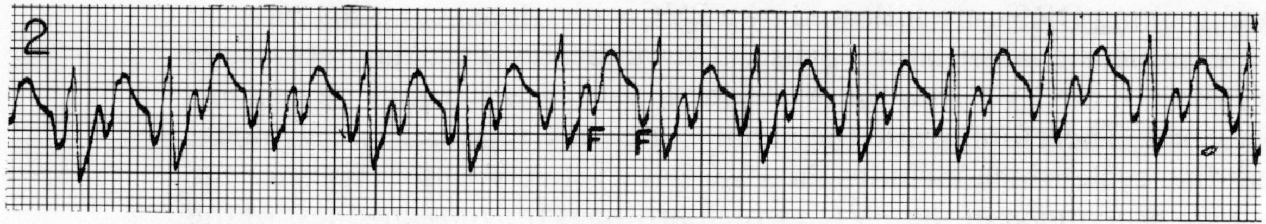

Fig. 29-B - Atrial flutter. Giant F waves in a patient with a congenital heart disease.

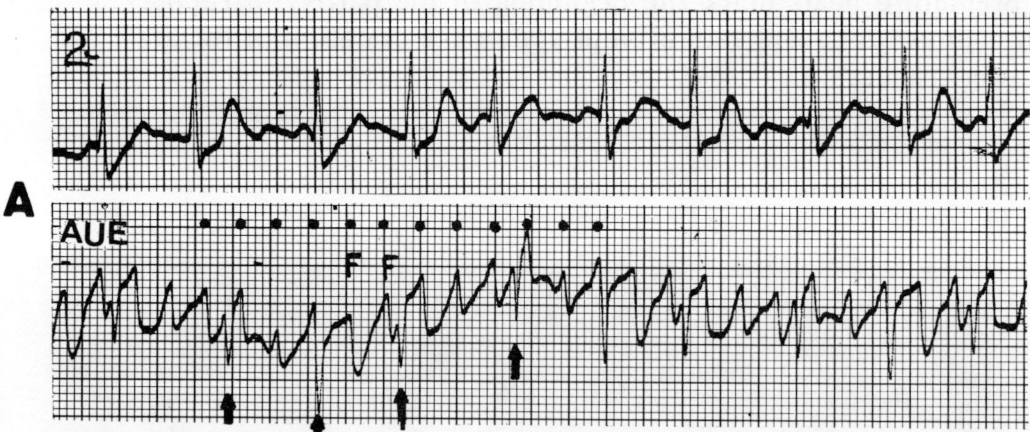

The control tracing and the unipolar atrial electrogram (UAE) are not simultaneous. Atrial flutter waves are evident (indicated by "F" and dots) and the irregular ventricular complexes are indicated by the arrows.

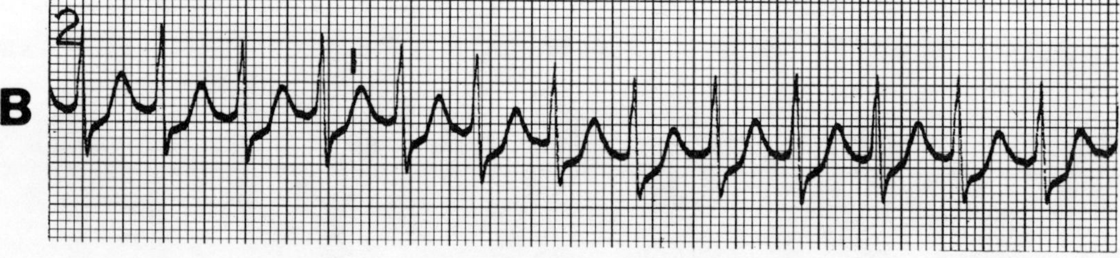

Fig. 29-C - Atrial flutter. Effect of Quinidine Sulfate on the A-V ratio (see text).

An *atrial flutter with a variable A-V block* is presented in fig. 29-A. In this tracing, the A-V ratio varies from 4:1 to 3:1 and 2:1 and determines an irregular ventricular rate (1000, 680, 560 msec.), simulating the ventricular response of an atrial fibrillation.

Fig. 29-B shows an atrial flutter with giant F waves, secondary to atrial dilatation in a patient with congenital heart disease. ·

Fig. 29-C illustrates the effect of Quinidine Sulfate on the conduction velocity of atrial impulses through the A-V junction. The tracing recorded in L2 and the atrial unipolar electrogram (AUE) show an atrial flutter with an atrial rate of 320/min. and a variable A-V block of 3:1 and 2:1 (A). A few hours after the oral administration of Quinidine Sulfate (B), the patient shows a tachyarrhythmia (ventricular rate = 150/min.) which was found to be an atrial flutter with a 2:1 A-V block. While it may decrease the frequence of formation of the atrial impulses. Quinidine Sulfate increases the conduction velocity through the A-V junction. Therefore, it may transform a flutter with a variable A-V block into one with a constant 2:1 A-V block (such as the case presented in fig. 29-C) or in a 1:1 A-V conduction. Quinidine Sulfate must always be associated with an adequate digitalization.

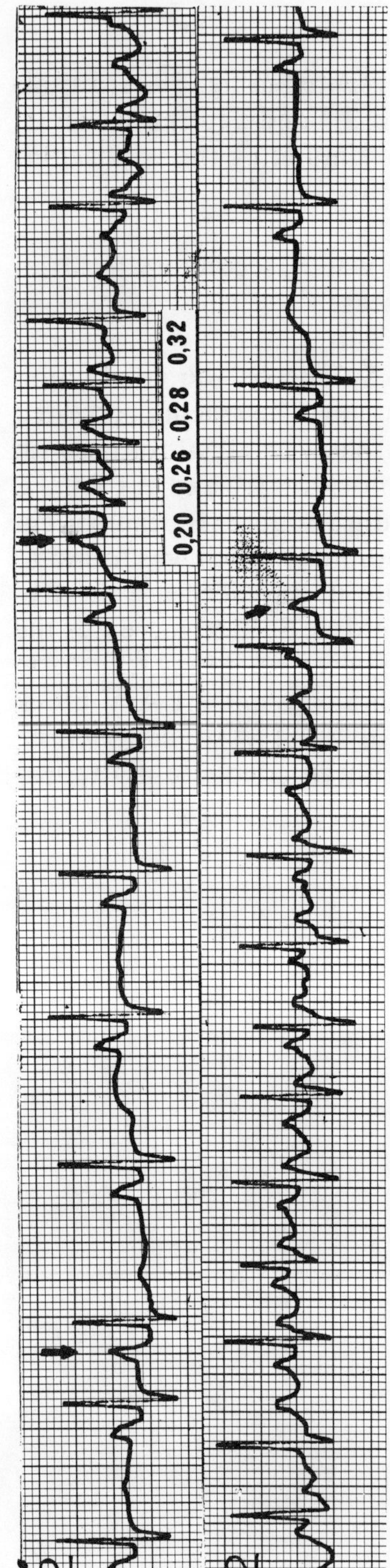

Fig. 30-A - Atrial flutter. Continuous recording of a paroxysmal atrial flutter which is initiated by a PAC (second arrow in the upper tracing). The atrial flutter shows initially an A-V Wenckebach phenomenon and later it stabilizes in a A-V block which varies from a 3:1 to a 2:1. Another PAC is present in the upper tracing (first arrow).

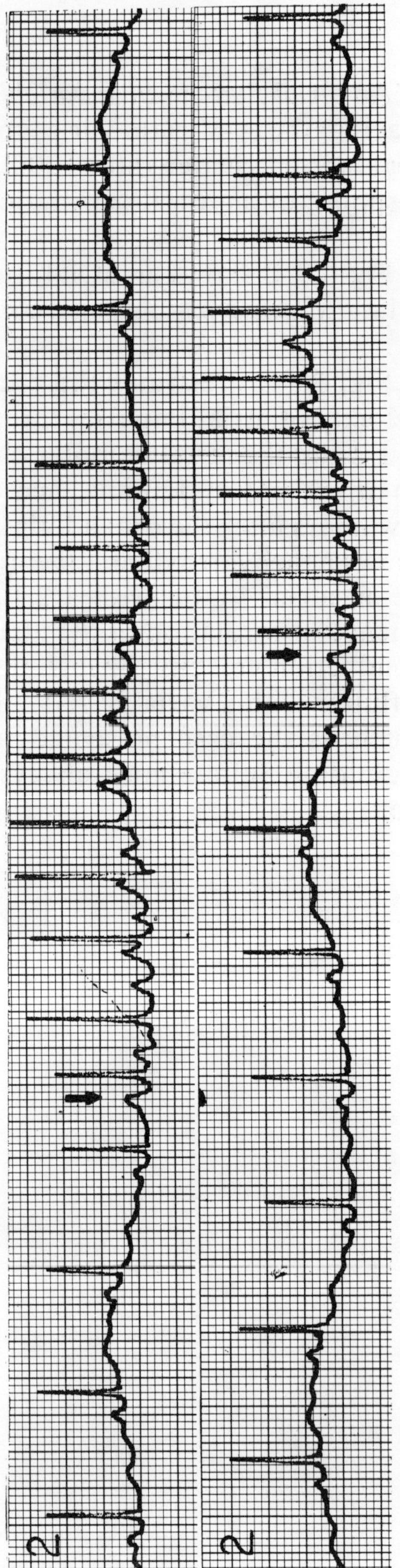

Fig. 30-B - Atrial flutter. Paroxysms of atrial flutter are present in the continuous tracing. In both cases the PAC which initiates the paroxysm is easily recognized (arrows).

ATRIAL FLUTTER

An atrial flutter, as any other type of tachyarrhythmia, may present itself in a paroxysmal form. The bursts usually start and cease abruptly. An atrial premature beat is almost always recognizable at the beginning of a paroxysm, and the arrhythmia usually appears in patients with persistent atrial extrasystoles, bigeminy or parasystoles.

Fig. 30-A shows a continuous recording of a very short burst of a *paroxysmal atrial flutter*. It is initiated by an atrial premature beat with a slight prolongation of the P^1-R interval. The first four beats of the paroxysm shows a 1:1 A-V conduction but, because of the high atrial rate, a Wenckebach mechanism (see page 164) comes immediately into action. The second, third and fourth F waves of the paroxysm are conducted to the ventricles with a gradual but always increasing prolongation of the F-R interval, while the fifth atrial wave is blocked and buried within the QRS. This is followed by a variable 3:1 and 2:1 A-V ratio. The paroxysmal atrial flutter terminates suddenly and the last F wave (arrow) enables the measurement of the F-R interval (0.28 sec.).

Two other brief paroxysms of atrial flutter are presented in fig. 30-B. Once again, two atrial extrasystoles mark the beginning of the arrhythmia and they are indicated by the arrows.

ARRHYTHMIAS DUE TO ABNORMAL IMPULSE FORMATION

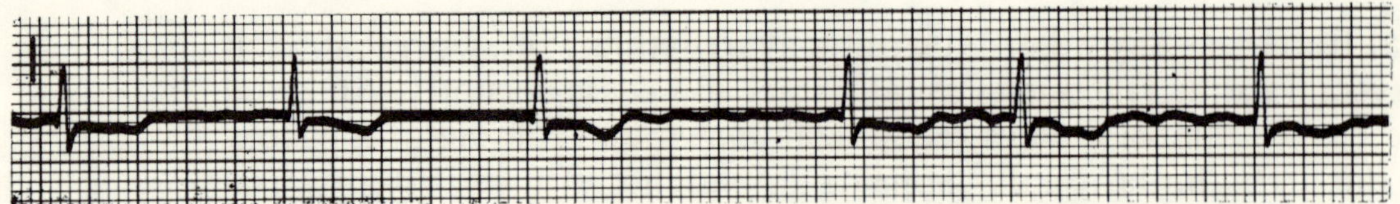

Fig. 31-A - Atrial fibrillation. A slight undulation of the baseline (f waves) and irregular ventricular response are the elements for the diagnosis of atrial fibrillation.

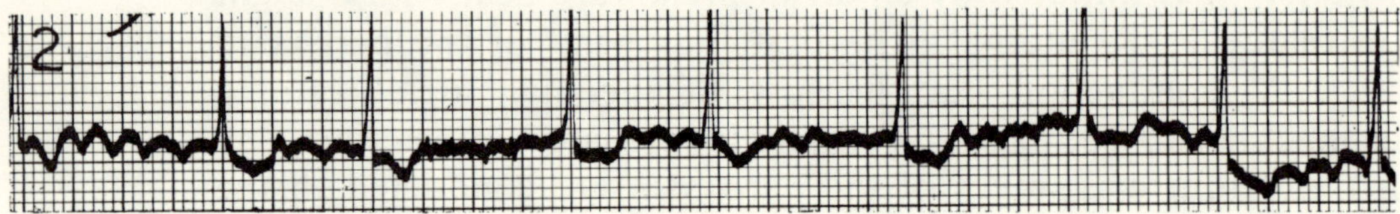

Fig. 31-B - Atrial fibrillation. Evident atrial fibrillatory waves (f waves).

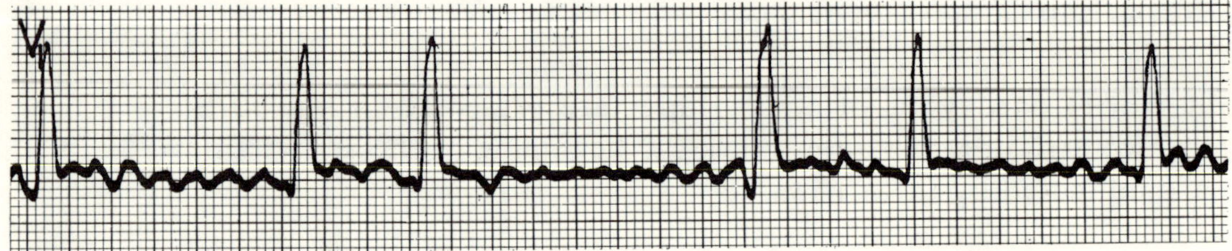

Fig. 31-C - Atrial fibrillation. The coarse f waves resemble those of an atrial flutter (F waves).

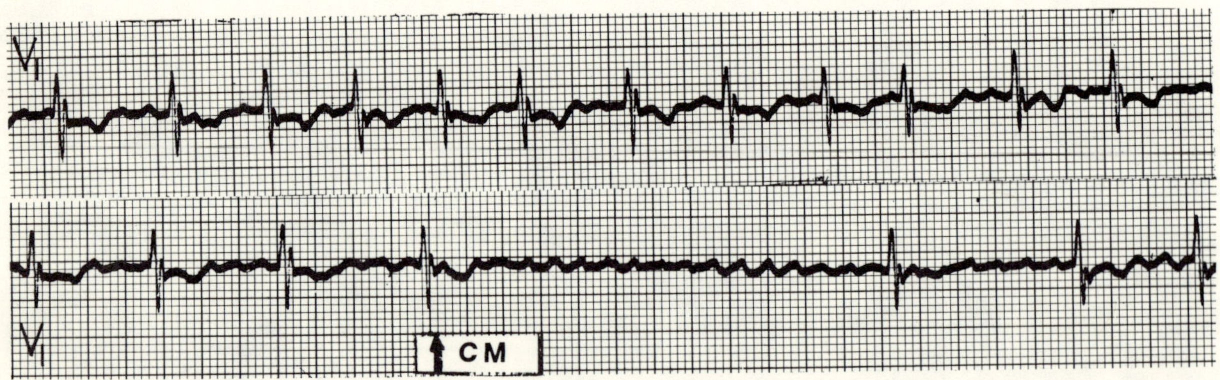

Fig. 31-D - Atrial fibrillation. In the upper tracing the mechanism of the arrhythmia is not clearly evident. The carotid sinus massage (CM) increases the A-V block and induces an asystolic pause. This permits the identification of the f waves.

ATRIAL FIBRILLATION

Atrial fibrillation is the most common of the atrial arrhythmias. It is diagnosed when an ECG tracing shows an irregular ventricular rate and the absence of P waves which are replaced by irregular undulations called *fibrillatory waves* (f waves). The leads where f waves are best recognized are V1, L2, L3 and AVF.

The amplitude of f waves may change from that of almost imperceptible undulations, (fig. 31-A) to that of coarse waves (fig. 31-B). Occasionally they may appear with an amplitude and a rate which resembles that of the F waves of an atrial flutter (fig. 31-C).

The QRS complexes of an atrial fibrillation may have a normal morphology (figs. 31-A and 31-B) or show a bundle branch block (fig. 31-C) or an aberrant ventricular conduction.

Sometimes, especially in the presence of a fast ventricular rate, it may be necessary to differentiate an atrial fibrillation from an atrial flutter with a variable A-V block. In these cases, a vagal stimulation may clearly reveal the atrial mechanism, as is shown in fig. 31-D. The carotid massage (CM) determines a temporary increase of the A-V block and a long asystolic pause which reveals the atrial fibrillatory waves.

ARRHYTHMIAS DUE TO ABNORMAL IMPULSE FORMATION

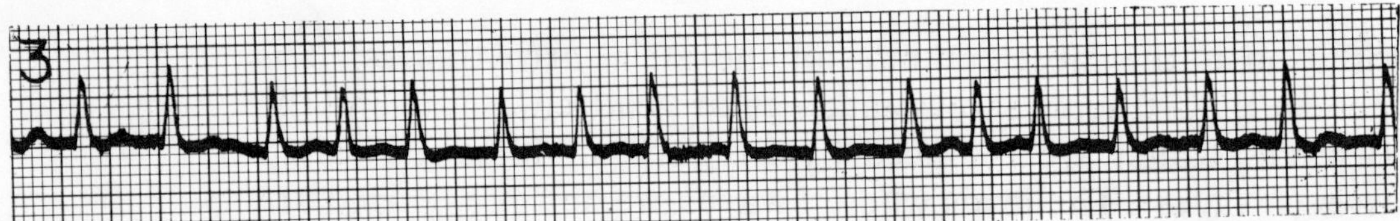

Fig. 32-A - Atrial fibrillation. The mean ventricular rate is 180/min.

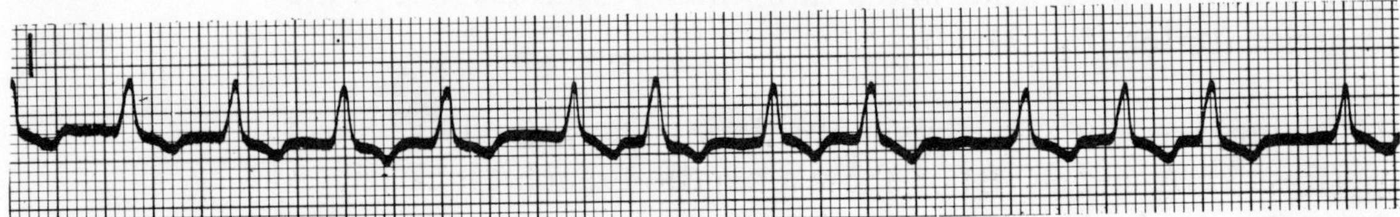

Fig. 32-B - Atrial fibrillation. The mean ventricular rate is 160/min.

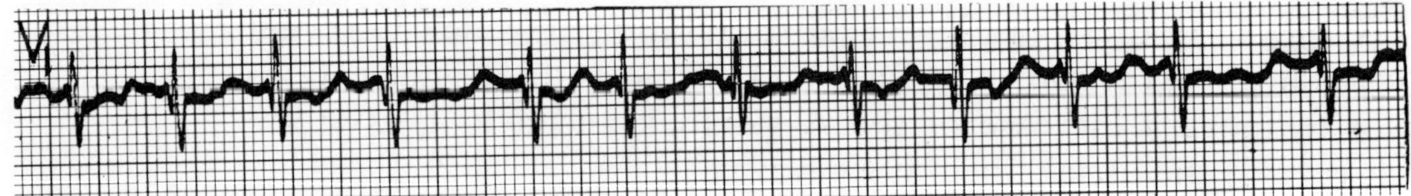

Fig. 32-C - Atrial fibrillation. The mean ventricular rate is 130/min.

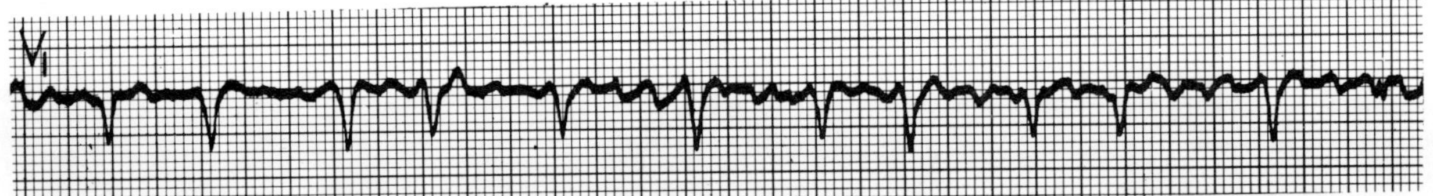

Fig. 32-D - Atrial fibrillation. The mean ventricular rate is 110/min.

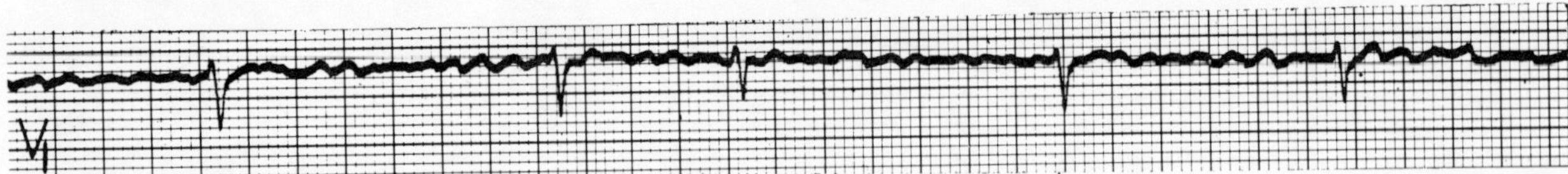

Fig. 32-E - Atrial fibrillation. The mean ventricular rate is 60/min.

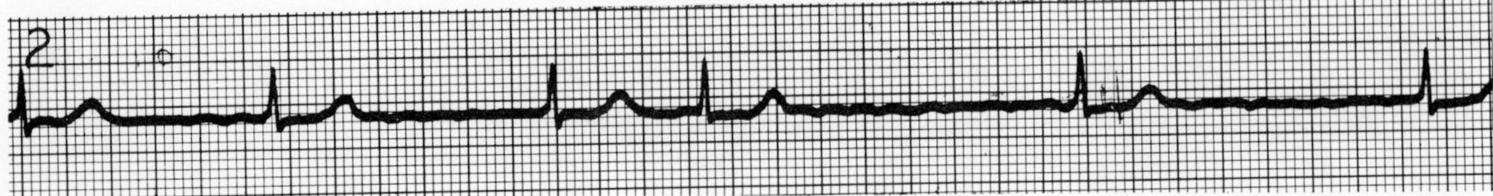

Fig. 32-F - Atrial fibrillation. The mean ventricular rate is 50/min.

VENTRICULAR RATE

The ventricular rate of an atrial fibrillation is determined by:
a)   the number of atrial impulses which bombard and penetrate through the A-V junction.
b)   the efficiency state of the A-V junction.

Figs. 32-A through 32-F show six cases of atrial fibrillation with different ventricular rates. They are in order: 180/min., 160/min., 140/min., 110/min., 60/min., 50/min.

While it is a common opinion that atrial tachycardias are caused by repetitive impulses from a single ectopic atrial focus, several theories have been proposed to explain the mechanism of atrial flutter and fibrillation.
1.   *Circular movement.* This theory maintains that a circular wave is established in a ring of atrial tissue around the vena cava and that, from the main wave, secondary waves are diffused in the remaining atrial myocardium.
2.   *Single ectopic focus.* This theory postulates the origin and propagation of the atrial impulses from a single atrial ectopic focus.
3.   *Multiple ectopic focus.* This theory admits the simultaneous presence of several active ectopic atrial foci which stimulate, simultaneously or sequentially, different areas of atrial myocardium.

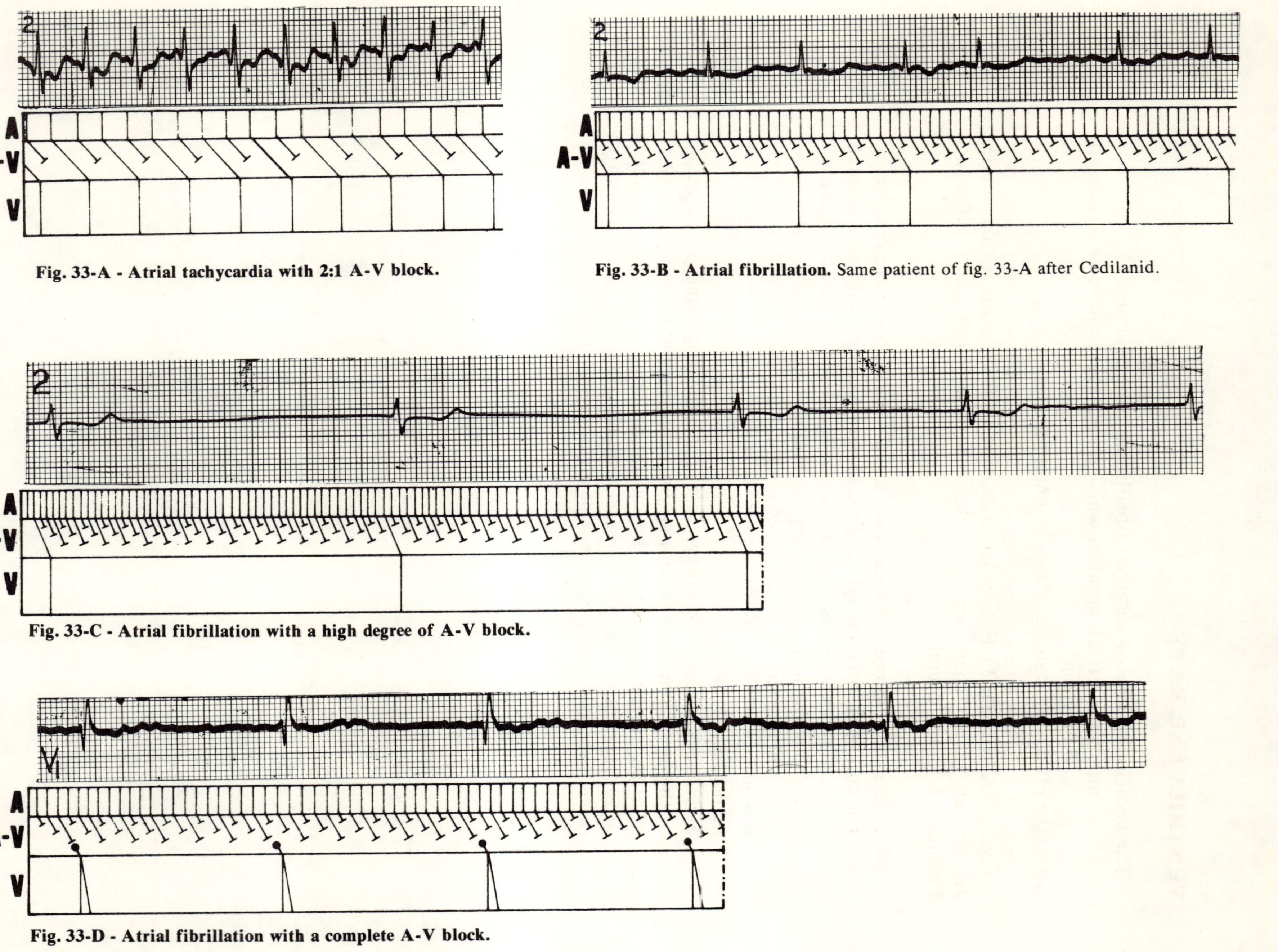

Fig. 33-A - Atrial tachycardia with 2:1 A-V block.

Fig. 33-B - Atrial fibrillation. Same patient of fig. 33-A after Cedilanid.

Fig. 33-C - Atrial fibrillation with a high degree of A-V block.

Fig. 33-D - Atrial fibrillation with a complete A-V block.

ATRIAL FIBRILLATION

A-V RATIO

Fig. 33-A presents an atrial tachycardia with a 2:1 A-V block. The ventricular rate is 180/min. After Cedilanid IV (fig. 33-B), the rhythm is transformed into an atrial fibrillation with an irregular but definitely slower, ventricular rate (mean rate = 85/min.). The digitalis has increased the rate of atrial impulses and, at the same time, decreased the conduction velocity through the A-V junction. Numerous atrial impulses penetrate, in a concealed fashion, the A-V junction, but only a few can filter through and capture the ventricles.

Fig. 33-C shows a slow and irregular ventricular rhythm. Atrial activity is not recorded but the irregularity of the QRS complexes suggest an atrial fibrillation. In this case, a high degree of A-V block is present in the transmission of impulses from the fibrillating atria.

Fig. 33-D records a fine undulation of the baseline, typical of the "f waves" of an atrial fibrillation. However, the ventricular rate is absolutely regular. The explanation of this seemingly paradoxical behavior is quite simple. A complete A-V block in the transmission of atrial impulses is in action and the ventricular rhythm is under control of a junctional pacemaker with ventricular aberration.

ARRHYTHMIAS DUE TO ABNORMAL IMPULSE FORMATION

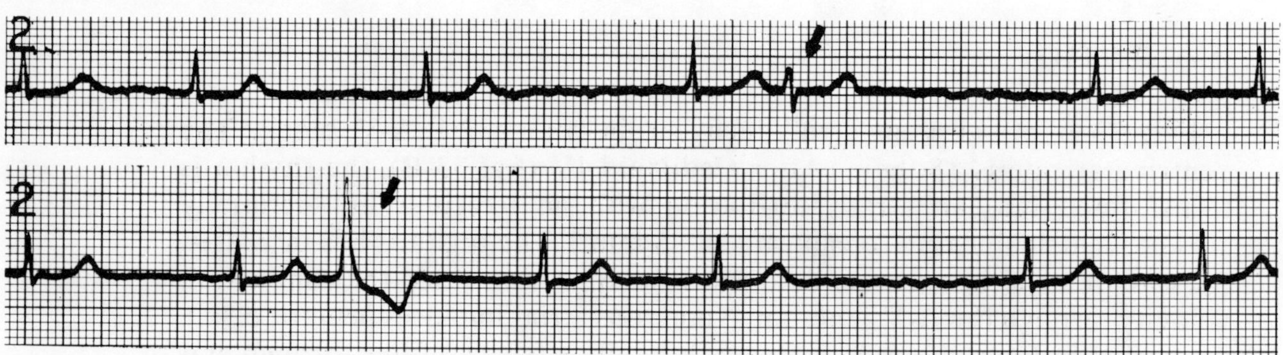

Fig. 34-A - Atrial fibrillation. The arrow in the upper tracing indicates an atrial beat with a slight aberration in the ventricular conduction. The arrow in the lower tracing indicates a PVC.

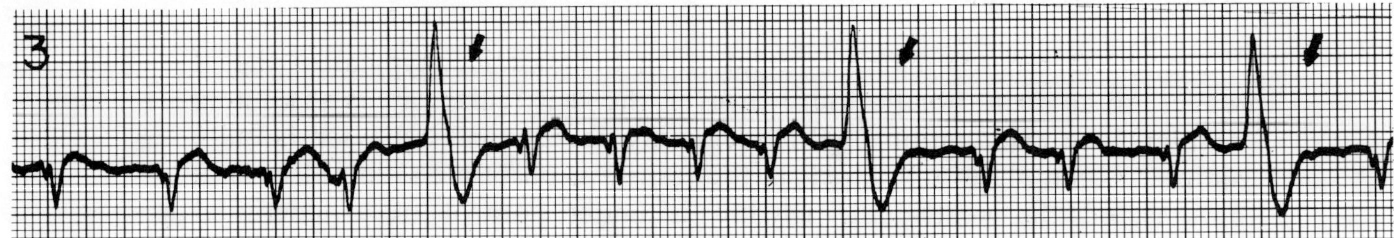

Fig. 34-B - Atrial fibrillation. Three PVC's, with a fixed coupling interval, are indicated by the arrows.

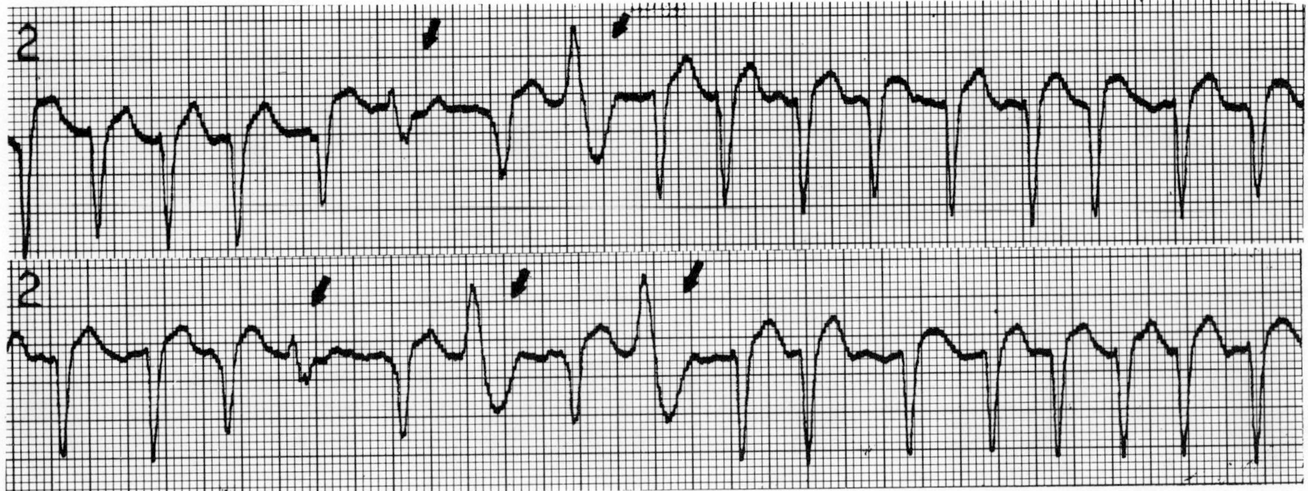

Fig. 34-C - Atrial fibrillation. Several ventricular extrasystoles are present in both tracings. The coupling interval is variable. In both tracings the morphology of the first extrasystole suggests a fusion beat.

ATRIAL FIBRILLATION

In the presence of an atrial fibrillation, the morphology of QRS complexes is normal unless a myocardial infarction or a conduction disturbance of one of the bundles is present. The possibility of atrial impulses conducted to the ventricles in an aberrant fashion must also be kept in mind. This is quite a common finding. The aberrant beats are often mistaken for PVC's and may, for example, determine the suspension of a digitalis therapy when it is mostly indicated.

With an atrial fibrillation it is not possible to "cherchez le P¹" and, therefore, one is deprived of an essential element in differentiating supra-ventricular beats with aberrant conduction versus PVC's (see page 16).

Fig. 34-A presents an atrial fibrillation with one beat showing *aberrant ventricular conduction* (top tracing) and a PVC (bottom tracing). Notice that the morphology of the aberrantly conducted beat is quite different from that of the PVC, while it is only slightly different from that of other QRS's.

Three ventricular extrasystoles are present in fig. 34-A, during an atrial fibrillation with a fast ventricular rate. They have a fixed coupling interval with the preceding QRS.

In fig. 34-C, the upper tracing shows two multifocal ventricular extrasystoles in a patient with atrial fibrillation. The coupling interval is variable. The lower tracing shows a brief salvo of ventricular bigeminy. It is interesting to note that the morphology of the extrasystoles follows the same sequence as in the top tracing. The first PVC has a configuration less bizarre than others and it is possible that this may be a fusion beat, suggesting the presence of a parasystolic focus (see page 144).

ARRHYTHMIAS DUE TO ABNORMAL IMPULSE FORMATION

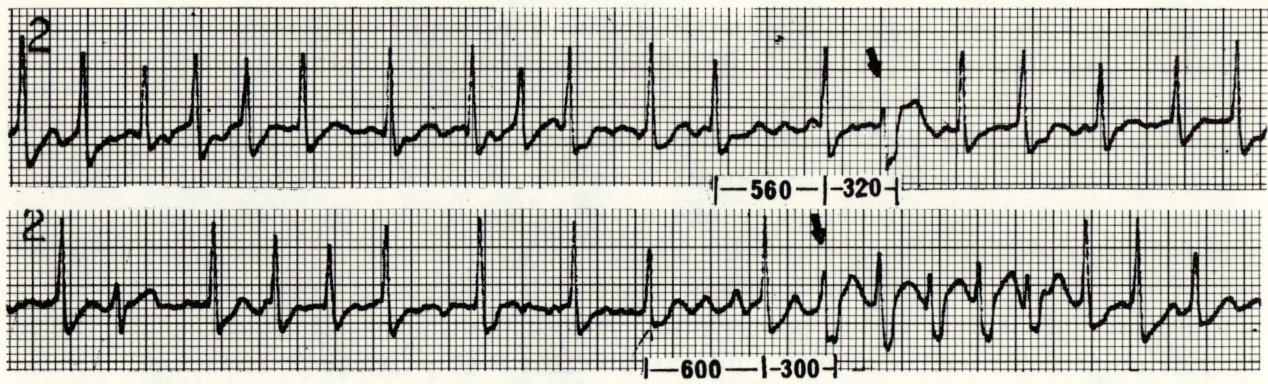

Fig. 35-A - Atrial fibrillation. The arrows indicate aberrantly conducted beats. In both tracings, these beats terminate a short cardiac cycle after a longer one. This is known as "Ashman phenomenon".

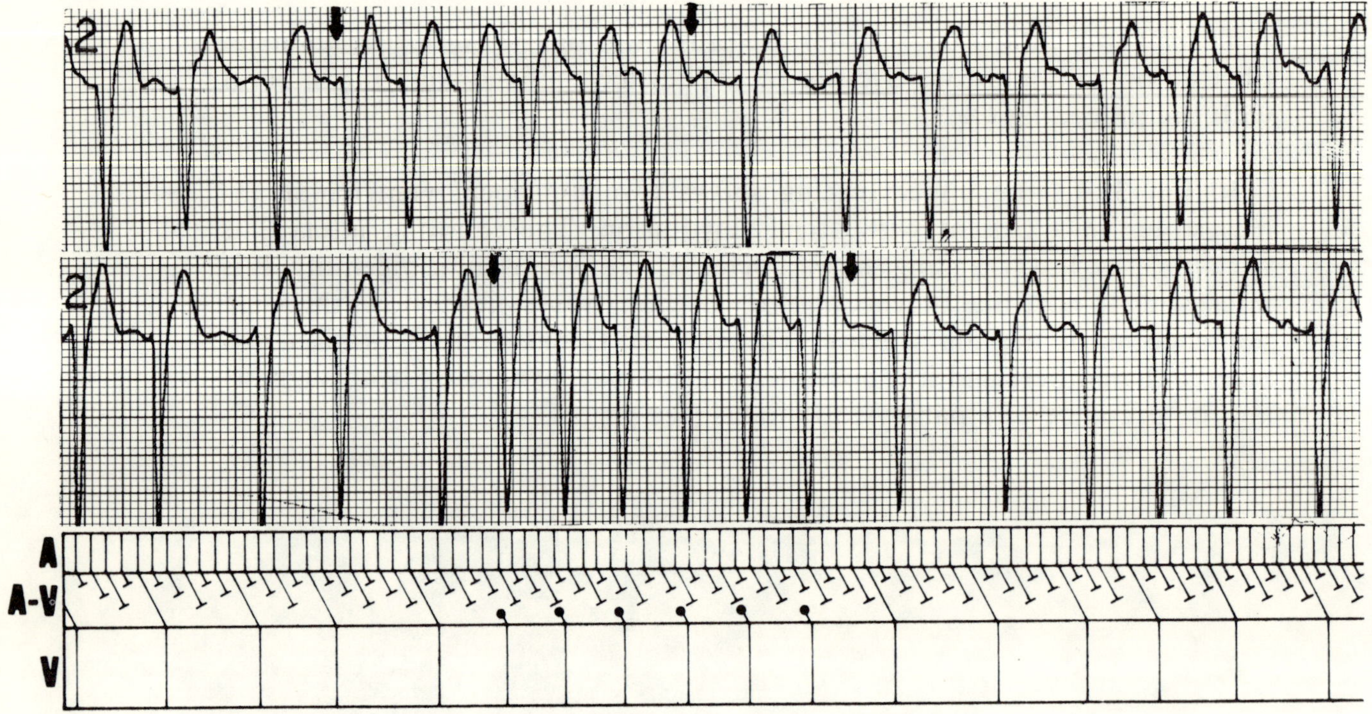

Fig. 35-B - Atrial fibrillation. In both tracings, the arrows enclose fast and regular beats within the context of a slower and irregular ventricular rate of an atrial fibrillation. They represent a junctional tachycardia with a transient A-V dissociation (as illustrated in the diagram).

The upper tracing of fig. 35-A shows an aberrantly conducted beat which closes a short cardiac cycle (320/msec.) after a preceding longer cycle (560 msec.). In the lower tracing a series of consecutive beats, with aberrant ventricular conduction, simulate a brief salvo of ventricular tachycardia. Notice that, again, the QRS's aberration starts with the beat which closes a short cardiac cycle following a longer one. *The sequence long-short cycle, which favors the aberrant ventricular conduction, is also known as Ashman phenomenon* (see page 186).

Fig. 35-B presents a case of atrial fibrillation with two episodes of rapid and regular ventricular rate due to salvos of a *junctional tachycardia*. The bursts of tachycardia momentarily determine an A-V dissociation (see page 120). The brief episodes of active junctional rhythm do not allow the penetration of atrial impulses into the A-V junction. The impulses coming from the atria find the A-V junction refractory for the simultaneous propagation of the junctional impulses. A similar situation is often encountered in patients with digitalis toxicity.

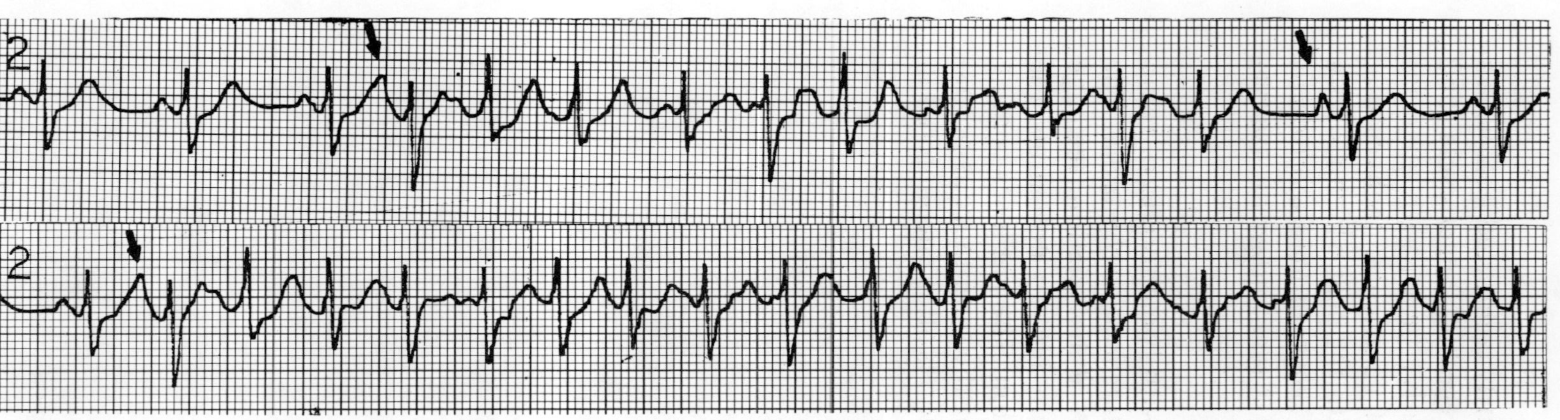

Fig. 36-A - Atrial fibrillation. Continuous recording of two paroxysms of atrial fibrillation. In both cases, the beat which initiates the paroxysm (arrows) shows an aberrant ventricular conduction (Ashman phenomenon). The basic rhythm is sinus.

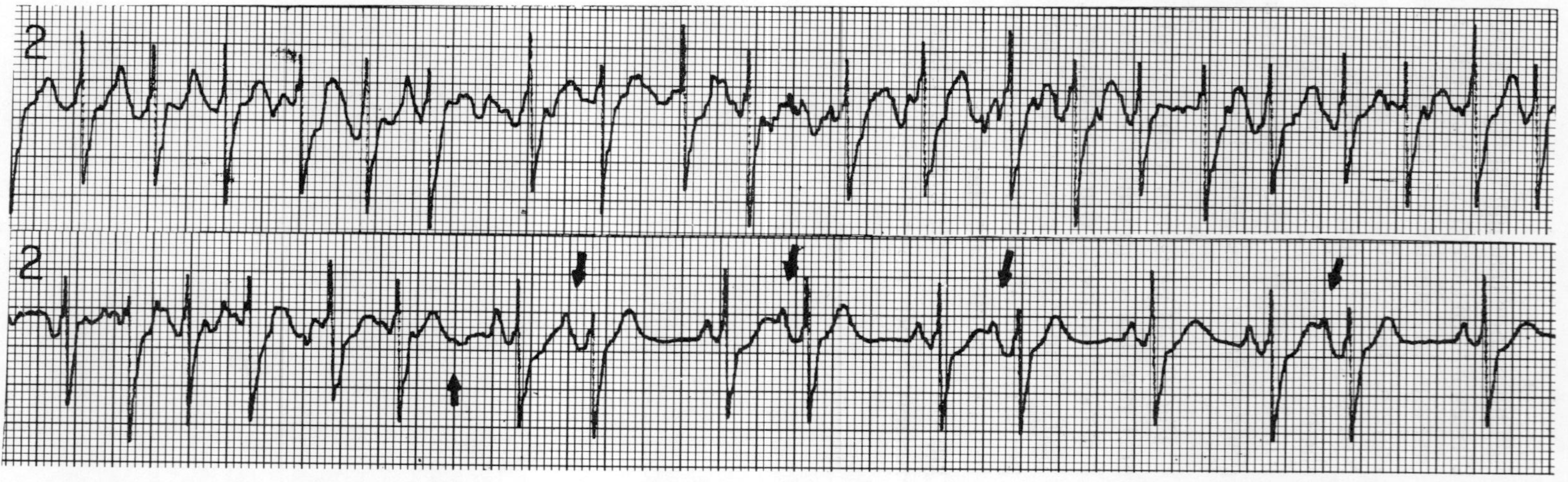

Fig. 36-B - Atrial fibrillation. PAC's, with a bigeminal behavior are present within the paroxysmal atrial fibrillation. A PAC initiates the paroxysmal arrhythmia.

Among the atrial tachyarrhythmias, atrial fibrillation has the highest tendency of self perpetuation; however it is not uncommon to find patients who present themselves with paroxysmal episodes of atrial fibrillation.

The upper tracing of fig. 36-A shows two paroxysms of atrial fibrillation with a fast ventricular response. In both episodes one can easily recognize the PAC which interrupts the sinus rhythm and which initiates the short burst of atrial fibrillation. Notice that the PAC's at the beginning of the atrial fibrillation clearly show an aberrant ventricular conduction. They terminate a short cardiac cycle after a longer one and suggest the presence of an *Ashman phenomenon*.

A paroxysmal atrial fibrillation may cease suddenly and spontaneously. It is quite common to find PAC's before and after the paroxysmal arrhythmia. In the case of fig. 36-B, the sinus rhythm following the cessation of the atrial fibrillation is uncertain and counterpointed by an atrial bigeminy.

ARRHYTHMIAS DUE TO ABNORMAL IMPULSE FORMATION

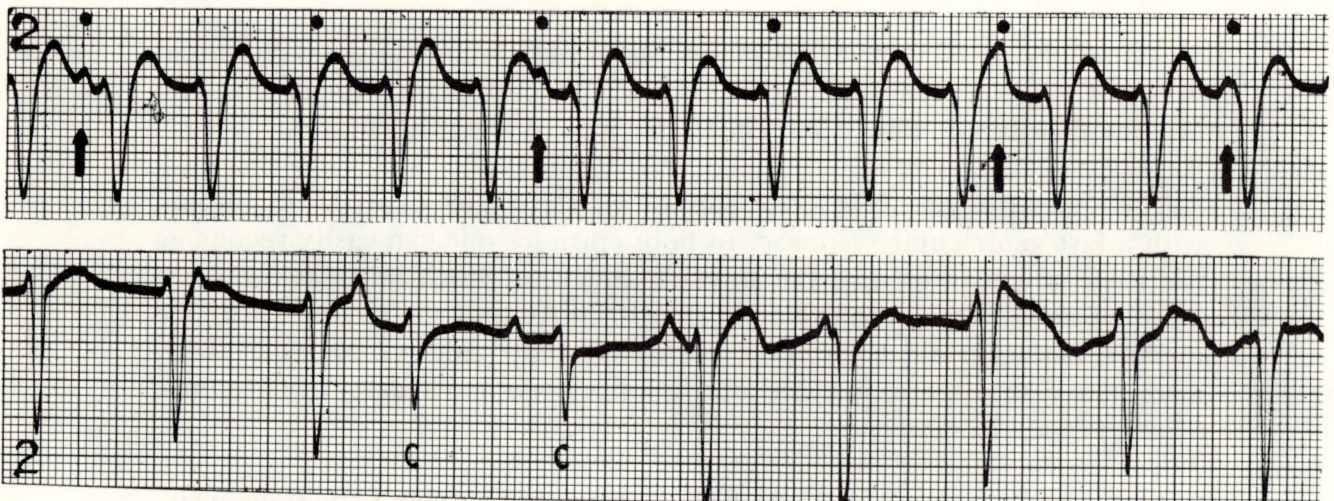

Fig. 37-A - Ventricular tachycardia. The dots in tracing "A" indicate sinus P waves which are independent from the QRS complexes. The arrows indicate P waves. In tracing B, the two sinus beats with ventricular capture (C) confirm the diagnosis of VT.

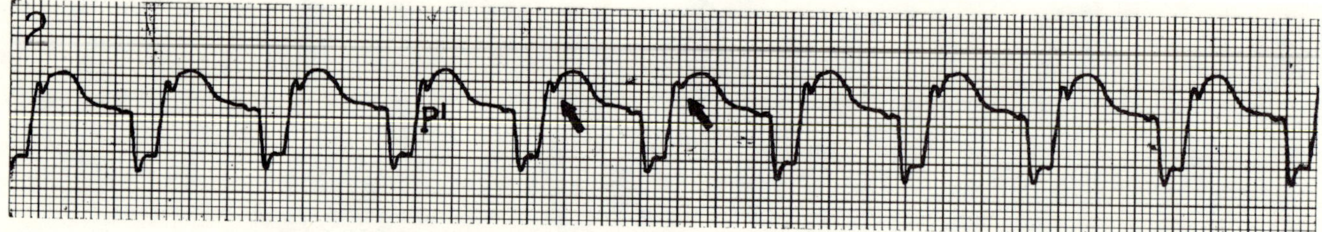

Fig. 37-B - Ventricular tachycardia with retrograde conduction to the atria. P^1 waves follow each ectopic QRS.

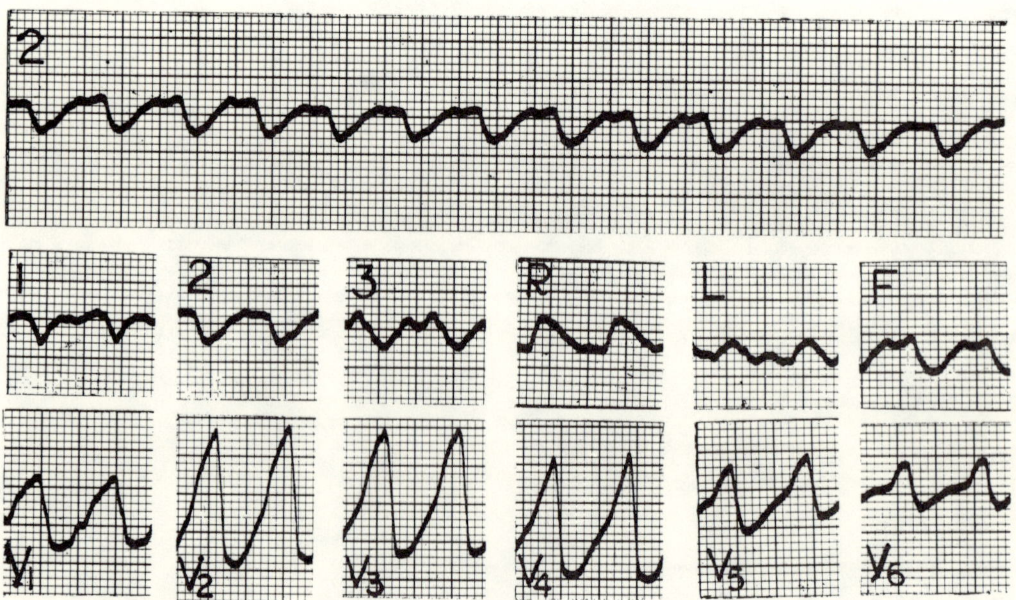

Fig. 37-C - Ventricular tachycardia. P^1 waves are not recognized. The monophasic appearance of the QRS complexes is particularly evident in the precordial leads, and is typical of a ventricular tachycardia.

VENTRICULAR TACHYCARDIA (VT)

Three or more ventricular extrasystoles in rapid succession represent a *ventricular tachycardia.* The term tachycardia signifies a cardiac rate above 100/min. In this broad sense, it has more of a clinical significance than an electrophysiologic one. The limit of 100/min., although it may be valid for the intrinsic automaticity of the sinus node, may not be applicable in reference to "active rhythms" with foci situated within the A-V junction or in the ventricles. The rate of impulse formation, which means the intrinsic automaticity, of secondary pacemakers usually fluctuates between 30 and 60 beats/min. Therefore, in the case of "idio-ventricular or junctional rhythms" the term *tachycardia* must be used anytime the ventricular rate is above 60/min.

The elements necessary for the diagnosis of a ventricular tachycardia are:
a) *the presence of A-V dissociation.* P waves and QRS's are independent and dissociated (atria and ventricles contract independently).
b) *the presence of fusion beats or of supraventricular beats that are conducted to the ventricles.*
c) *the differential diagnosis with a supraventricular tachycardia with aberrant ventricular conduction.*

Tracing A of fig. 37-A shows a ventricular tachycardia with an A-V dissociation. Independent and regular sinus waves, with P-P interval equals 1 sec., may be traced among the QRS complexes. They are indicated by dots. Only two P waves are clearly visible (first two arrows); however, a careful examination of the tracing brings out two additional P waves (last two arrows), one buried in the ST segment, and one immediately preceding the last QRS. The last two P waves can not be conducted to the ventricles because they are too close to the QRS complexes and, therefore, they suggest the presence of an A-V dissociation (see page 120).

Tracing B of fig. 37-A is obtained a few minutes later and shows the same tachycardic focus, with a slower rate, penetrating through the A-V junction with two sinus beats conducted to the ventricles (*ventricular capture beats*). The ventricular capture is facilitated by a slight increase of the sinus rate (P-P = 860 msec.). The following P waves are again blocked and dissociated with the VT focus. *Ventricular capture beats* (C) have the same meaning of fusion beats. They give information about the presence of two pacemakers situated into different cardiac chambers, atria and ventricles.

It is not unusual to find a situation like that presented in fig. 37-B. Bizarre and widened QRS complexes, typical of an ectopic ventricular focus, are clearly followed by small, negative waves which indicate a retrograde conduction to the atria (P[1]). The QRS-P[1] interval is equal to 0.20 sec. and is within the normal limits of the ventriculo-atrial conduction time. The *retrograde conduction to the atria,* when it is present, invalidates that important element in the recognition of VT that is represented by the presence of an A-V dissociation. This is because the sinus node is continuously suppressed by the retrograde atrial depolarization.

When P or P[1] waves are not recognized, the QRS morphology in the 12 ECG leads may be useful in defining the arrhythmia. Fig. 37-C shows a tachycardia recorded in L2. P[1] waves are not visible. The dominant monophasic R waves, particularly evident in all the precordial leads (V1 - V6), are highly indicative of an ectopic origin of the tachycardia.

ARRHYTHMIAS DUE TO ABNORMAL IMPULSE FORMATION

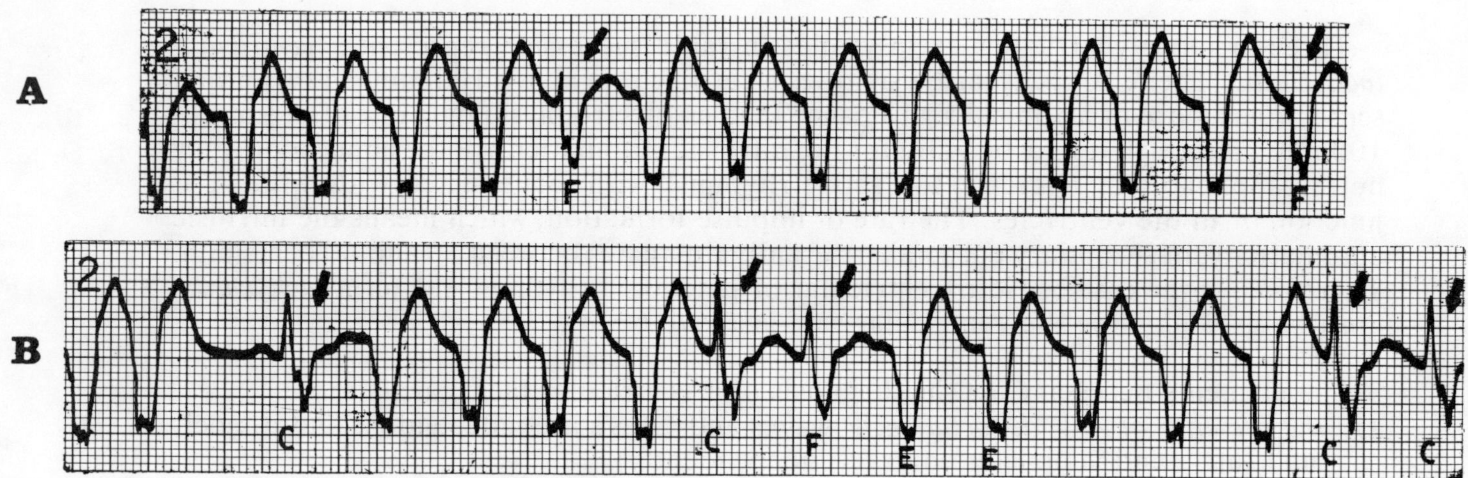

Fig. 38-A - Ventricular tachycardia. The arrow in tracing "A" indicates a QRS complex which is clearly different from the bizarre and widened QRS's of a VT. In "B" the QRS complexes show three different morphologies. B = ventricular beats. C = supraventricular beats conducted to the ventricles. F = fusion beats. The presence of fusion beats confirm the diagnosis of ventricular tachycardia.

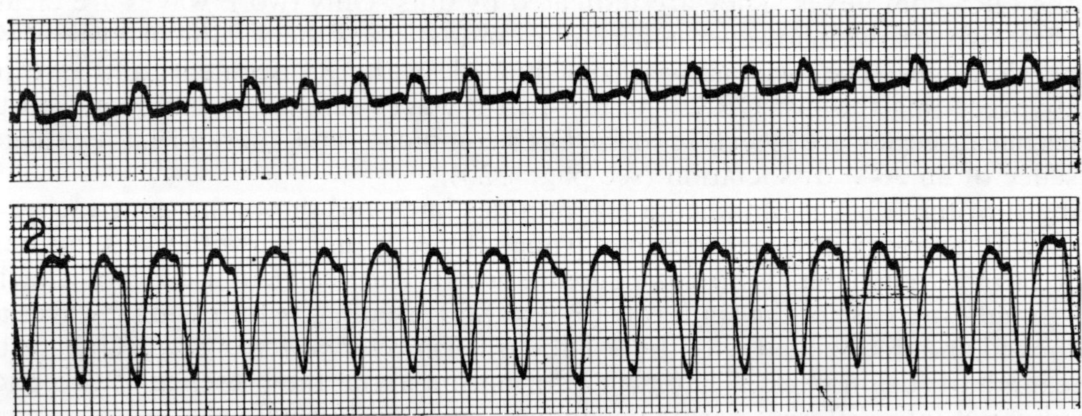

Fig. 38-B - Supraventricular tachycardia with left bundle branch block. The QRS morphology and the rapid heart rate would lead one to think of a ventricular tachycardia.

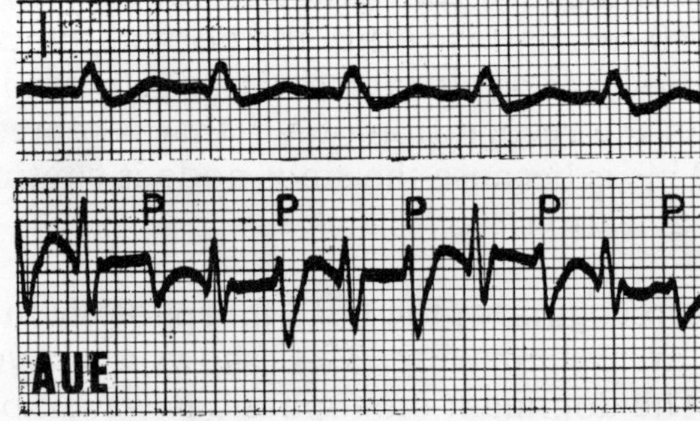

Fig. 38-C - The atrial unipolar electrogram (AUE) reveals a sinus tachycardia with a prolongation of the P-R interval. L1 is not simultaneous and shows an aberration of left bundle branch block type similar to that of fig. 38-B.

74

One important element in confirming the ventricular origin of a tachycardia is represented by the presence of *"fusion beats"* (see page 180).

Fig. 38-A presents a tachycardia with wide and aberrant complexes (tracing A). The two beats indicated by the arrows in the upper tracing have a narrower and slightly different configuration. Although P waves are not clearly visible, the beats indicated with "F" originate from sinus impulses which share the ventricular depolarization with the VT focus (F = fusion beats). By indicating an independent atrial and ventricular activation, the fusion beats confirm the ventricular origin of the tachycardia.

This is seen again in tracing B of the same patient, recorded a few seconds later. The third and eighth QRS's are clearly preceded by sinus P waves and are sinus beats conducted to the ventricles (C). The ninth QRS complex has an intermediate morphology (fusion beat = F) between that of a sinus beat and that of a QRS of ectopic ventricular origin (E). The last two QRS's of the lower tracing are again sinus beats conducted to the ventricle (C).

Fig. 38-B presents a patient with a fast heart rate and QRS complexes with a left bundle branch block morphology. P[1] waves are not clearly seen and this fact suggests a ventricular tachycardia. Fig. 38-C was recorded from the same patient a few hours later. While L1 shows the same ventricular aberration of left bundle branch block type, the atrial unipolar electrogram (AUE) clearly reveals the nature of the rhythm (see page 209). The rhythm is a sinus tachycardia with a prolongation of the P-R interval. This confirms that the tachycardia of fig. 38-B is of a supraventricular origin and with a left bundle branch block aberration.

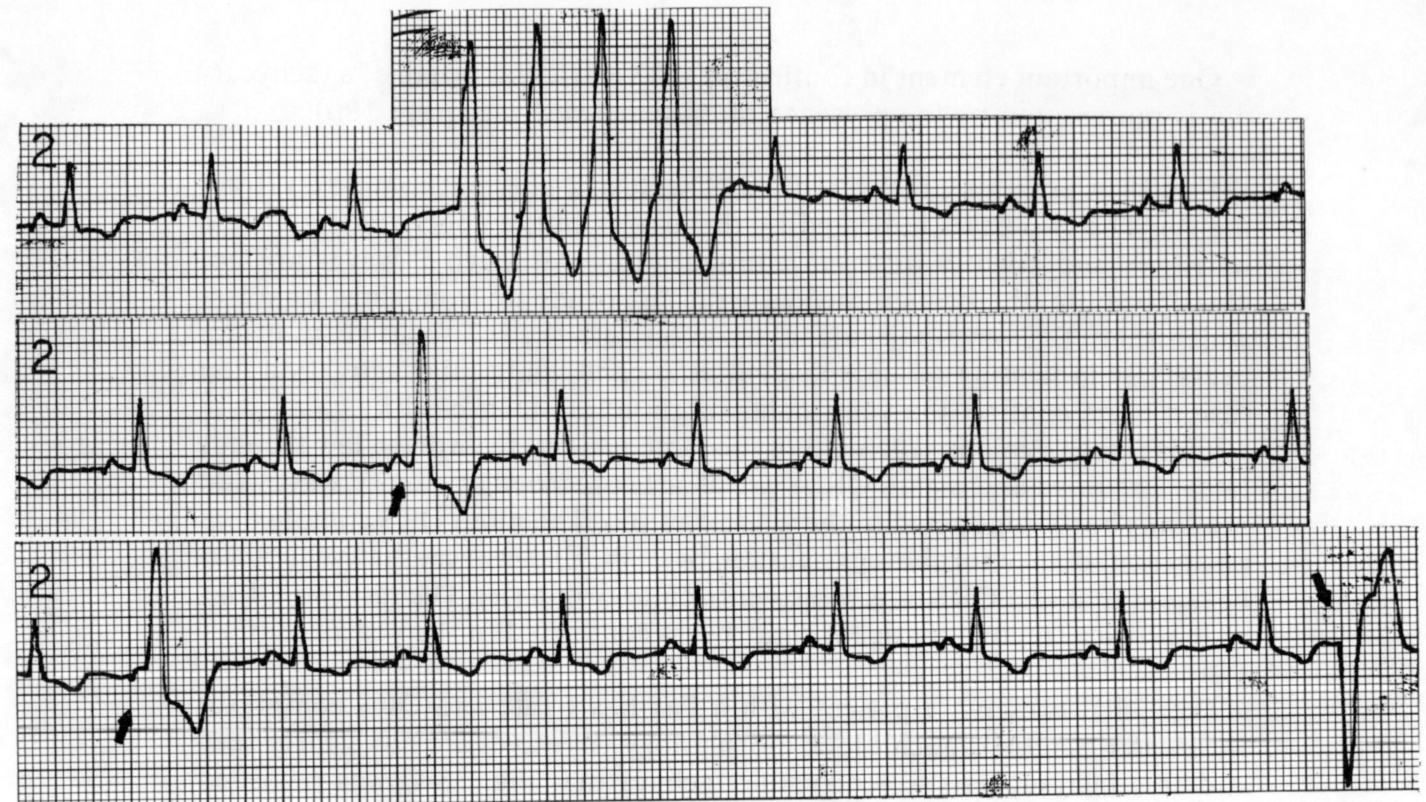

Fig. 39-A - Ventricular tachycardia. A rapid salvo of PVC's is present in the upper tracing. Multifocal PVC's, with variable coupling interval, are present in the lower tracings.

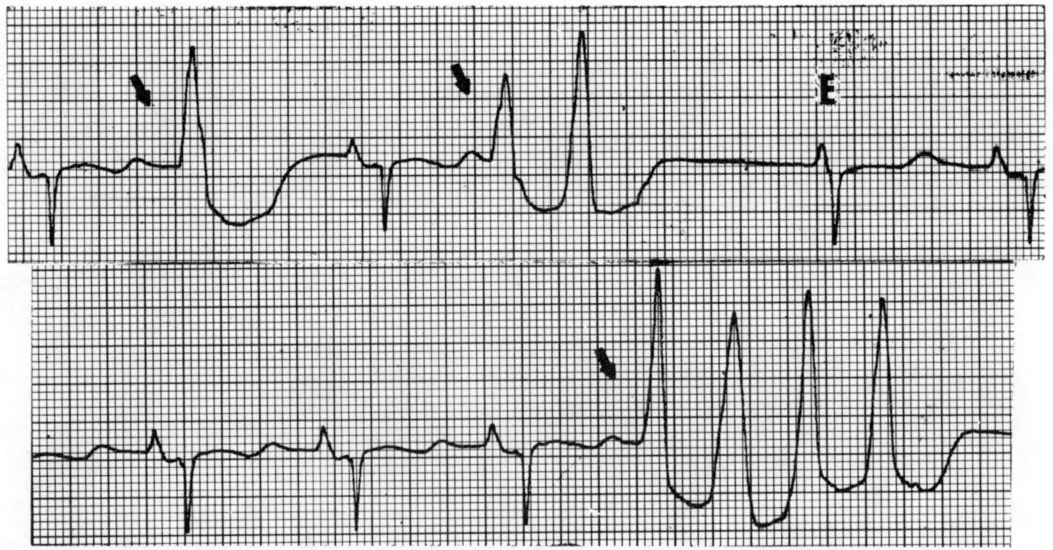

Fig. 39-B - Ventricular tachycardia. The PVC's show variable coupling intervals. They determine repetitive salvos of ventricular tachycardia. "E" is a junctional escape beat.

VENTRICULAR TACHYCARDIA

Two examples of short runs of paroxysmal ventricular tachycardia are presented in figs. 39-A and 39-B. Fig. 39-A shows a brief salvo of VT in a patient with frequent endiastolic, multifocal, ventricular extrasystoles with variable coupling intervals.

A similar case is presented in fig. 39-B where, again, the ventricular extrasystoles have variable coupling intervals and degenerate into VT (repetitive phenomenon). The arrhythmia is probably facilitated by the prolongation of the Q-T intervals of sinus beats. In the top tracing, an escape beat (E) follows two ventricular extrasystoles (see page 112).

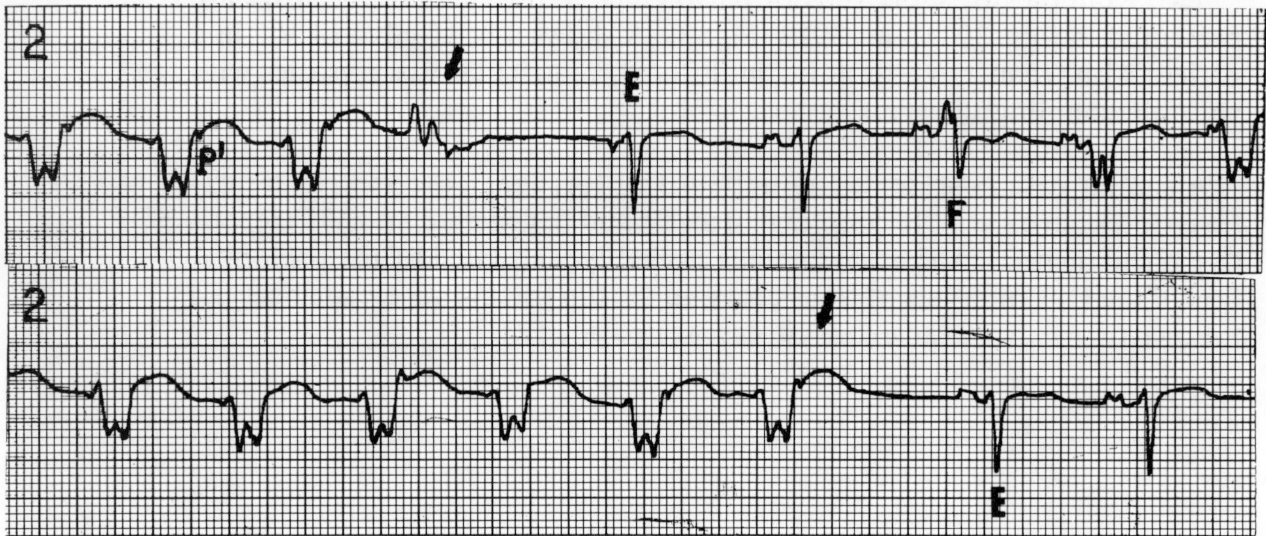

Fig. 40-A - Ventricular tachycardia. Continuous recording of two episodes of VT. The PVC in the upper tracing (arrow) is followed by a junctional escape beat (E) and the emergence of a sinus beat. The next beat is a fusion beat (F) which confirms the diagnosis of VT. The tachycardia stops suddenly in the lower tracing and it is followed by an escape (E) and a sinus beat.

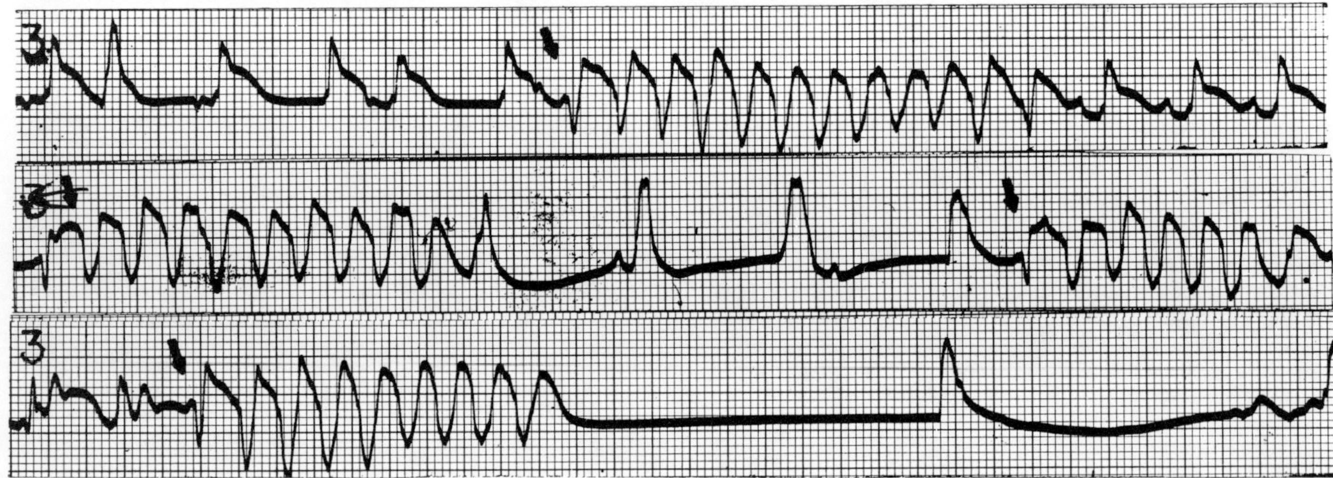

Fig. 40-B - Chaotic cardiac action. The episodes of ventricular tachycardia are always initiated by the same extrasystole (arrow). Long asystolic pauses are present in the bottom tracing.

VENTRICULAR TACHYCARDIA

Fig. 40-A begins with three ectopic beats of ventricular origin and with retrograde conduction to the atria (P^1). A PVC from a different focus (arrow) interrupts the sequence and induces a junctional escape beat ("E" - see page 112). This is followed by a sinus and a fusion beat ("F" - see page 180) and, again, by a brief sequence of VT. The arrhythmia ceases abruptly and is followed by an escape (E) and a sinus beat. The two escape beats show different P waves configurations which are dissimilar from that of sinus P waves. The P-R intervals are shorter than those of sinus beats and, therefore, the *escape beats* must be of *atrial* or *high junctional origin*.

Fig. 40-B presents several paroxysms of ventricular tachycardia in an agonal type of tracing. Notice that it is always the same ventricular premature beat which initiates the paroxysms. In the middle tracing, the R-R intervals of the slow idioventricular rhythm, alternating with the tachycardia, suggest the development of a cardiac arrest. This type of rhythm is also called *"chaotic atrial activity."*

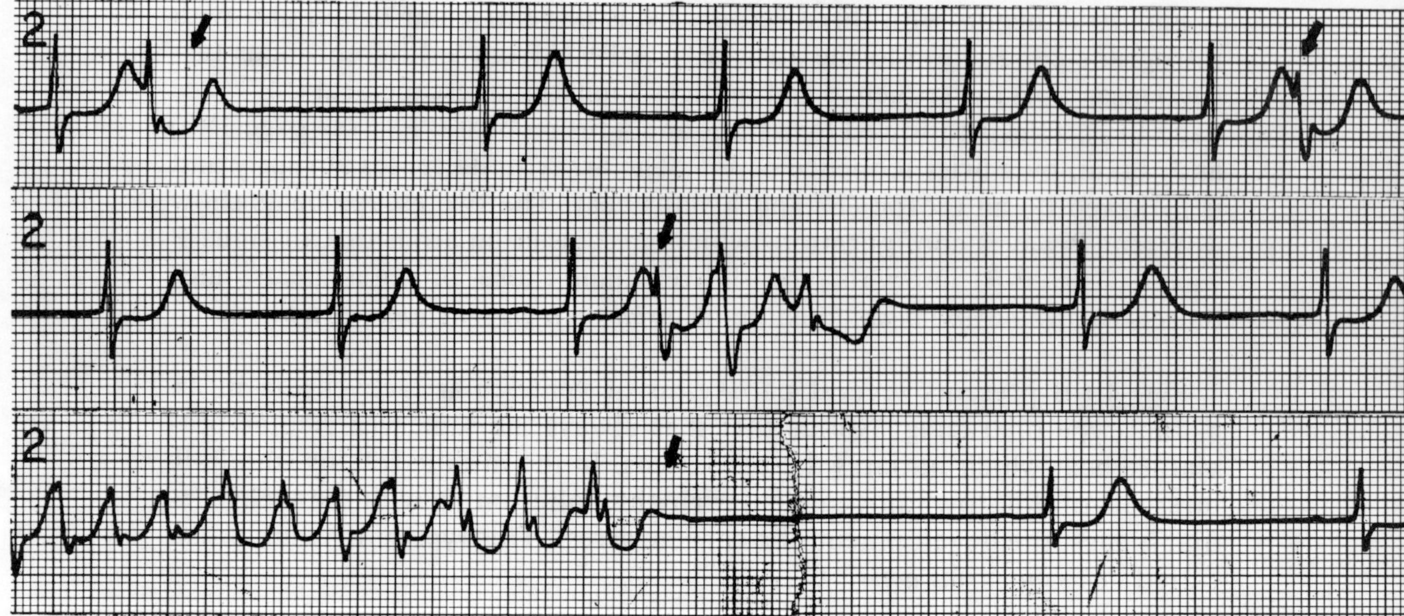

Fig. 41-A - Ventricular tachycardia and "R on T phenomenon." The PVC's with early coupling interval land on the descending branch of the preceding T waves. In the middle tracing they originate a brief salvo of VT. The VT stops suddenly and is followed by the reappearance of a sinus rhythm.

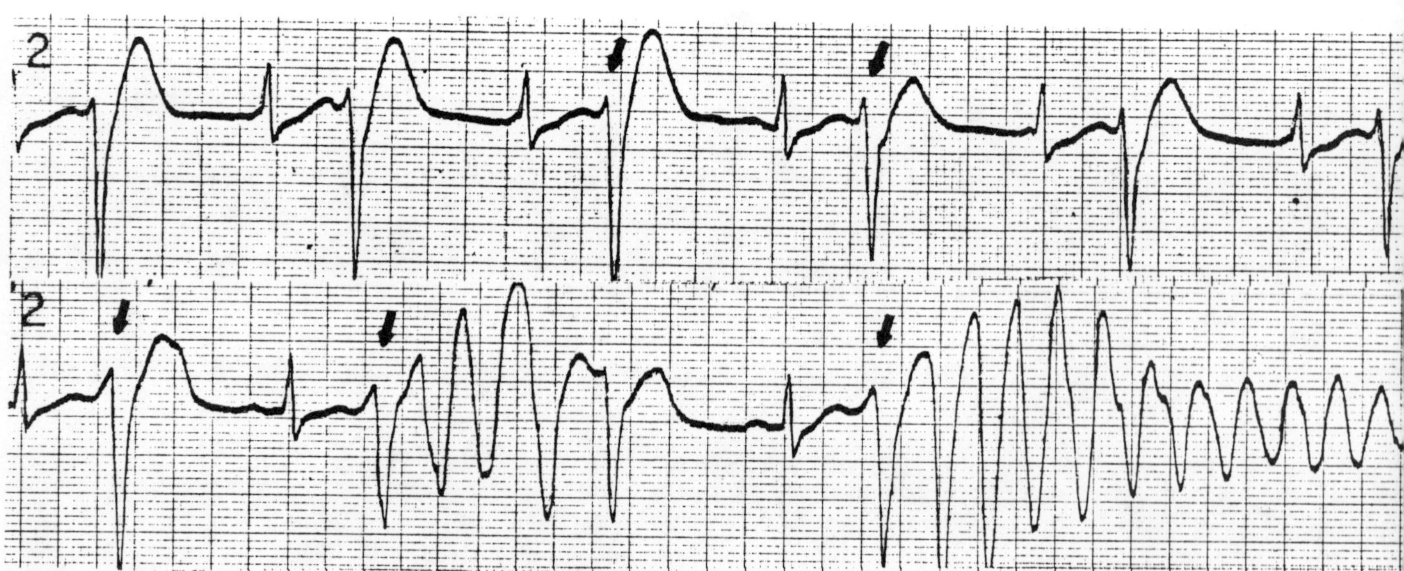

Fig. 41-B - Ventricular tachycardia and "R on T phenomenon." A ventricular bigeminy, with PVC's interrupting the descending branch of the T waves, generates a short burst of VT. This is followed by a VT which degenerates into a ventricular fibrillation.

EXTRASYSTOLIC VENTRICULAR TACHYCARDIA
("R on T Phenomenon")

It is not unusual to find ventricular extrasystoles falling on the descending limb of the preceding T waves. This type of extrasystoles are sinisterly bound to repetitive phenomena and salvos of ventricular tachycardia and fibrillation. Since they interrupt the descending branch of the T wave, the extrasystoles may fall within the vulnerable period of ventricular repolarization and may develop into a sustained ventricular rhythm (ventricular tachycardia) or degenerate into a ventricular fibrillation. The repetitive phenomena are also facilitated by bradycardic rhythms and prolongation of the QT intervals.

Fig. 41-A shows a typical *"R on T phenomenon."* The ventricular extrasystoles have a fixed and early coupling interval and land into the descending branch of the preceding T waves. A brief salvo of repetitive PVC's heralds more serious problems (second tracing). The last tracing records a ventricular tachycardia (the QRS complexes of the VT are similar to the extrasystolic QRS's) which ceases spontaneously and, after a prolonged period of asystole, is followed by a sinus bradycardia.

Fig. 41-B shows a ventricular bigeminy with fixed coupled PVC's falling on the descending branch of the preceding T waves *(R on T phenomenon)*. In the bottom tracing, both the brief salvo and the sustained ventricular tachycardia, which degenerates in ventricular fibrillation, are induced from VPC's falling in the vunerable period of ventricular repolarization.

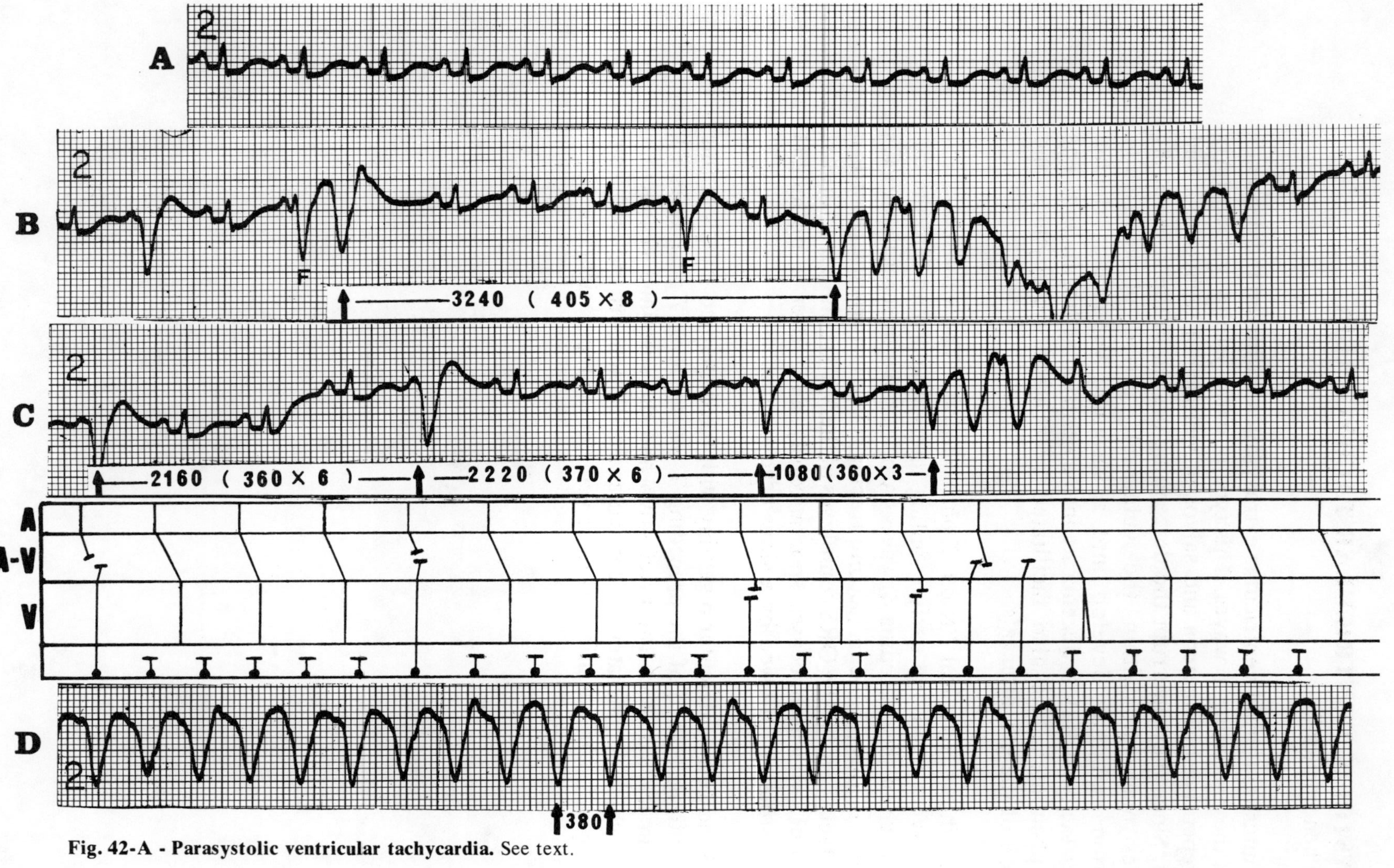

Fig. 42-A - Parasystolic ventricular tachycardia. See text.

PARASYSTOLIC VENTRICULAR TACHYCARDIA

More often than is usually thought VPC's, with variable coupling intervals and arising from a ventricular parasystolic focus, may degenerate into a ventricular tachycardia (see page 144). The diagnosis of *parasystolic ventricular tachycardia* is made when:

a) the extrasystoles do not have a fixed coupling interval;

b) paroxysms of repetitive VPC's are present with different coupling intervals;

c) the interectopic interval (see page 144) between the last beat of one paroxysm and the first beat of the next one is a multiple of the cardiac cycle during the ventricular tachycardia.

A beautiful example of parasystolic ventricular tachycardia is illustrated in fig. 42-A. Tracing A shows the patient during a normal sinus rhythm. Tracing B shows several PVC's with variable coupling intervals. Fusion beats are also recognizable(F). The tracing terminates with a paroxysm of VT, followed again by sinus beats. Tracing C again shows VPC's with variable coupling intervals and one salvo of VT. Tracing D shows the patient, a few minutes later, during a long episode of sustained ventricular tachycardia. This case has all the necessary elements for the diagnosis of ventricular parasystole (fusion beats, variable coupling intervals, an interectopic interval common denominator). In fact, the interval between the two arrows in tracing B (3240 msec.) is a multiple of a cardiac cycle of the ventricular tachycardia (380 msec.). This confirms the theory that a ventricular parasystole is nothing else than a latent ventricular tachycardia (see pages 84, 144, 148, and 184).

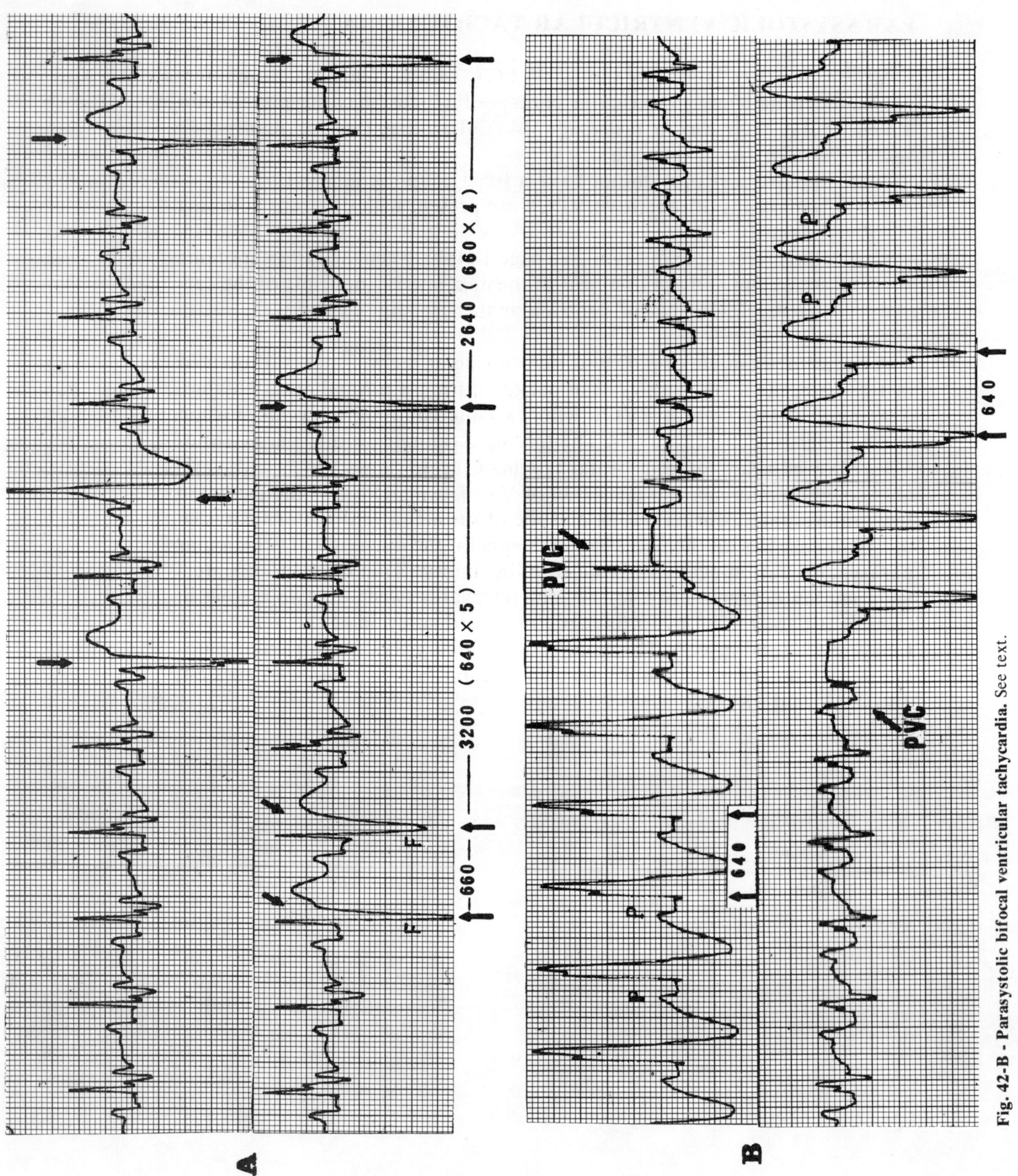

Fig. 42-B - Parasystolic bifocal ventricular tachycardia. See text.

VENTRICULAR TACHYCARDIA

Again, a case of parasystolic ventricular tachycardia is presented in fig. 42-B. In tracing A, the patient shows multiform or multifocal endiastolic ventricular extrasystoles with variable coupling intervals (arrows). Two fusion beats (F) in tracings "A", confirm the diagnosis of ventricular parasystole. The common denominator interectopic interval is equal to 640-660 msec.

Tracings "B" are of the same patient and show the continuous recording of a *bifocal parasystolic ventricular tachycardia*, interrupted by eleven sinus beats. The QRS complexes of the paroxysms show two totally different configurations: one of RBBB type and the other of LBBB type. The first paroxysm is suddenly interrupted by a PVC and followed by sinus beats. The sinus rhythm is again interrupted by a PVC which signals the appearance of a VT from a different focus.

Sinus P waves precede the tachycardic QRS's. This may suggest an alternative diagnosis of a sinus rhythm with alternating right and left bundle branch block (see page 106). A careful examination of the tracings reveals that the P-R interval of the aberrant beats is shorter than that of sinus beats, and that their QRS morphology resembles that of the multifocal PVC's of tracing A. This confirms the diagnosis of bifocal parasystolic VT. For a coincidence the rate of both parasystolic foci is almost similar to the sinus rate. This explains the presence of undisturbed sinus P waves preceding each QRS of the tachycardia.

ARRHYTHMIAS DUE TO ABNORMAL IMPULSE FORMATION

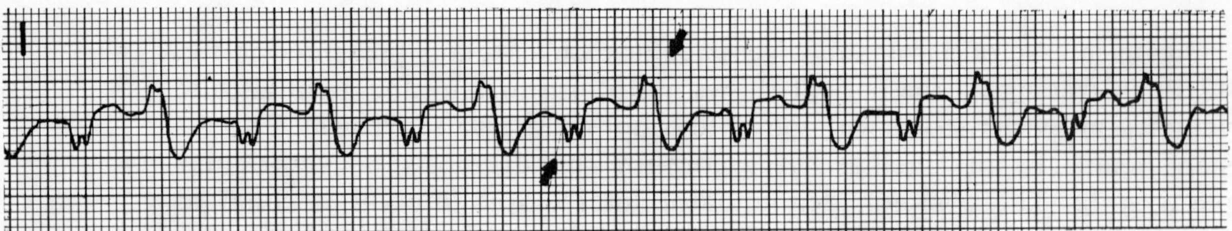

Fig. 43-A - Bifocal ventricular tachycardia. Bizarre and widened QRS complexes alternate in polarity in the same lead.

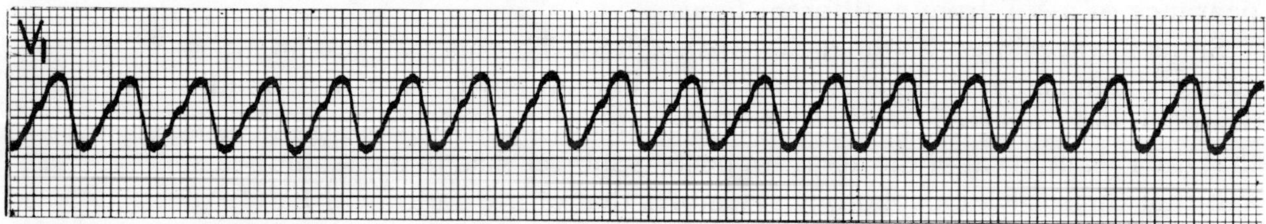

Fig. 43-B - Ventricular flutter. "Saw-tooth" appearance of the QRS complexes.

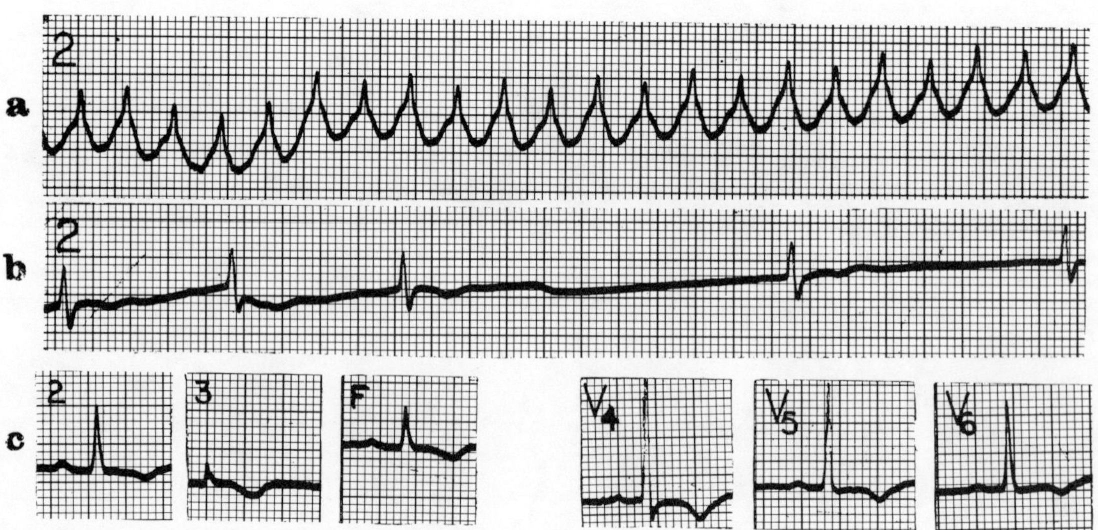

Fig. 43-C - Post-tachycardia syndrome. The ventricular tachycardia (a) is promptly controlled with drugs (b). Ischemic type of abnormalities are present in the post-tachycardia tracing (c). These abnormalities are frequent and usually transitory.

VENTRICULAR TACHYCARDIA

When a ventricular tachycardia shows bizarre and wide QRS complexes alternating in polarity in a same lead, it is called *bifocal or bidirectional ventricular tachycardia* (fig. 43-A). However, it may be difficult to distinguish this type of tachycardia from a supraventricular tachycardia with an alternating ventricular aberration, or in association with a ventricular bigeminy.

When the heart rate is fast and the QRS complexes and T waves are not clearly separable one from another and assume a "zig-zag" or "saw-tooth" pattern, the rhythm is often called *ventricular flutter*. This is presented in fig. 43-B.

Fig. 43-C shows a rapid and quite regular ventricular tachycardia in a 19 year old patient with an otherwise normal heart. The tachycardia was secondary to an antidepressant overdose (a); the post-conversion tracing (b) was obtained immediately after the paroxysm and shows T wave abnormalities which may suggest myocardial ischemia (c). ST segment and T wave changes may be present after a supraventricular or a ventricular tachycardia and do not necessarily indicate coronary artery disease (*post-tachycardia syndrome*). Two days later the ECG of the patient of fig. 43-C returned to normal.

ARRHYTHMIAS DUE TO ABNORMAL IMPULSE FORMATION

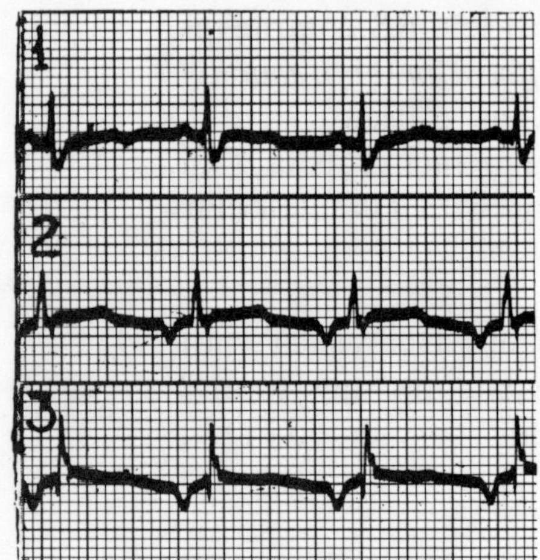

Fig. 44-A - Coronary sinus rhythm.

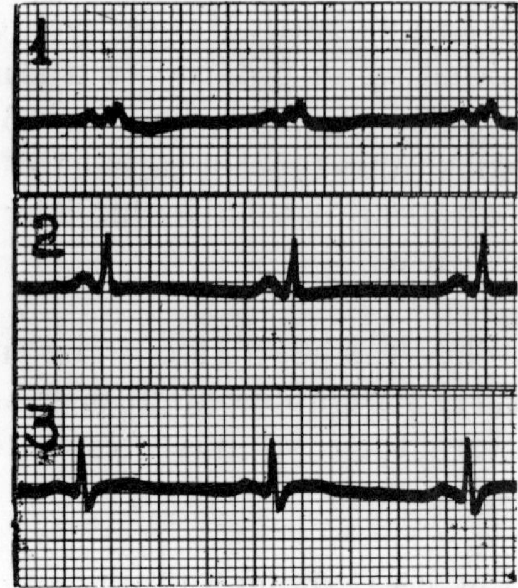

Fig. 44-B - Coronary nodal rhythm.

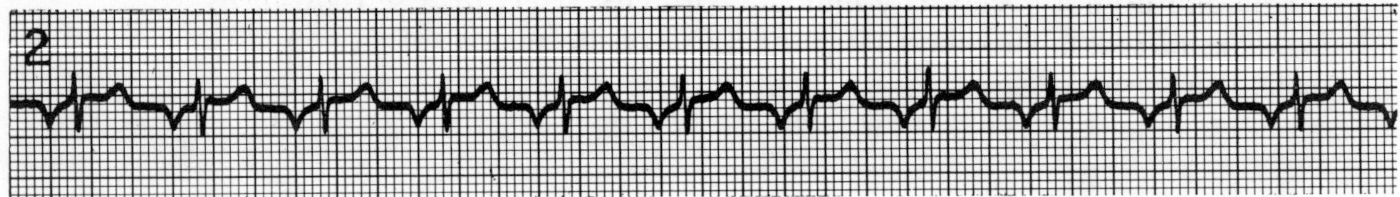

Fig. 44-C - Accelerated coronary sinus rhythm.

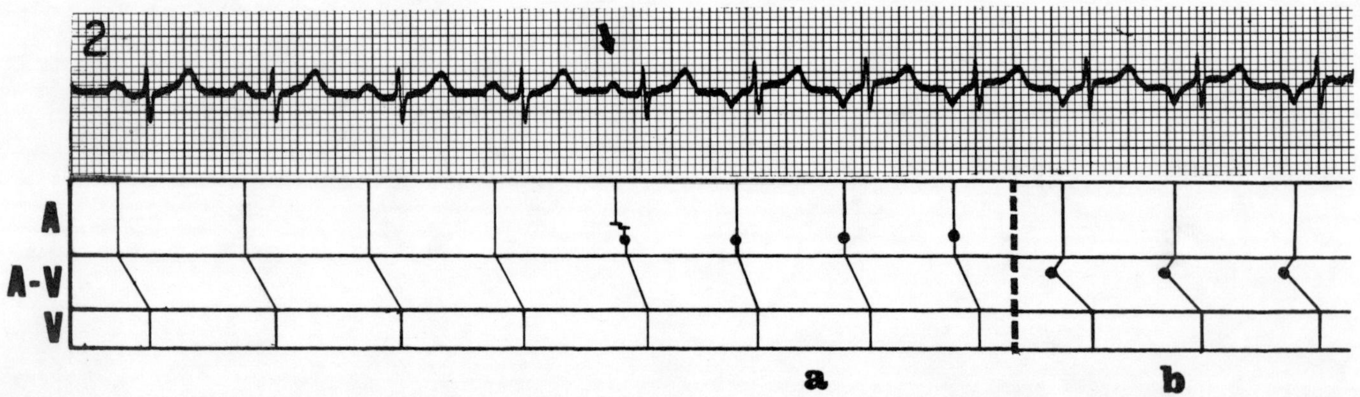

Fig. 44-D - Transition from a sinus rhythm into a coronary sinus rhythm. The arrow indicates an "atrial fusion beat." Section "b" of the diagram suggests an alternative explanation on the origin of the rhythm (junctional pacemaker with a normal conduction to the atria and a delayed conduction to the ventricles).

CORONARY SINUS RHYTHM

CORONARY NODAL RHYTHM

LEFT ATRIAL RHYTHM

These terms are mainly descriptive and apply to supraventricular rhythms other than sinus or A-V junctional as suggested by the different P wave morphologies and by P-R intervals of variable length.

A *coronary sinus rhythm* is a rhythm such as the one of fig. 44-A where P¹ waves of junctional type are followed by normal P¹-R intervals (more than 0.12 sec.).

A *coronary nodal rhythm* is the one of fig. 44-B, where P¹ waves of sinus type are associated with definitely short P-R intervals (less than 0.12 sec.). Patients with coronary nodal rhythms seem to have a high incidence of paroxysmal atrial tachycardias (Lown-Ganong-Levine syndrome).

A *left atrial rhythm* is the one with inverted P¹ waves in L1 and positive P¹ waves in L2 and L3.

Fig. 44-C shows an *accelerated coronary sinus rhythm*. P¹ waves are clearly negative in L2 and the P¹-R interval is 0.18 sec.

The transition from a sinus rhythm into a coronary sinus rhythm is presented in fig. 44-D. The first four beats are clearly of sinus origin. The morphology of the fifth P wave is something in between that of sinus P waves and that of the negative P waves of a coronary sinus rhythm. Therefore, this is an *atrial fusion beat* (see part "a" of the diagram).

At this point, it is necessary to state that a coronary sinus rhythm may represent nothing else than a high junctional rhythm with a normal retrograde conduction to the atria and a delay in the anterograde conduction to the ventricles (see "b" of the diagram of fig. 44-B). A coronary nodal rhythm (fig. 44-B) may also be explained as an accelerated conduction of sinus impulses within the atria. To further complicate the picture, it has been recently demonstrated that impulses coming from the coronary sinus or the left atrium (where pacemaker cells have also been found) may determine P¹ waves in L2, L3 and aVF, totally similar to those coming from the A-V junction. These findings, therefore, invalidate the morphology of P¹ waves as a differential criteria for these different type of rhythms.

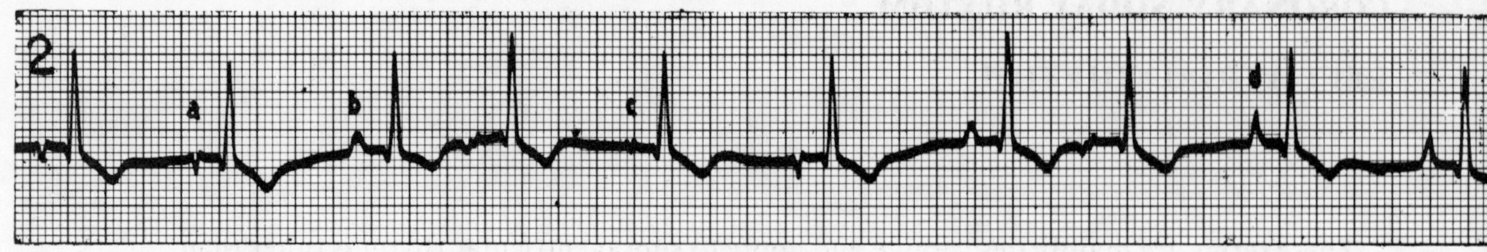

Fig. 45-A - Wandering pacemaker. Four different atrial foci (a b c d) compete for the control of the heart rhythm. The pacemaker migrates from one to the other determining an irregular ventricular rhythm. The P¹ waves have a different morphology.

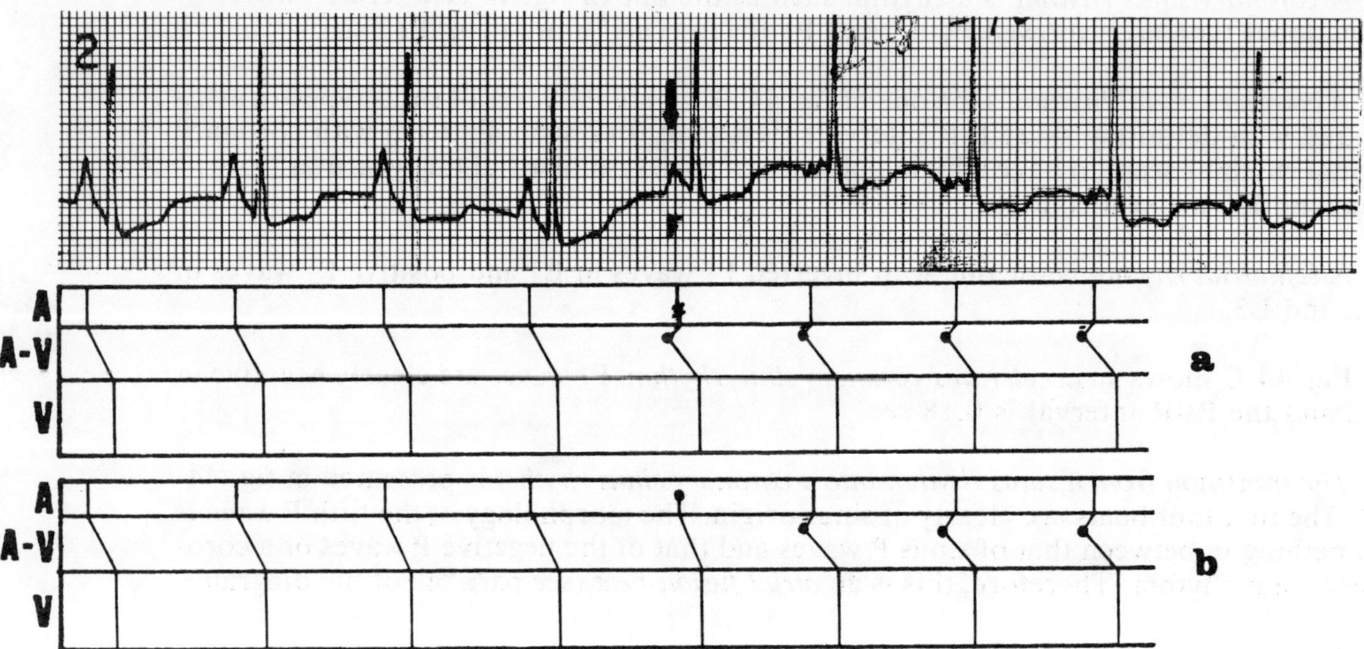

Fig. 45-B - Wandering pacemaker. The cardiac pacemaker migrates from the S-A node into the A-V junction. The transition is marked by beat F. (see text).

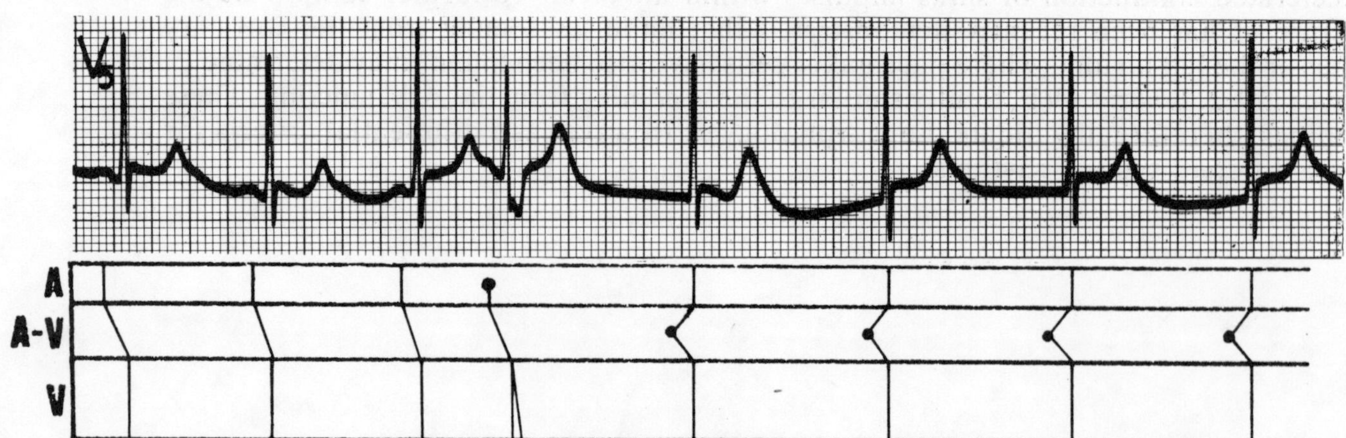

Fig. 45-C - Wandering pacemaker. The transition from a sinus rhythm into a "mid"-junctional rhythm occurs through a PAC with aberrant ventricular conduction.

WANDERING PACEMAKER

At the bedside examination, a *wandering pacemaker* may be easily mistaken for a sinus arrhythmia or an atrial fibrillation. Not uncommonly, several ectopic foci are simultaneously present in the atria and they share the control of the cardiac rhythm.

The basic rhythm is irregularly irregular, because of the intrinsic automaticity of the different pacemakers or because atrial extrasystoles may complicate the picture. In a same lead, P^1 waves may show different morphologies and the P^1-R intervals may vary in length, suggesting that the pacemakers have different origin and distance from the A-V junction.

Fig. 45-A presents a pacemaker which migrates among four different ectopic atrial foci (a, b, c, d).

More commonly, the pacemaker moves back and forth between the sinus node and the A-V junction. In typical cases, sinus P waves are replaced, after some beats, by P^1 of A-V origin. Often, between these two types of waves (P and P^1) there are intermediate morphologies (F waves of fig. 45-B). These waves may have two explanations:

a) atrial fusion beats, formed partly by the sinus impulse, and partly by the simultaneous retrograde junctional impulse (diagram a).

b) beats originating in foci localized half way from the S-A node and the A-V junction (diagram b).

The transition from one pacemaker into another is often facilitated by atrial or ventricular extrasystoles. Fig. 45-B shows a migration of a sinus into a mid-junctional pacemaker (see page 119). This occurs after an atrial extrasystole with ventricular aberration.

ARRHYTHMIAS DUE TO ABNORMAL IMPULSE CONDUCTION

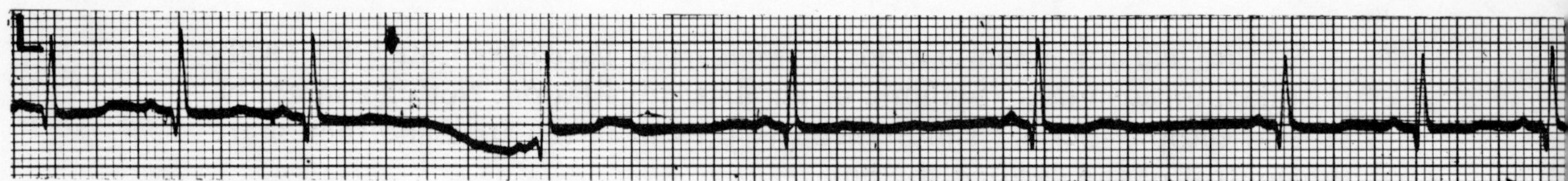

Fig. 46-A - Sino-atrial block. The sudden halving of the heart rate is due to a 2:1 sino-atrial block.

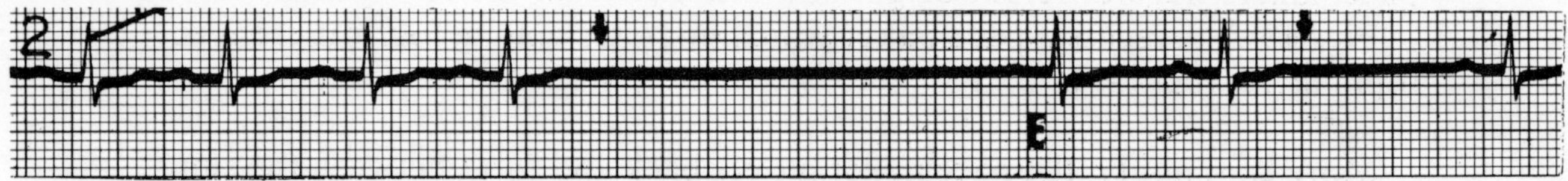

Fig. 46-B - S-A block. The longer asystolic pause, determined by a high degree of S-A block, terminates with an atrial escape beat (E). The shorter pause is due to a 2:1 S-A block.

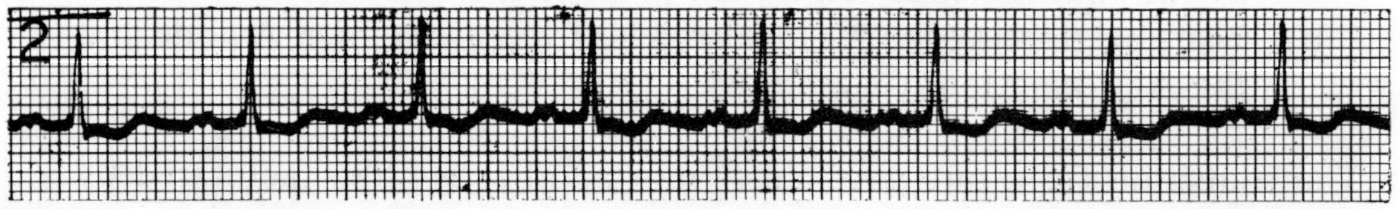

Fig. 46-C - Intra-atrial block. Notched P waves, with a duration longer than 0.10 sec., indicate a delay in the intra-atrial conduction of sinus impulses.

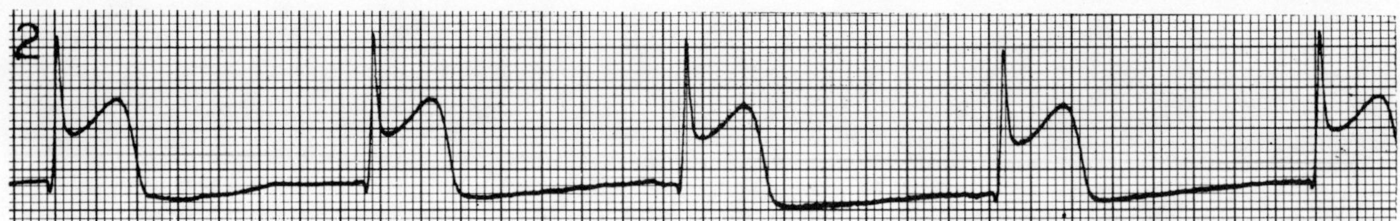

Fig. 46-D - Sinus arrest. Absence of atrial activity in the presence of obvious findings of an acute myocardial infarction.

ARRHYTHMIAS DUE TO ABNORMAL IMPULSE CONDUCTION

SINO-ATRIAL BLOCK, INTRA-ATRIAL BLOCK, SINUS ARREST

The conduction of the impulse between the sinus node and the surrounding atrial tissue does not leave a visible trace on the surface EKG. Therefore, it can only be determined indirectly by referring to P waves and P-P^1 intervals.

When the impulse from the S-A node is not conducted to the atria or is conducted with some delay, the resulting rhythm disturbance is called *sino-atrial block*.

If the sinus impulse is transmitted to the atrial myocardium with a constant delay, the situation is indicated as a *first degree sino-atrial block*. This conduction disturbance can not be recognized on the surface ECG, because there is no way of determining the interval of time between the formation of the impulse in the S-A node and the appearance of the P wave on the surface ECG.

A Wenckebach phenomenon in the sino-atrial node is present when the conduction between the sinus node and the atrial myocardium is progressively delayed until an impulse is blocked (see page 176).

If asystolic pauses appear during regular cardiac cycles and are equal to two sinus cycles they usually indicate a *second degree sino-atrial block*. When the asystolic pause halves the cardiac rate, it indicates a 2:1 S-A block. S-A blocks of 3:1, 4:1 etc. are possible if the pauses are multiples of the sinus cycle.

Fig. 46-A shows a sinus rhythm with a rate suddenly changing from 100/min. (first three beats) to 52/min. in the following four beats, and then again increasing suddenly to 100/min. The rate changes are too sudden (the sinus rate halves and doubles suddenly) to suggest the phasic changes of a sinus arrhythmia. In fact, a *2:1 S-A block* is present in the conduction of sinus impulses. The pauses determined by the block are usually shorter than multiples of sinus cycles, because the P wave which terminates the pause may have an accelerated S-A conduction time, which is not visible on the surface ECG.

In fig. 46-B, the fourth and sixth beats are followed by asystolic pauses. The first pause is almost four times longer than a sinus cycle while the second is exactly twice. The configuration of the P wave which terminates the longer pause appears different than others and it indicates an *atrial escape beat* (E). It is not unusual that an S-A block may induce the escape of atrial, junctional or ventricular beats. When escape beats are present the asystolic pause is never a multiple of sinus cycles.

The impulse conduction within the atria may be delayed, particularly when the atria are enlarged and dilated and their activation is delayed. When P waves are notched and longer than 0.10 secs. *(P mitrale)* or biphasic with a delay in the inscription of terminal forces in V1 and V2, they indicate an *intra-atrial block* (fig. 46-C).

When P waves are absent, there is a *complete sino-atrial block* or a *sinus arrest* as in fig. 46-D, where the cardiac rhythm is under control of a junctional pacemaker. The QRS's show clear evidence of an acute myocardial infarction.

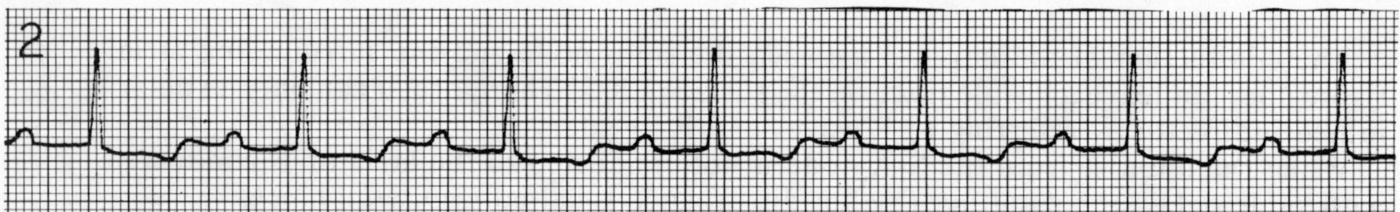

Fig. 47-A - First degree A-V block. P waves are conducted to the ventricles with a P-R interval longer than 0.20 secs.

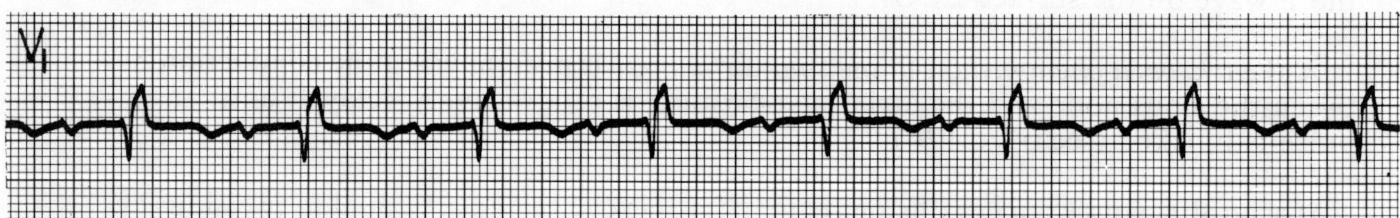

Fig. 47-B - First degree A-V block.

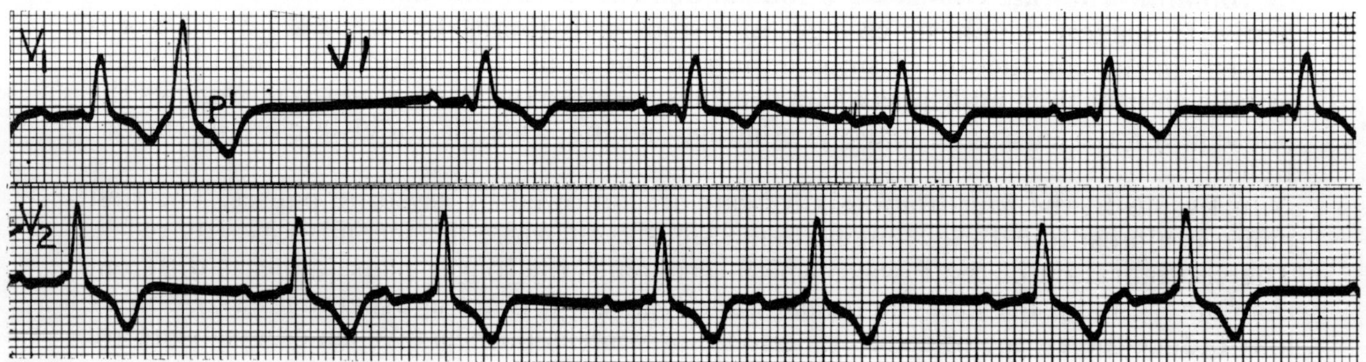

Fig. 47-C - First degree A-V block. The retrograde conduction of the PVC's through the A-V junction is normal (R-P¹ = 0.26). The bigeminal PAC, in the bottom tracing, shows a P¹-R interval longer than that of sinus beats.

FIRST DEGREE A-V BLOCK

When a P-R interval is longer than 0.20 secs. it indicates a *first degree A-V block*. In this situation there is a delay in the A-V conduction of sinus impulses which, however, are still able of reaching the ventricles.

Occasionally, first degree A-V blocks may have P-R intervals of 0.80 - 1 sec. This indicates a high degree of delay but all P waves still reach the ventricles.

Figs. 47-A and 47-B present two cases of first degree A-V block with P-R intervals of 0.40 and 0.32 secs.

Fig. 47-C also shows a sinus rhythm with a first degree A-V block. The P-R interval is 0.24 secs. In the upper tracing a ventricular premature beat shows a retrograde conduction to the atria (P^1). The retrograde ventriculo-atrial conduction (R-$P^1 = 0.26$ sec.) does not show any signs of delay. In the lower tracing, the same patient exhibits an atrial bigeminy. It may be noted that the P-R interval of the atrial extrasystole is prolonged when compared to that of sinus beats. This indicates that the already fatigued A-V junction (first degree A-V block) conducts with a further delay the premature atrial impulses to the ventricles.

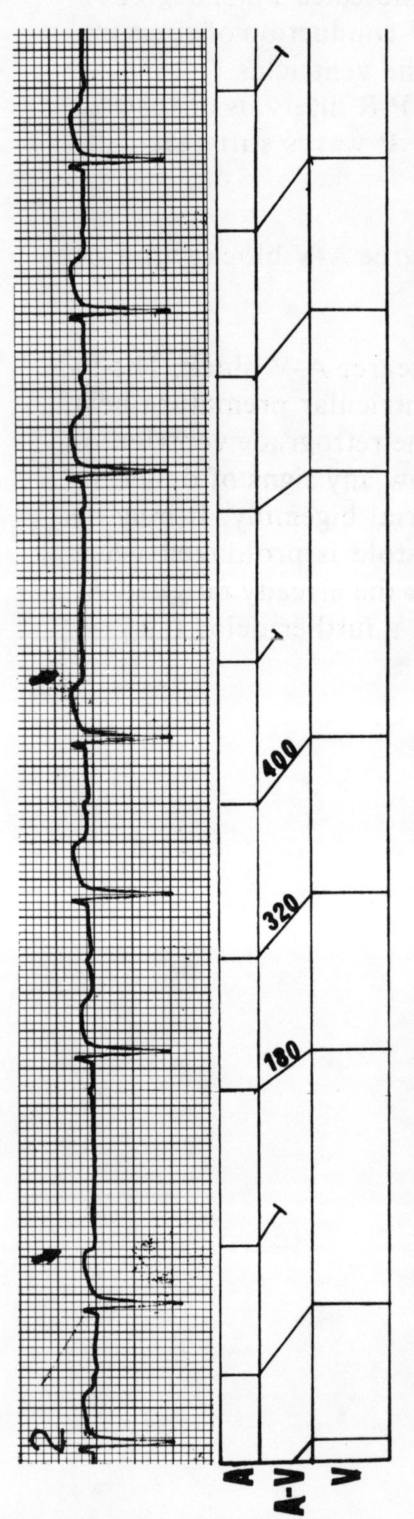

Fig. 48-A - Second degree A-V block Mobitz type I. (Wenckebach period of 4:3). The sinus beats show a progressive delay in the P-R intervals until the fourth P wave is blocked in the A-V junction.

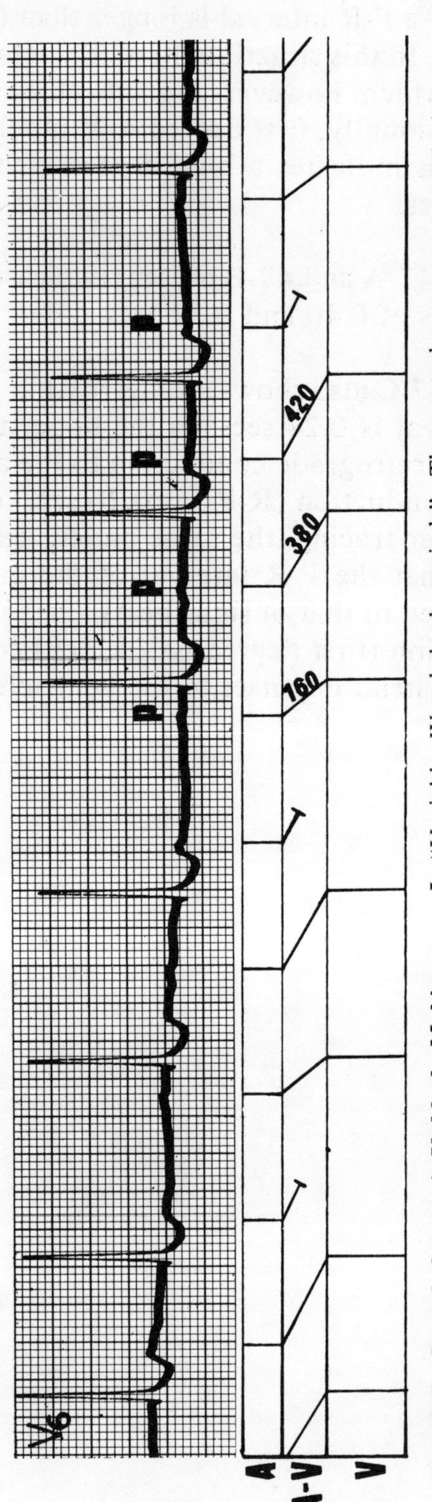

Fig. 48-B - Second degree A-V block Mobitz type I. "Variable Wenckebach periods". The central sequence presents two Wenckebach periods of 3:2 and 4:3.

SECOND DEGREE A-V BLOCK

During a second degree A-V block, the conduction of atrial impulses is intermittently blocked in the A-V junction. The *second degree A-V block* is divided, according to the Mobitz classification, into two types:

MOBITZ TYPE I: most common, when a *P wave is blocked after a progressive prolongation of the P-R intervals.* The sequence is also called *"Wenckebach period."*

MOBITZ TYPE II: less common, when a *sinus P wave is intermittently blocked within an otherwise regular sinus rhythm.* The P-R intervals may be normal or prolonged.

SECOND DEGREE A-V BLOCK MOBITZ TYPE I

Fig. 48-A shows a sinus rhythm with a progressive delay in the A-V conduction (P-R = 180-320-400 msec.) until the fourth P wave is blocked within the A-V junction. This determines a pause and the next sinus beat shows the shortest P-R interval. This is, therefore, a *second degree A-V block Mobitz type I*, with "Wenckebach periods of 4:3" (which means that for each four P waves, three are conducted to the ventricles while one is blocked).

Another example of *second degree A-V block Mobitz type I,* with variable Wenckebach periods, is presented in fig. 48-B. The P-R intervals get progressively longer until a P wave is blocked. The central sequences show Wenckebach periods of 3:2 and 4:3. Notice that, again, P waves are not easily recognized and the rhythm may simulate the irregular ventricular response of an atrial fibrillation (cherchez le P).

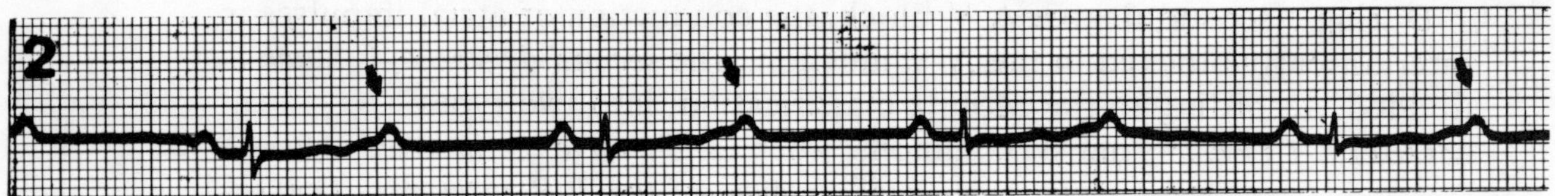

Fig. 49-A - Second degree A-V block Mobitz type II. The A-V ratio is of 2:1. The arrows indicate blocked P waves.

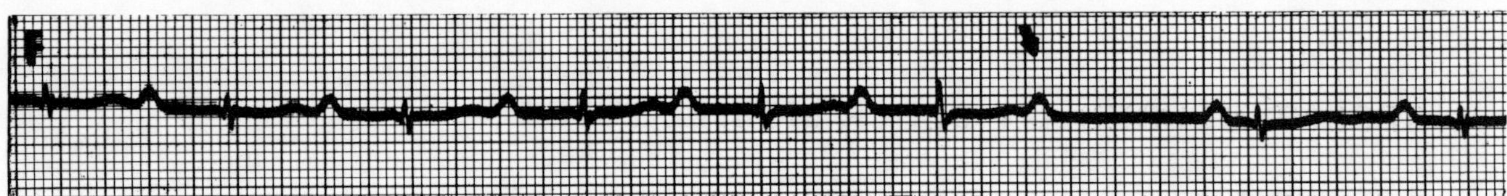

Fig. 49-B - Second degree A-V block Mobitz type II. A P wave is suddenly blocked in the contest of a sinus rhythm with prolonged P-R interval.

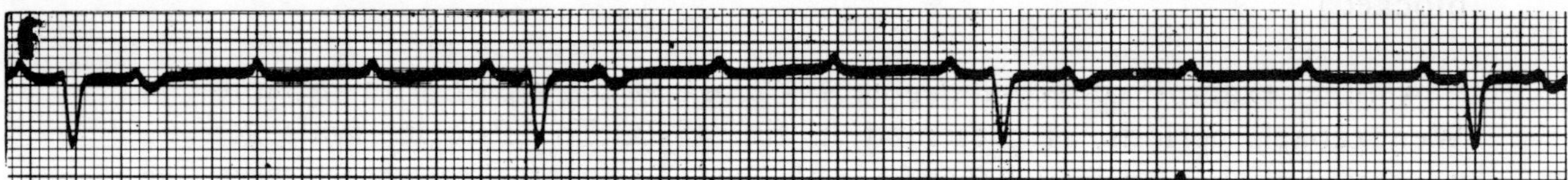

Fig. 49-C - Second degree A-V block Mobitz type II. The A-V ratio is 4:1.

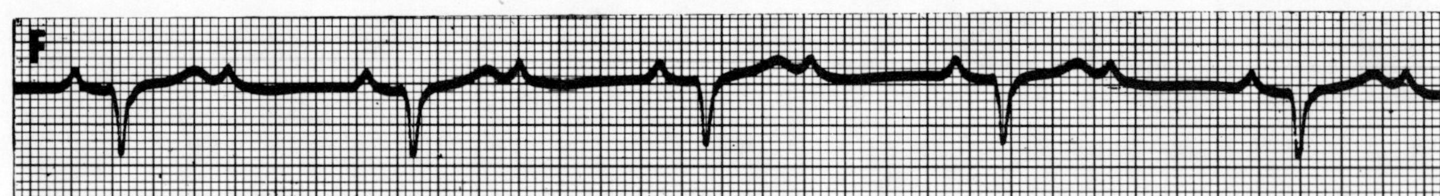

Fig. 49-D - Second degree A-V block Mobitz type II.

SECOND DEGREE A-V BLOCK MOBITZ TYPE II

In this situation, a P wave is intermittently blocked within an otherwise regular sinus rhythm and with a constant P-R interval. The P-R intervals may have either a normal or prolonged duration.

Fig. 49-A shows a *second degree A-V block Mobitz type II* with an A-V ratio of 2:1. One P wave is conducted to the ventricles with a prolonged P-R interval (240 msec.), while the following is blocked within the A-V junction.

Compare fig. 49-A with fig. 49-B where the sinus P waves are conducted to the ventricles with a progressive A-V delay until a blocked P wave. The P-R interval of the sinus beat following the blocked P wave has the shortest P-R interval which again is prolonged in the following beat. The tracing indicates the presence of a *second degree A-V block Mobitz type I*. The pause offers a longer recovery time to the A-V junction and this improves the conduction of the following sinus impulse.

A case of sinus tachycardia with a *second degree A-V block Mobitz type II* is presented in fig. 49-C. The atrial rate is 120/min., the ventricular is about 30/min.; the A-V ratio is, therefore, 4:1. In such a circumstance it is not uncommon to observe an improvement of the ventricular rate after a slowing of the atrial rate. The A-V ratio of a second degree A-V block is in relation both to the number of atrial impulses/min. and to the residual functional state of the A-V junction.

Again, a *second degree A-V block Mobitz type II* is presented in fig. 49-D. The sinus rhythm is regular and the A-V ratio is of a 2:1 type.

ARRHYTHMIAS DUE TO ABNORMAL IMPULSE CONDUCTION

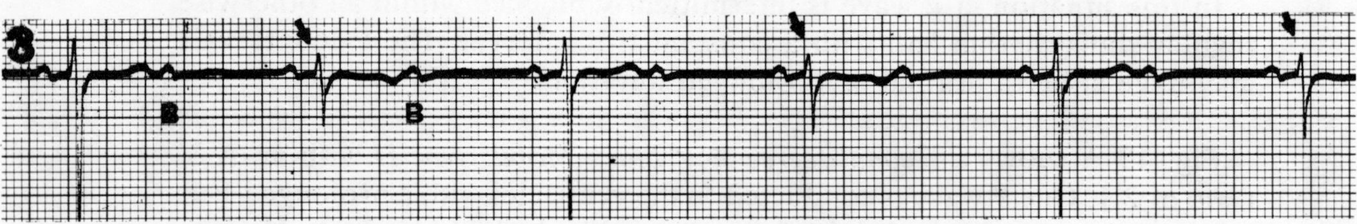

Fig. 50-A - Second degree A-V block Mobitz type II with ventricular electrical alternance. Small amplitude QRS's (arrows) alternate with normal QRS's. B = blocked P waves.

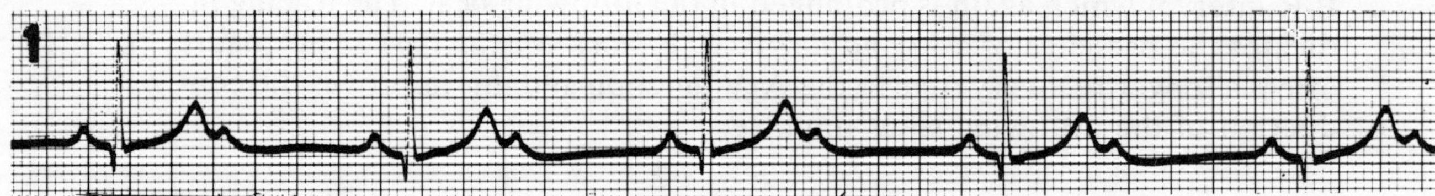

Fig. 50-B - Second degree A-V block Mobitz type II. The A-V ratio is of a 2:1 type.

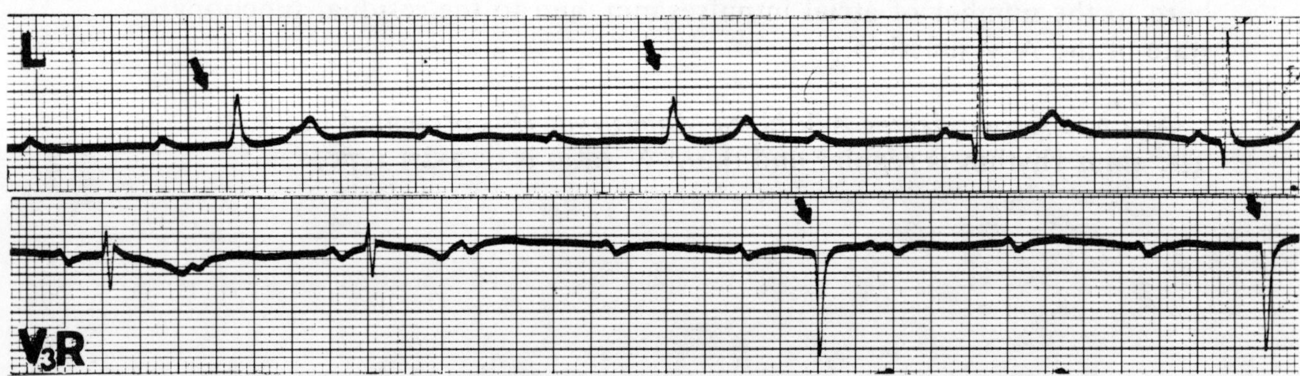

Fig. 50-C - Second degree A-V block Mobitz type II and complete A-V block. The patient is the same as in fig. 50-B. Arrows indicate idio-ventricular QRS complexes emerging during episodes of complete A-V block.

SECOND DEGREE A-V BLOCK MOBITZ TYPE II

In fig. 50-A, every other QRS complex shows a significantly reduced amplitude. The rhythm is a normal sinus with a second degree A-V block Mobitz type II and *electrical ventricular alternance*. There is not yet a satisfactory explanation for the electrical ventricular alternance, but it is possible that it may represent an intra-ventricular conduction disturbance of minor significance. It must not be confused with the mechanical ventricular alternance of relevant hemodynamic significance.

Figs. 50-B and 50-C are recorded from the same patient. They show a progressive deterioration of the A-V conduction into an advanced type of A-V block. Fig. 50-B presents a normal sinus rhythm, with a normal P-R interval in the conducted beats, and a second degree A-V block Mobitz type II. The A-V ratio is 2:1.

Fig. 50-C illustrates the same patient a few days later. Leads aVL and aVR show two different QRS morphologies. The rate of the first and second QRS's (arrows) is equal to 25/min. and the QRS morphology is different from that of beats with a 45/min. rate. Furthermore, the slower QRS's do not have any relation with sinus P waves, while the faster QRS complexes are preceded by P waves, with a constant P-R interval, and followed by a blocked P wave. There is, therefore, an *alternating second degree A-V block Mobitz type II*, and with a 2:1 A-V ratio, and a *third degree or complete A-V block* (see page 102).

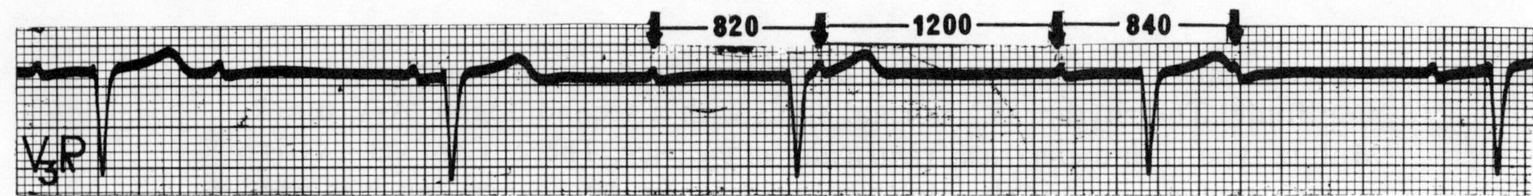

Fig. 51-A - Third degree A-V block (complete). Ventriculo-phasic sinus arrhythmia. Some of the P-P intervals are indicated by the arrows. The short P-P interval includes the QRS of the subsidiary junctional pacemaker.

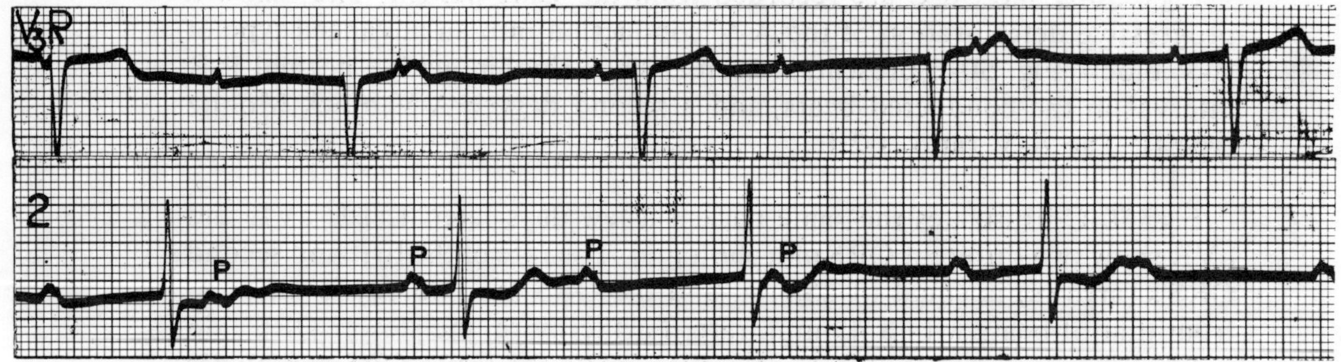

Fig. 51-B - Third degree A-V block (complete A-V block). The tracing is recorded from the same patient of fig. 51-A, a few days later. The rate of the idio-ventricular pacemaker is slightly faster.

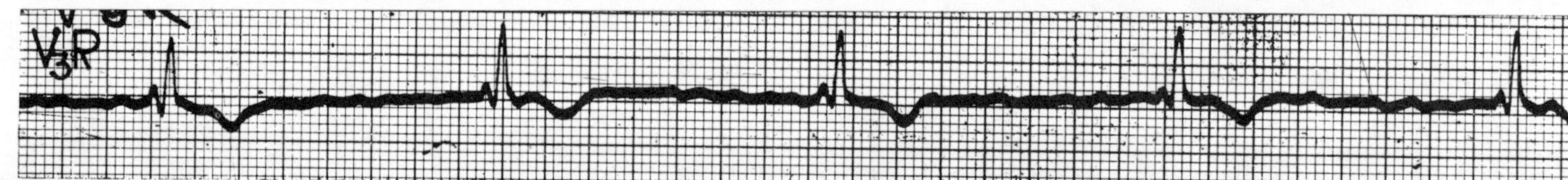

Fig. 51-C - Third degree A-V block and atrial fibrillation. Atrial fibrillatory waves are recognizable (f waves). The ventricular rate is regular. The pacemaker is either idio-ventricular or junctional with ventricular aberration.

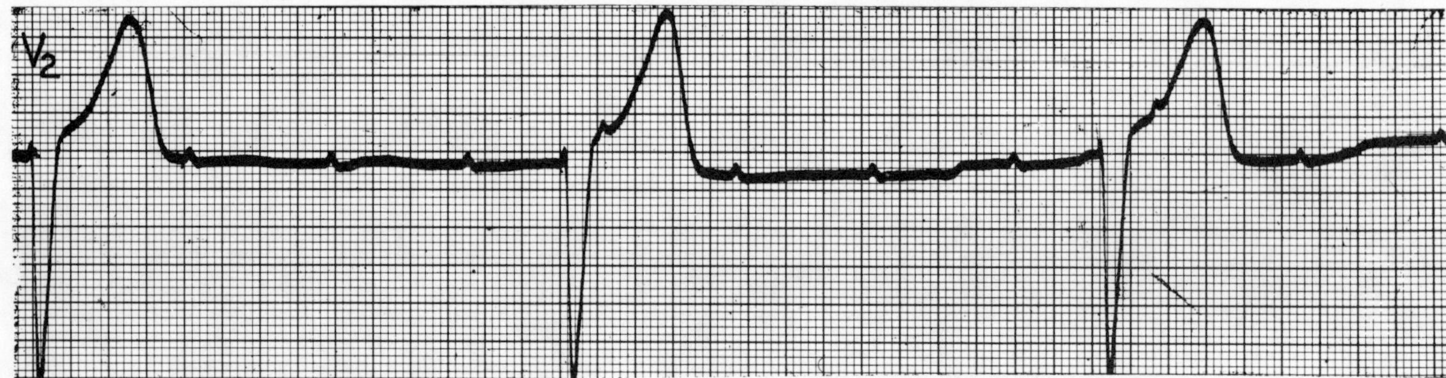

Fig. 51-D - Third degree A-V block. The subsidiary pacemaker is located in the ventricles. Notice the marked difference in rate between the atrial and the independent ventricular rhythm.

THIRD DEGREE A-V BLOCK (Complete A-V block)

When P waves and QRS's have no relation to each other and the atria contract independently from the ventricles, the conduction disturbance is called *third degree or complete A-V block* (the term A-V dissociation *must not* be used as a synonym of third degree A-V block).

Fig. 51-A shows a patient with a third degree A-V block. The P waves are clearly independent and without any fixed relationship to the QRS's. The atrial rate is 63/min., while the ventricular is 33/min. The ventricular activation occurs in a normal fashion (since the QRS complexes have a normal morphology) and this suggests that the subsidiary pacemaker, which controls the ventricular rhythm, must be localized above the His bundle. Furthermore, it may be observed that the sinus P wave falling immediately after the QRS is, in some way, "attracted" by the preceding beat. This determines a shortening of the P-P interval which encloses the QRS and a prolongation of the following P-P interval.

This type of sinus arrhythmia, which is frequently found in third degree A-V blocks, is called *ventriculo-phasic sinus arrhythmia*. It seems to be related to:

a) an improved coronary circulation and, therefore, an increased S-A node blood supply following a ventricular contraction. This in turn determines an improvement in the rate of formation of sinus impulses.

b) a mechanical effect of the ventricular contraction on the S-A node which delivers the next impulse slightly prematurely.

Tracings of fig. 51-B are recorded from the same patient of fig. 51-A only after a few days. This example shows that: 1) in a third degree A-V block the rate of a subsidiary pacemaker is not fixed but it may be variable, especially if the secondary pacemaker is of a junctional type; 2) the chronotropic effect of the ventricular systole on the sinus rhythm (ventriculo-phasic sinus arrhythmia) may not be clearly recognized in standard leads. In L2 the P waves "attracted by the QRS" are buried within the ST segment and this could alter the measurement of the effective atrial rate.

The rapid impulses of an atrial fibrillation may be all blocked within the A-V junction because of the presence of a *third degree A-V block*. This is the case of fig. 51-C where, in spite of the presence of an atrial fibrillation, the ventricular rate is regular. This is because the ventricular rhythm is due to an idio-ventricular pacemaker (or by a junctional pacemaker with aberrant ventricular conduction) for the presence of a complete A-V block.

In a third degree A-V block, the control of the ventricular rhythm is usually undertaken by idio-ventricular foci, as is the case of fig. 51-D. In this tracing the QRS is wide, bizarre, aberrant and, therefore, typical of an idio-ventricular ectopic focus. However, remember that, while the rate of formation of impulses of a junctional pacemaker fluctuates between 40 and 60 beats/min. and is usually constant, that of an idio-ventricular focus may be unstable and it is usually slower (25-40/min.).

ARRHYTHMIAS DUE TO ABNORMAL IMPULSE CONDUCTION

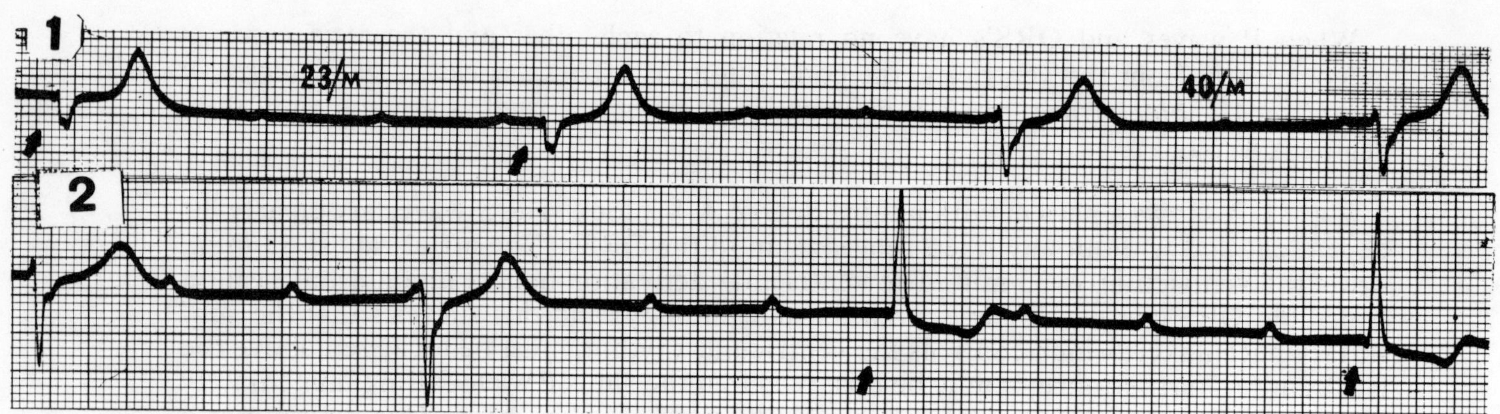

Fig. 52-A - Third degree A-V block. Two different ventricular pacemakers share the control of the ventricular rhythm. The arrows indicate the slower ventricular pacemaker, which comes into action when the faster ventricular pacemaker fails.

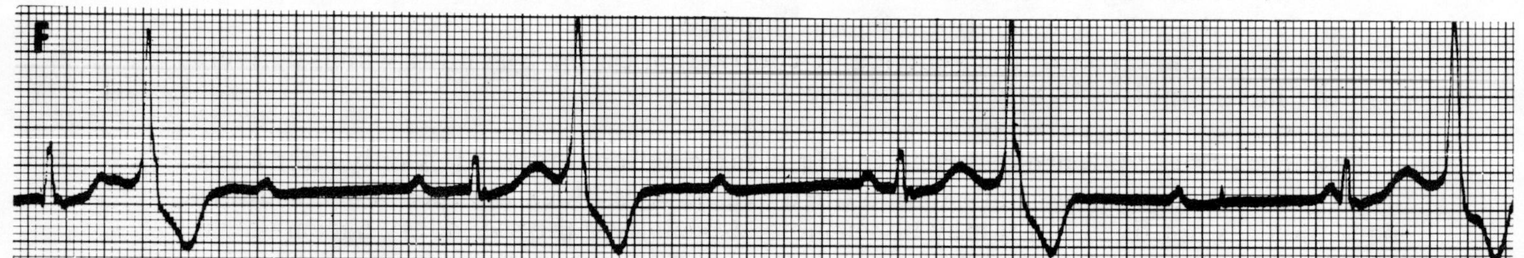

Fig. 52-B - Third degree A-V block and ventricular bigeminy. The bigeminy may be "facilitated" by the bradycardic ventricular rhythm secondary to a complete A-V block.

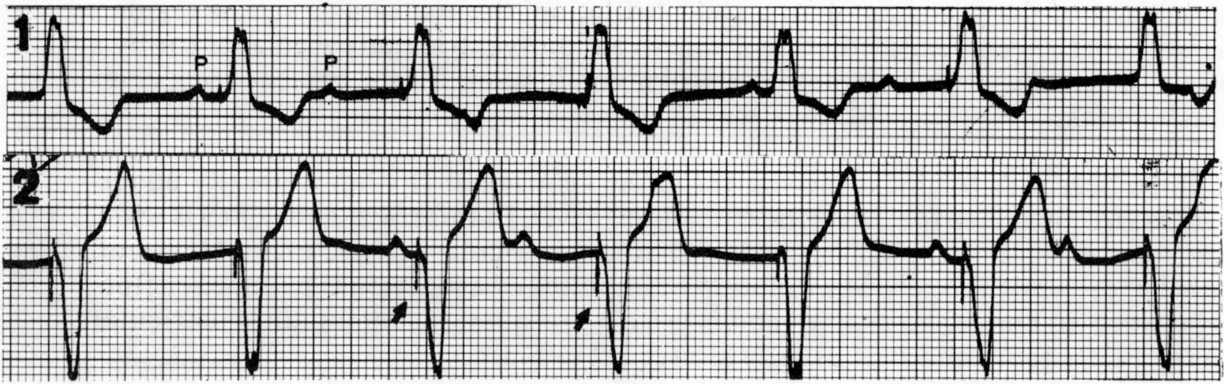

Fig. 52-C - Third degree A-V block. Artificial pacemaker. Notice the spikes of the artificial pacemaker best seen in L2.

THIRD DEGREE A-V BLOCK (Complete A-V block)

Occasionally, in the presence of a third degree A-V block two idio-ventricular pacemakers may compete for the control of the cardiac rhythm. Fig. 52-A shows a sinus rhythm with a rate of 95/min. and a third degree A-V block. With a careful observation of the tracings it appears that the first, second, and last two QRS's (indicated by the arrows) have a rate and a morphology different than other QRS complexes. The ventricles are controlled by the faster idio-ventricular pacemaker (40/min.), but when this subsidiary pacemaker fails, a second idio-ventricular focus escapes and maintains a slower cardiac rhythm (23/min.).

In the presence of a third degree A-V block the bradycardic rhythm of a subsidiary pacemaker is usually a good substrate for the appearance of ventricular extrasystoles. Fig. 52-B shows a sinus rhythm with a complete A-V block, a junctional subsidiary pacemaker and bigeminal PVC's. bigeminal PVC's.

In fig. 52-C, the P-waves are independent from the QRS's which are bizarre, wide, and with a rate slower than the atrial rate. The rhythm seems to be a third degree A-V block with a subsidiary idio-ventricular pacemaker. With a careful examination of the tracings, however, it can be noticed that rapid impulses of very short duration (1-2 msec.) are present just at the beginning of each QRS. They are more evident in L2 and are due to an artificial pacemaker (see page 196) which also determines the aberrant QRS's. The amplitude of the artificial impulses is different in the two leads because of the different vectorial representation of the pacemaker impulses. This type of tracing is encountered more often because of the increasingly greater role of electronics in today's medicine.

ARRHYTHMIAS DUE TO ABNORMAL IMPULSE CONDUCTION

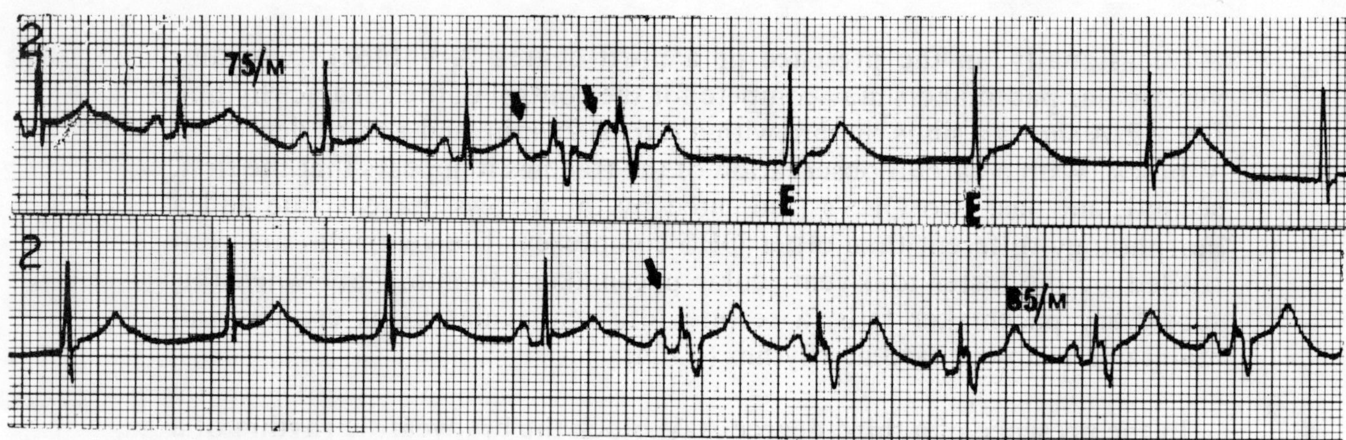

Fig. 53-A - Right bundle branch block. The PAC's of the upper tracing are conducted to the ventricles with a right bundle branch block aberration. They are followed by a short episode of a junctional escape rhythm (E) and by a faster sinus rhythm (85/min.). The rate of 85/min. induces a complete right bundle branch block and, therefore, is a "critical rate for the right bundle."

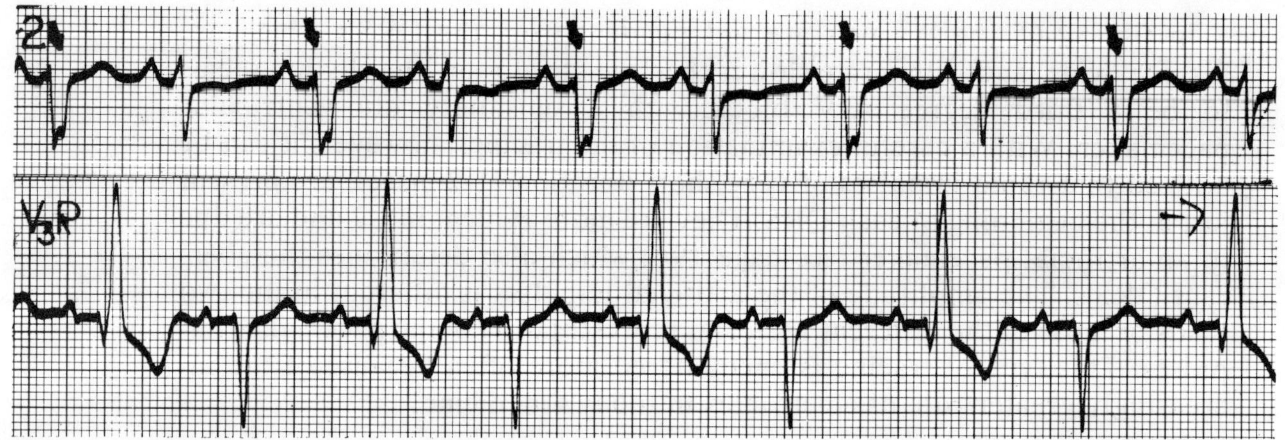

Fig. 53-B - Intermittent right bundle branch block. The block is of a 2:1 type. For each two QRS's, one is conducted to the ventricles with aberration of the right bundle branch block type. In this case the RBBB is not related to a "critical cardiac rate."

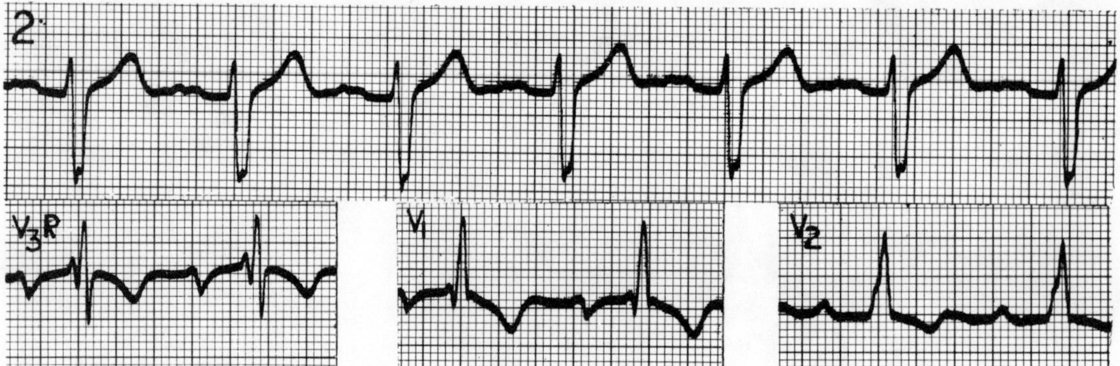

Fig. 53-C - Right bundle branch block. A first degree A-V block (prolonged P-R interval) and an intra-atrial conduction delay (notched P waves in L2 and biphasic in V1) are also present.

RIGHT BUNDLE BRANCH BLOCK (RBBB)

It has already been seen how ventricular aberration of RBBB type may be present in premature beats falling into the absolute refractory phase of the right bundle (see page 16). This is a *physiologic block* of the right bundle, caused by the prematurity of the impulse and the repolarization time of the right bundle, which is the longest of the A-V conduction system.

Fig. 53-A illustrates a case of a sinus rhythm with a rate of 75/min. (first four beats) and two premature atrial beats with aberrant ventricular conduction of RBBB type. The suppression of the sinus pacemaker by the extrasystoles is followed by the escape of a brief junctional rhythm (E) with simultaneous activation of the atria and ventricles. The *escape rhythm* lasts only for eight beats (the last two beats show the reappearance of P waves and A-V dissociation) and is followed by a sinus rhythm with ventricular capture. However, it may be observed that the sinus rate is slightly faster (85/min.) than the escape rhythm and that the sinus QRS's show a RBBB configuration similar to the PAC's of the upper tracing. The ventricular aberration of right bundle branch block type appears with only a slight increase of the cardiac rate. This happens during the premature atrial beats and with the faster sinus rhythm (rate increase from 75/min. to 85/min.). The minimal cardiac rate which induces the bundle branch block aberration (in this case 85/min.) is called *critical cardiac rate*. A RBBB at a critical cardiac rate of 85/min. is not the expression of a normal electrophysiological phenomenon, but indicates a latent A-V conduction disturbance which is manifested by the sudden rate increase.

Fig. 53-B presents an interesting tracing. Normal appearing QRS complexes alternate with beats with a RBBB configuration. The P-R interval is constant and the sinus rate is regular. The tracing shows a *2:1 right bundle branch block;* one of the sinus impulses is normally conducted to the ventricles while the other is blocked within the right bundle. An *intermittent right or left bundle branch block* is not a rare finding. Most of the time it is related to a critical cardiac rate or to premature supraventricular beats, but it may be also present with a perfectly regular sinus rhythm, as in the case of fig. 53-B.

Fig. 53-C shows multiple conduction disturbances localized in different cardiac areas. The sinus impulse has a long journey before reaching the ventricles. An *intra-atrial block* is present, as indicated by the configuration of the P waves in L2 (see page 92). It is followed by a *first degree A-V block* (P-R = 30 sec.) and a *complete right bundle branch block*.

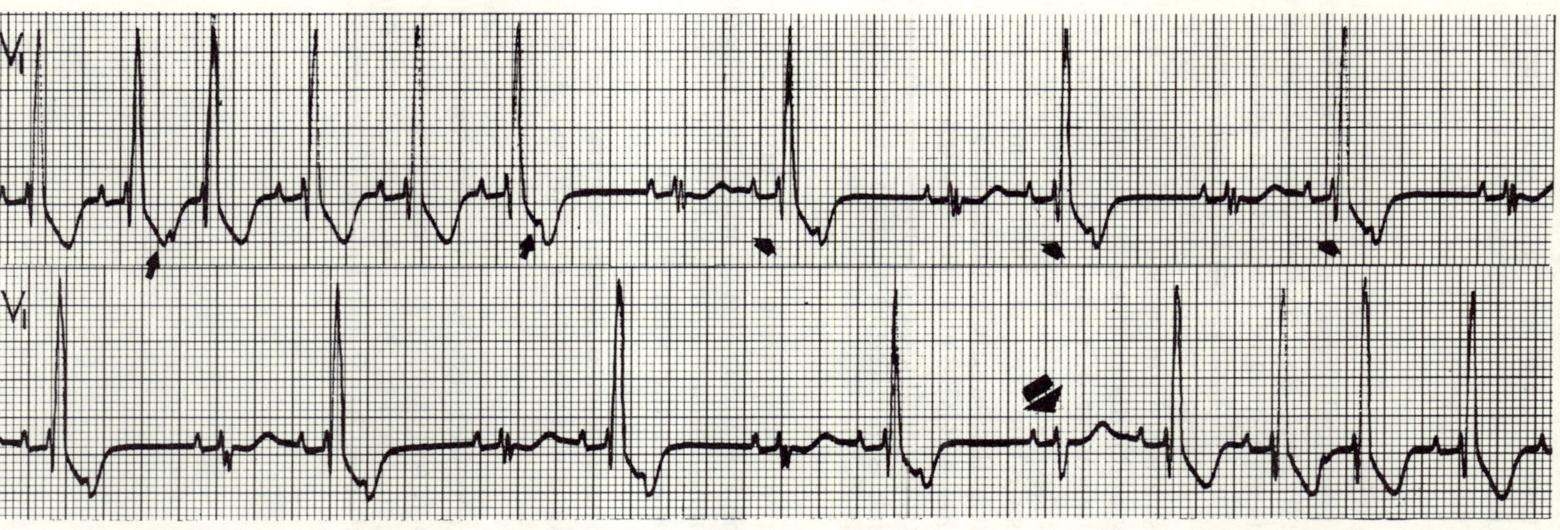

Fig. 54-A - Complete and incomplete right bundle branch block. The tracings are continuous. The pause determined by the blocked PAC, in the upper tracing (second arrow), allows for a better conduction of the following sinus beat (incomplete bundle branch block). This is followed again by a beat completely blocked in the right bundle. The sequence is repeated and creates a "bigeminal" rhythm. The beat indicated by the arrow (lower tracing) shows a normal ventricular conduction.

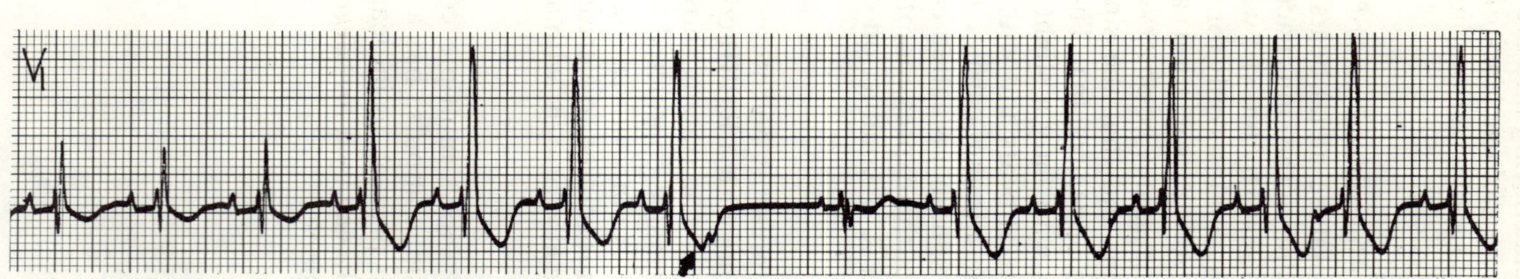

Fig. 54-B - Incomplete and complete right bundle branch block. The first three beats show an incomplete right bundle branch block; the following beats are conducted with a CRBBB. The blocked PAC (arrow) allows for a better conduction of the following sinus beat.

RIGHT BUNDLE BRANCH BLOCK

Tracings of fig. 54-A and 54-B show interesting cases of bundle branch block of different degrees. Fig. 54-A shows a sinus rhythm with a complete right bundle branch block. Atrial extrasystoles are present (arrows). While the first one is conducted to the ventricles with a slight prolongation of the P^1-R interval, others are blocked within the A-V junction. The sinus beat following the blocked extrasystole is conducted to the ventricles with an *incomplete right bundle branch block type* of aberration (rsr^1), while the next sinus beat is totally blocked in the right bundle. A blocked PAC (arrow) follows and the sequence is repeated several times, producing a bigeminal rhythm. The arrow in the bottom tracing points to a normally conducted sinus beat.

Fig. 54-B is recorded from the same patient. Here the *incomplete* right bundle branch block (first three beats) is transformed into a *complete* right bundle branch block in the following beats. The pause which follows the blocked PAC (arrow) allows for a better repolarization of the right bundle. Again, the following sinus beat is conducted with only a slight RBBB aberration.

Tracings of figs. 54-A and 54-B clearly illustrate the possibility of conduction disturbances of different degrees in a specific bundle branch. For the sake of simplicity, these conduction abnormalities are called *incomplete or complete right bundle branch block*. They may appear after pauses determined by extrasystoles, in relation to "critical cardiac rates", or for no obvious reasons. An *incomplete* bundle branch block which becomes *complete* indicates a progressive fatigue within that specific bundle branch to the point of complete block in the transmission of supraventricular impulses.

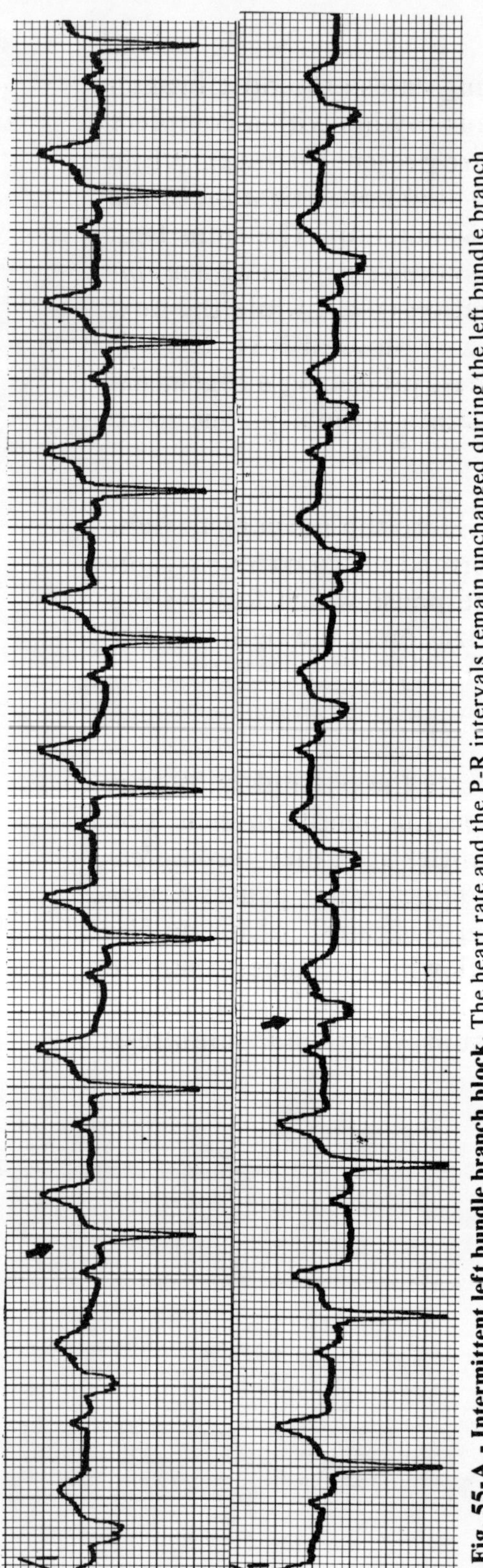

Fig. 55-A - Intermittent left bundle branch block. The heart rate and the P-R intervals remain unchanged during the left bundle branch block.

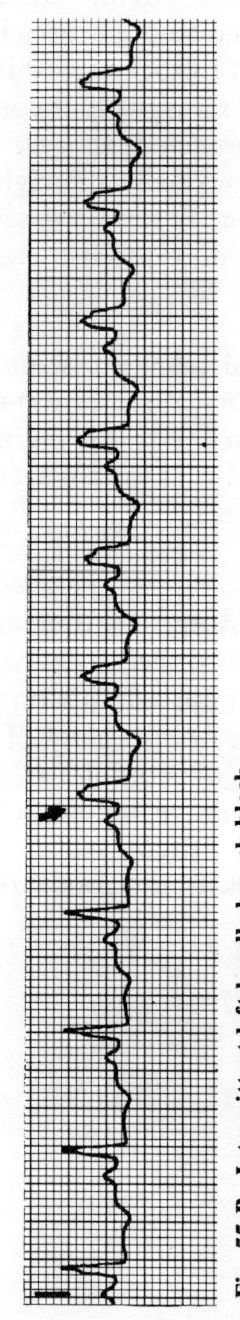

Fig. 55-B - Intermittent left bundle branch block.

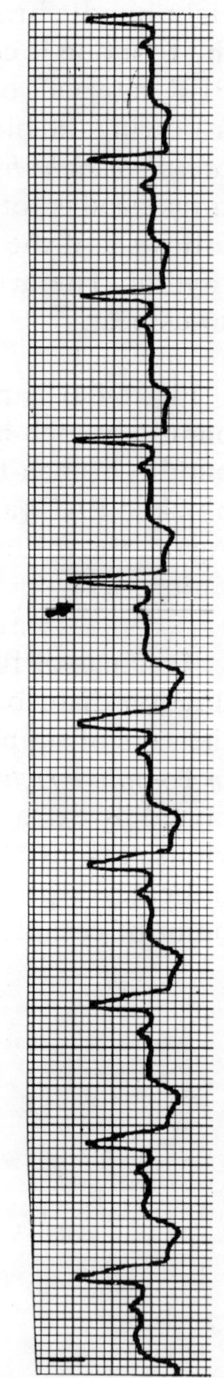

Fig. 55-C - Intermittent left bundle branch block. The beat indicated by the arrow is a transitional beat with an incomplete left bundle branch block.

Three examples of *intermittent left bundle branch block* are presented in figs. 55-A, 55-B, and 55-C.

Two sinus beats with a ventricular aberration of left bundle branch block type open the rhythm of fig. 55-A. They are followed (arrows) by a series of 12 beats with a normal QRS morphology and duration and, again, by sinus beats conducted to the ventricles with left bundle branch block (second tracing). The appearance of LBBB, in this sequence, is related to a "critical cardiac rate" almost unappreciable to the eye. The P-R interval is the same, both in the beats with left bundle branch block and in those with normal conduction.

Fig. 55-B again records the transition from a sinus rhythm, with a normal ventricular conduction, into a sinus rhythm with a *complete left bundle branch block*. Once again, the P-R interval and the sinus rate do not show appreciable variations.

Fig. 55-C shows the transition of a rhythm with a left bundle branch block into a rhythm with a normal conduction. The beat indicated by the arrow is a transitional beat with a *partial or incomplete left bundle branch block,* before the restoration of a normal intraventricular conduction.

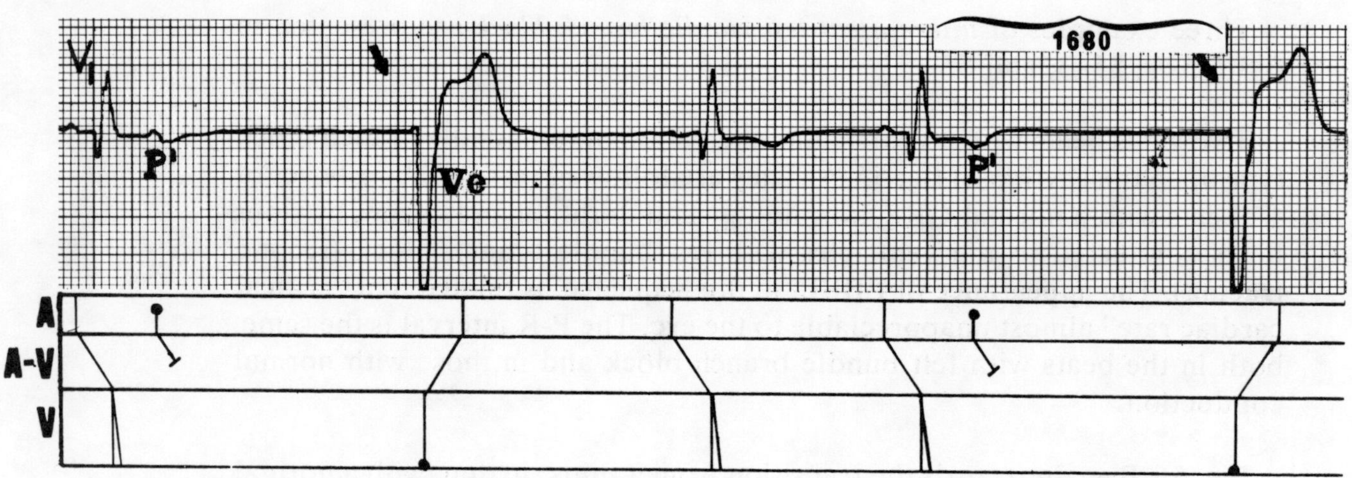

Fig. 56-A - Escape beat. P[1] indicates the blocked PAC which after a pause of 1680 msecs. is followed by a ventricular escape beat (ve).

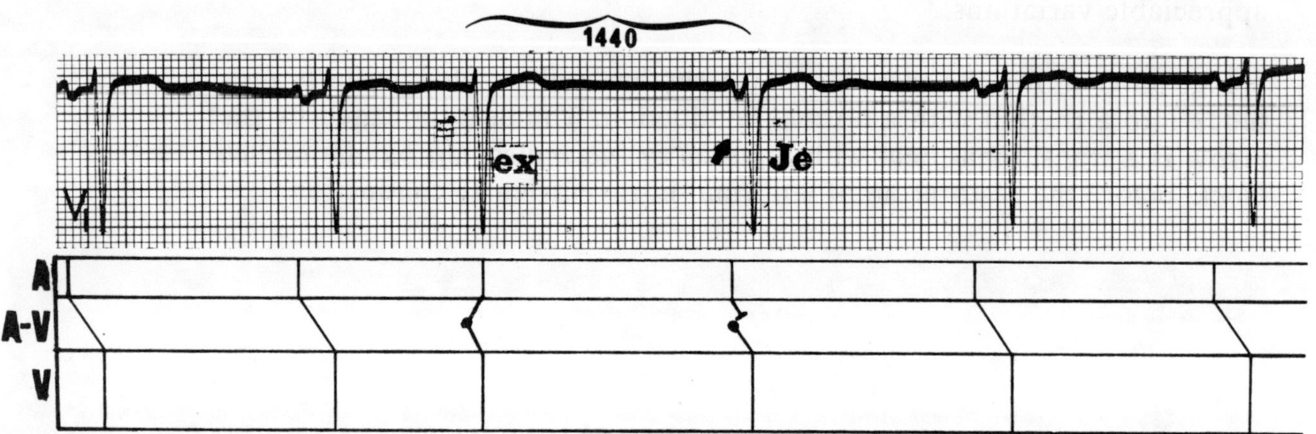

Fig. 56-B - Escape beat. A junctional extrasystole (ex.) is followed by a junctional escape beat (je) at a moment when the next sinus impulse reaches the A-V junction.

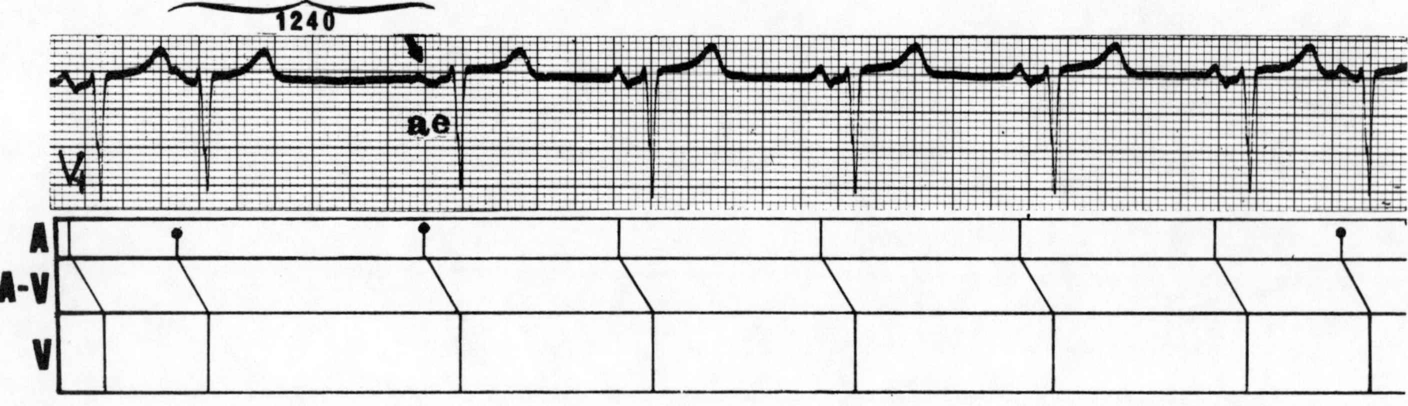

Fig. 56-C - Escape beat. The PAC is followed, after 1240 msecs., by a beat with a P wave markedly different than sinus P waves. This indicates an atrial escape beat (ae).

ARRHYTHMIAS SECONDARY TO ABNORMAL IMPULSE FORMATION AND CONDUCTION

ESCAPE BEATS

If, for any reason, there is a failure in the formation of a sinus impulse or if, once formed, the impulse is blocked in its trip to the ventricles, a secondary pacemaker comes into action and *"escapes"* from a normal sinus control. Beats having such an origin are called *escape beats*. The subsidiary pacemaker most commonly called into emergency action is the A-V junction. Less commonly, escape beats originate from the atria or ventricles. They are easily recognized because *they always appear after an asystolic pause longer than the basic cardiac cycle.* An entire family of arrhythmias exists that does not originate from "active mechanisms", such as ectopic foci which take command over the S-A node automaticity, but from "passive mechanisms," which come into action when the main cardiac pacemaker fails or when the sinus impulse is blocked in its trip to the ventricles.

Fig. 56-A shows a sinus beat, with right bundle branch block, followed by a blocked atrial extrasystole (P[1]). The long asystolic pause which follows the PAC is terminated by a *ventricular escape beat*, (ve). The sequence repeats itself with two sinus beats, followed again by a blocked PAC, a long pause and a ventricular escape beat.

The QRS's of the ventricular escape beats are bizarre and widened and resemble those of ventricular extrasystoles. However, *they are not PVC's but emergency beats;* they are not secondary to an increased ventricular excitability, but to automatic impulses of subsidiary pacemakers liberated by long periods of cardiac inactivity (*escape beats*).

Fig. 56-B presents two sinus beats followed by a "mid" junctional extrasystole and an asystolic pause. When the next sinus impulse propagates into the atrium, a simultaneous junctional impulse escapes and depolarizes the ventricles. Although a P wave precedes the QRS of the *junctional escape beat* (je), the sinus and the junctional impulses are dissociated. The P-R interval is very short and it indicates a block of the P wave within the A-V junction for the simultaneous formation of the junctional escape impulse.

Fig. 56-C presents a sinus beat followed by an atrial extrasystole and by an asystolic pause. The beat after the pause has a P wave and a P-R interval different than those of sinus beats. This is an *atrial escape beat* (ae). The interval of time separating the escape beat from the preceding QRS is called *escape interval*. In the cases presented, it is equal to 1680, 1440, 1240 msecs.

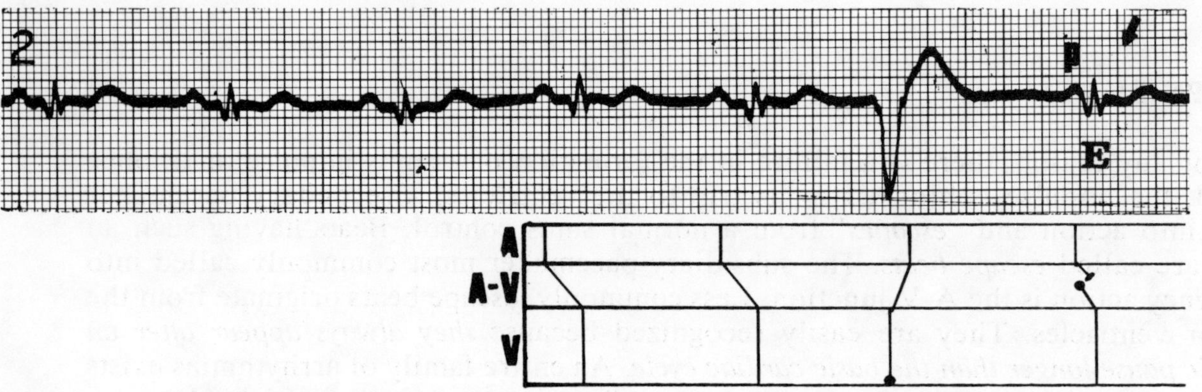

Fig. 57-A - Escape beat. The ladder diagram illustrates a ventricular extrasystole, with a retrograde atrial depolarization, and a junctional escape beat with a temporary A-V dissociation.

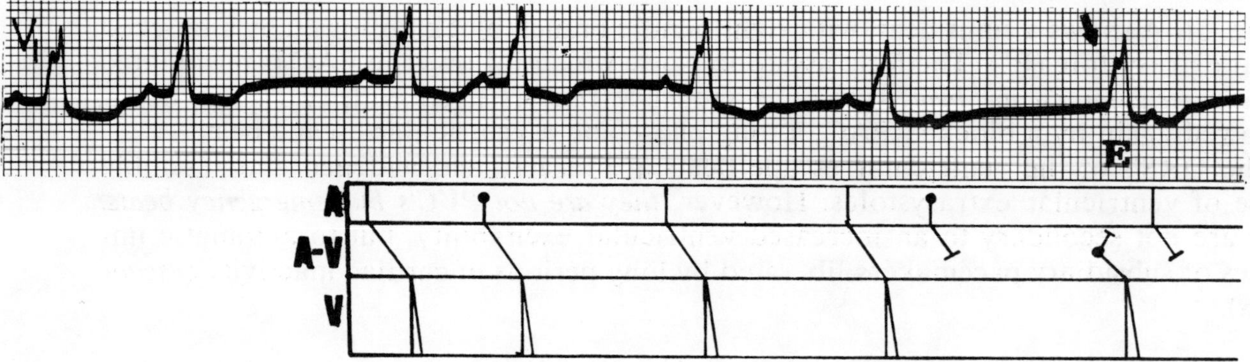

Fig. 57-B - Escape beat. The last PAC is blocked. The premature beat induces a pause which is terminated by the appearance of a junctional escape beat.

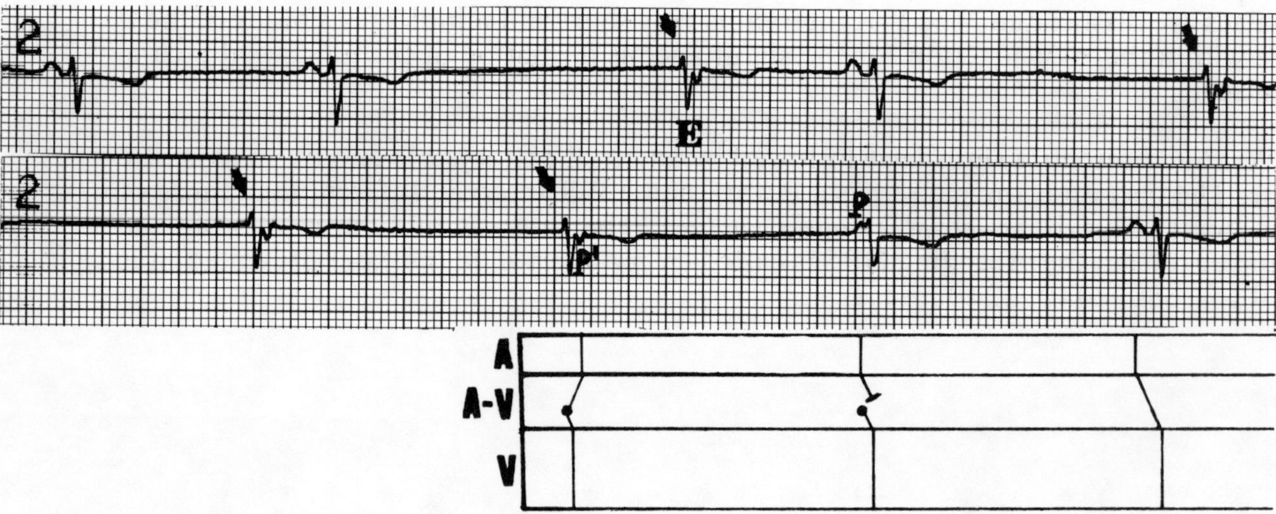

Fig. 57-C - Escape beat. The continuous tracing shows junctional escape beats with a retrograde atrial activation. The diagram shows a junctional escape beat with A-V dissociation and, finally, a sinus beat.

The ventricular extrasystole in fig. 57-A is followed by an incomplete compensatory pause which indicates that the PVC has suppressed the sinus pacemaker in a retrograde fashion. This pause allows for an A-V junctional *escape* (E) before the next sinus P wave could reach the ventricles. Therefore, during the propagation of the *junctional escape beat* there is a transient A-V dissociation (see page 120).

Fig. 57-B shows a sinus rhythm with PAC's in a patient with a right bundle branch block. One of the extrasystoles is blocked and is followed by an emergence beat (E) with a QRS similar to that of a sinus beat, but not preceded by a P wave. Therefore, this is a *junctional escape beat*. The following sinus P wave finds the A-V junction refractory and is again blocked.

The recording of fig. 57-C is continuous and shows a sinus bradycardia and the emergence of a "low" junctional beat (E). A P^1 wave follows the escape QRS and indicates a retrograde atrial depolarization. The next sinus beat is again followed by three *"low" junctional escape beats with retrograde activation of the atria* (P^1 waves.) The S-A node control reappears in the last two beats. Only the last sinus P wave reaches the ventricles, while the one immediately preceding is blocked in the A-V junction for the simultaneous propagation of the escape beat. Again, a transient A-V dissociation is present between the atrial and ventricular depolarization.

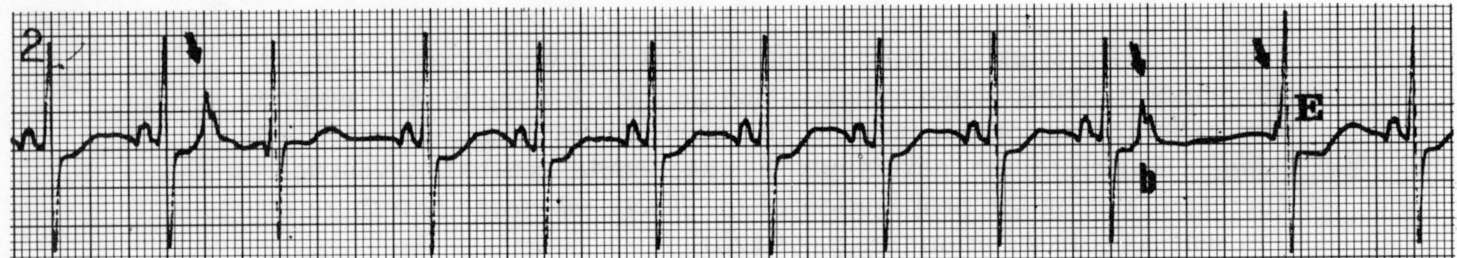

Fig. 58-A - Escape beat. One PAC (first arrow) is conducted to the ventricles with a prolonged P-R interval while a second PAC (second arrows) is blocked. The following pause is terminated by a junctional escape beat and by the reappearance of a sinus rhythm.

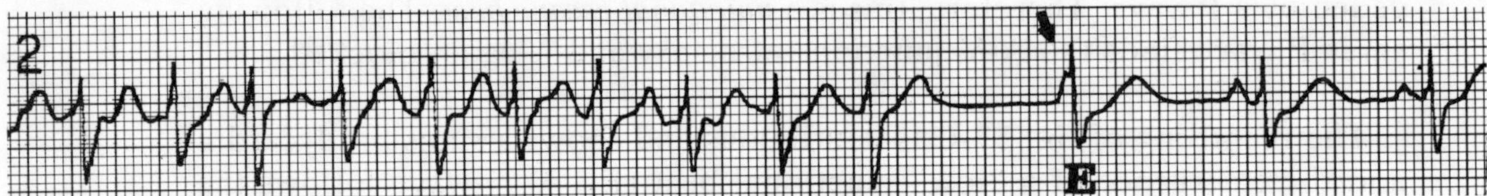

Fig. 58-B - Escape beat. The termination of the PAT is followed by a junctional escape beat and the reappearance of a sinus rhythm.

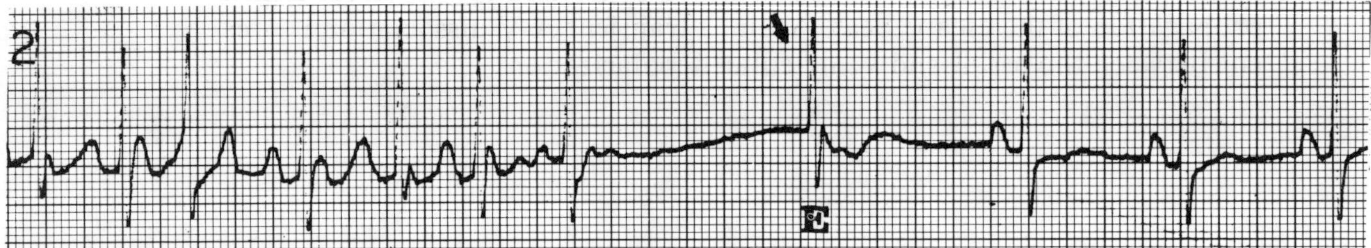

Fig. 58-C - Escape beat. The abrupt cessation of the atrial flutter is followed by a pause. This determines the "escape" of a junctional beat. A normal sinus rhythm follows.

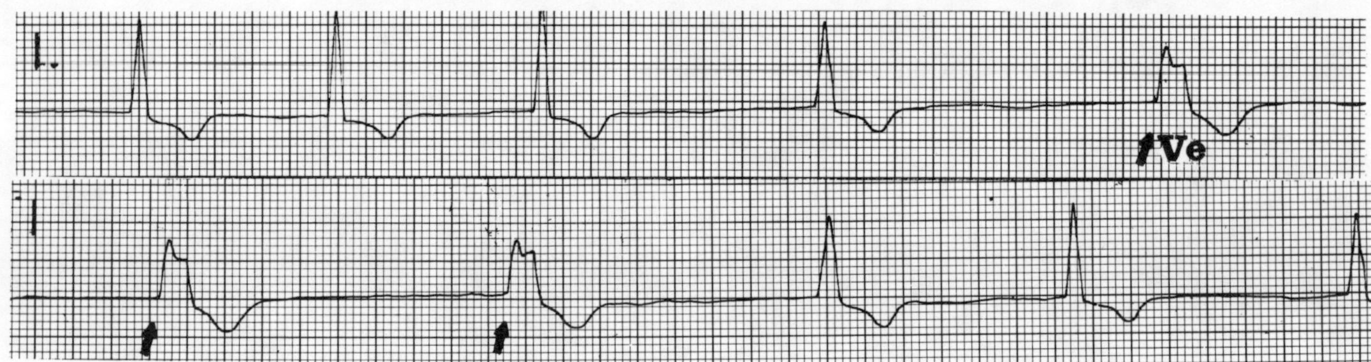

Fig. 58-D - Escape beat. Because of the atrial fibrillation, the ventricular rhythm is irregular. The arrows indicate ventricular escape beats which appear when the conduction of atrial impulses through the A-V junction is blocked.

Fig. 58-A presents a sinus rhythm interrupted by two atrial extrasystoles. The first one is conducted to the ventricle with a markedly prolonged P^1-R interval while the second is blocked (b). The following short asystolic pause is terminated by a junctional escape beat (E) dissociated from a sinus P wave which is buried within the QRS complex of the escape beat.

It is not unusual to find a paroxysmal atrial tachycardia followed by a pause and by the emergence of a junctional escape beat (E). This is illustrated in fig. 58-B. In this instance, the sinus P wave, merging into the escape QRS, is blocked within the A-V junction.

Fig. 58-C shows a similar situation at the end of a paroxysmal atrial flutter. An escape junctional beat (e) follows the cessation of the paroxysm and anticipates the reappearance of a normal sinus rhythm.

Fig. 58-D is a case of atrial fibrillation. The fifth, sixth and seventh QRS's are wide, bizarre and suggest an ectopic ventricular origin. They are separated by regular intervals; the first beat (ve) appears after a particularly long cardiac cycle. Therefore, the rhythm is an atrial fibrillation with periods of complete A-V block and ventricular escape beats *(idio-ventricular escape rhythm)* before an adequate A-V conduction is re-established (final three QRS's of the bottom tracing).

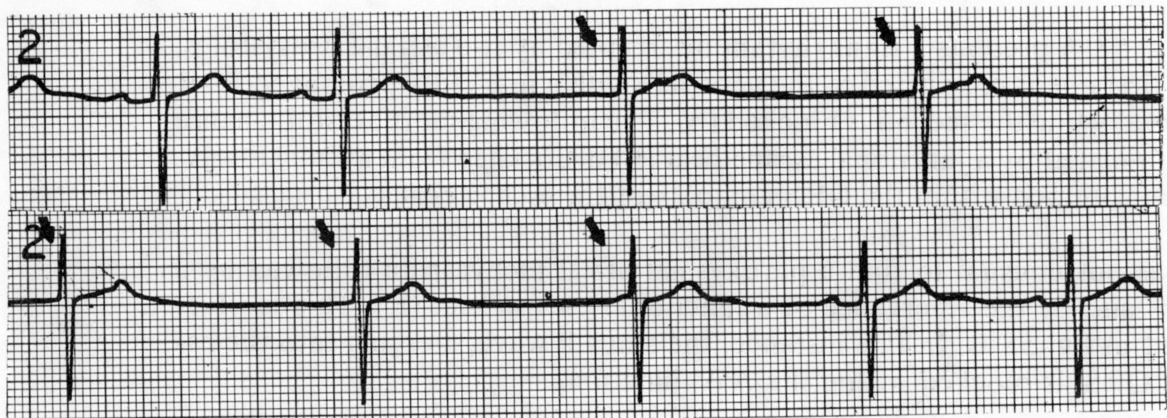

Fig. 59-A - Junctional rhythm. The arrows indicate a series of escape junctional beats which originates from a "mid-junctional pacemaker."

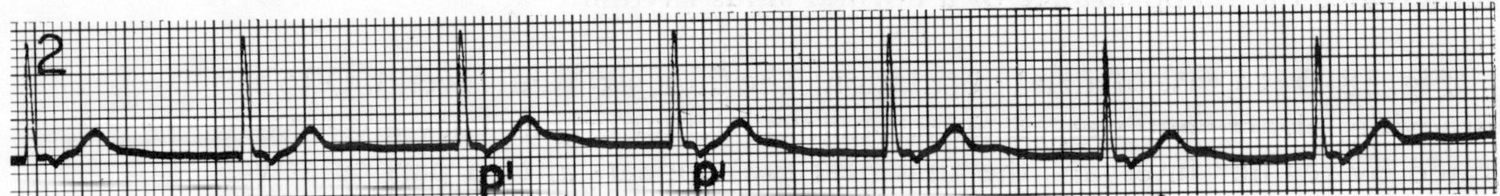

Fig. 59-B - Junctional rhythm. P^1 waves indicate a retrograde atrial depolarization following the ventricular one. Therefore, the rhythm is a "low" junctional rhythm.

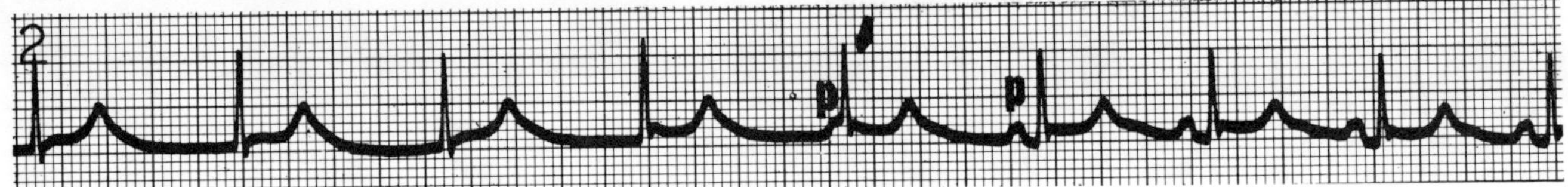

Fig. 59-C - Junctional rhythm. The transition between a junctional and a sinus rhythm is marked by a dissociation of a junctional QRS and a sinus P wave.

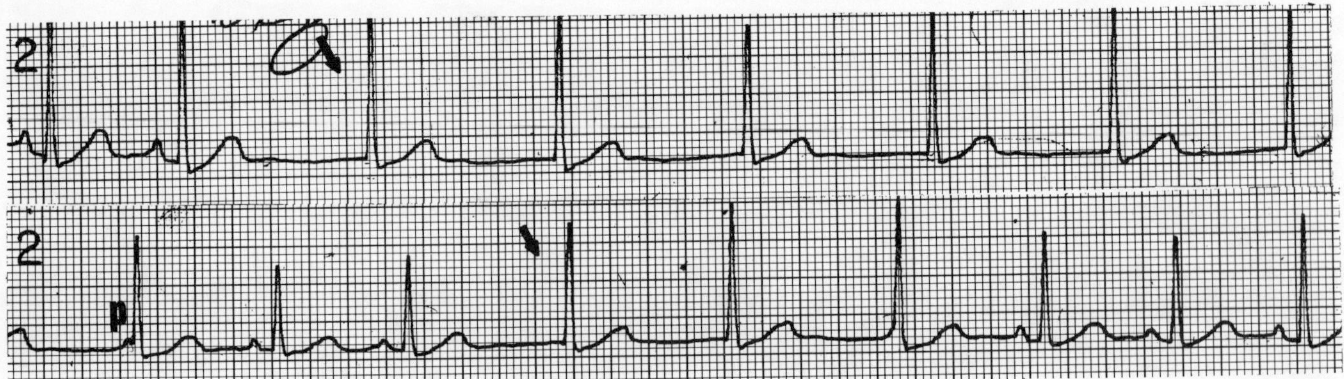

Fig. 59-D - Junctional rhythm and sinus arrhythmia. The phasic slowing of the sinus rate during inspiration allows for the escape of junctional beats. The expiratory phase is made of sinus beats.

JUNCTIONAL RHYTHM (A-V nodal)

When several junctional escape beats follow each other, activating almost simultaneously both atria and ventricles, they produce a *junctional rhythm*. A junctional rhythm may be of "high", "mid", or "low" type, according to the P^1-QRS ratio; however, it must be remembered that, more than to the anatomical site of the pacemaker, the A-V ratio is due to the anterograde and retrograde conduction velocity of the impulse into the A-V junction. The intrinsic automaticity of a junctional secondary pacemaker fluctuates between 40-60 beats/minute. In the presence of fast junctional rates, the rhythm will not be indicated as a junctional rhythm (which means a passive escape rhythm) but as a *junctional tachycardia* (which is an active rhythm due to an increased excitability of a secondary pacemaker, as seen on page 37).

Fig. 59-A presents a sinus rhythm that is substituted, after the first two beats, by a slower mid-junctional rhythm. The pause originating the escape of the five junctional beats is, in this case, due to a sino-atrial block or a marked sinus arrhythmia. (A sinus arrhythmia from increased vagal tone may give rise to salvos of junctional beats in people with otherwise normal hearts.)

A *"low" junctional rhythm,* with P^1 waves following the QRS's, is shown in fig. 59-B. Both atria and ventricles are activated by the junctional pacemaker.

During the transition from a junctional into a sinus rhythm, it is almost a rule to find one or more beats with P waves buried within the QRS and, therefore, with a temporary A-V dissociation. This is clearly illustrated in fig. 59-C, where the fifth beat, still of a junctional origin, anticipates a sinus P wave blocked within the A-V junction.

At the bedside examination, a rhythm such as the one presented in fig. 59-D may be easily interpreted as a sinus arrhythmia. Faster sinus rates alternate with slower cardiac cycles (junctional rhythm). Even in normal individuals, the bradycardic phase of a respiratory sinus arrhythmia may often be replaced by a series of junctional escape beats (as in the case of figs. 59-A and 59-B).

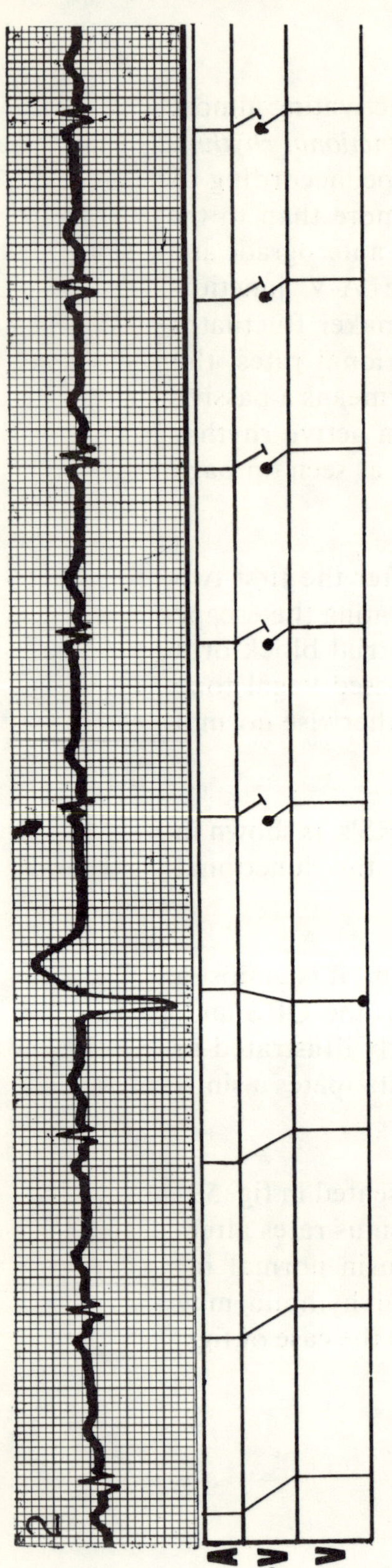

Fig. 60-A - A-V dissociation. A dissociation between atria and ventricles follows the ventricular extrasystole. Since the sinus and junctional pacemaker rates are very similar, the sinus P waves are partially buried within the QRS complexes.

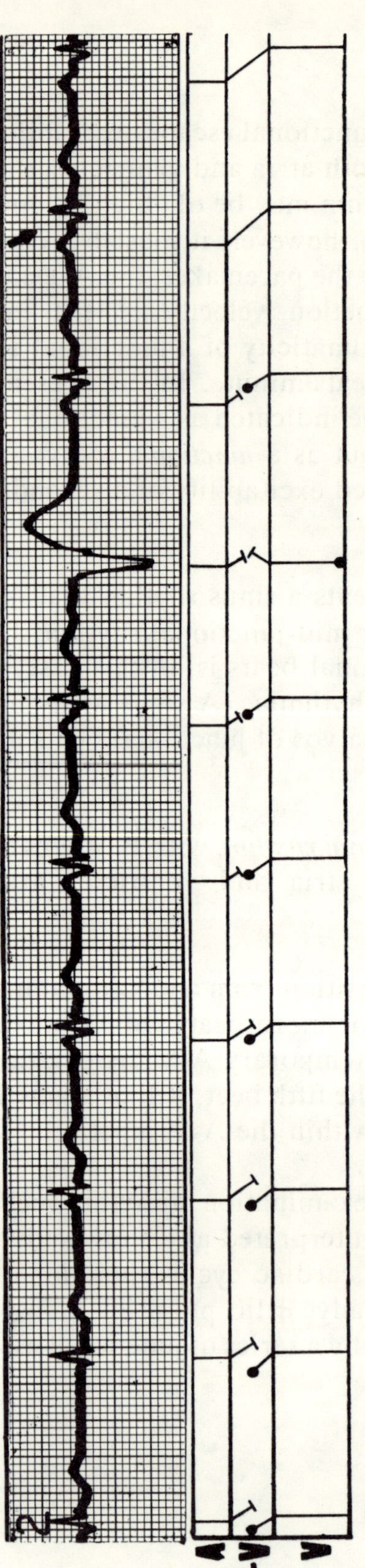

Fig. 60-B - A-V dissociation. The sequence is interrupted by a PVC which is followed by the reappearance of a sinus rhythm (arrow).

ATRIO-VENTRICULAR (A-V) DISSOCIATION

When a series of escape beats follow each other regularly but the atria remain under sinus control, the resulting rhythm is called *atrio-ventricular dissociation*. This is the most common form of A-V dissociation, ("passive A-V dissociation") and is determined by a slowing or a temporary suppression of the primary cardiac pacemaker. A temporary A-V dissociation has been already encountered in PVC's which do not alter the sinus rhythm (see page 19), during escape beats without retrograde conduction to the atria (see pages 114-116), and during the transition from a junctional into a sinus rhythm and vice-a-versa (see pages 116-118).

Although the term *"A-V dissociation"* indicates that the atria and ventricles are responding to two different pacemakers, *it will not be used as a synonim of complete or third degree A-V block*. However, an A-V dissociation may also be secondary to an "active rhythm." This means that a subsidiary pacemaker takes command of the ventricles, while the atria are independently activated by the S-A node. A-V dissociation is usually present during a ventricular tachycardia (see page 72) and may also be found during a junctional tachycardia.

Fig. 60-A presents a typical case of A-V dissociation. After three sinus beats, a PVC with retrograde conduction to the atria induces an incomplete compensatory pause long enough for the *escape of a junctional rhythm*. The rate of the junctional pacemaker is almost similar to that of the sinus node and this determines an *A-V dissociation*. The atria and the ventricles are almost simultaneously activated by two different and independent pacemakers. The junctional subsidiary pacemaker delivers its impulse just at the moment of arrival of the sinus impulse. The latter is blocked because it finds the junctional tissue already depolarized and, therefore, refractory. On the other hand, the junctional impulse can not propagate in a retrograde fashion to the atria which already have been activated by the sinus impulse. The P waves are first preceded, then buried, and finally follow the QRS complexes because of the slight difference in rates between the two pacemakers. This situation, where there is a collision of impulses of two pacemakers propagating almost simultaneously, is also called *"interference dissociation"*.

Only a few seconds have elapsed between the recording of fig. 60-A and that of fig. 60-B. The firing rates of the two pacemakers are almost similar and P waves gradually reappear before the QRS's. Again a ventricular extrasystole interrupts the sequence of fig. 60-B. The PVC is followed by three beats with P waves clearly preceding the QRS's. The first P-R interval is shorter than the following intervals and therefore, an *A-V dissociation* is still present during this beat. The arrow indicates the reappearance of a normal A-V conduction of the sinus impulses.

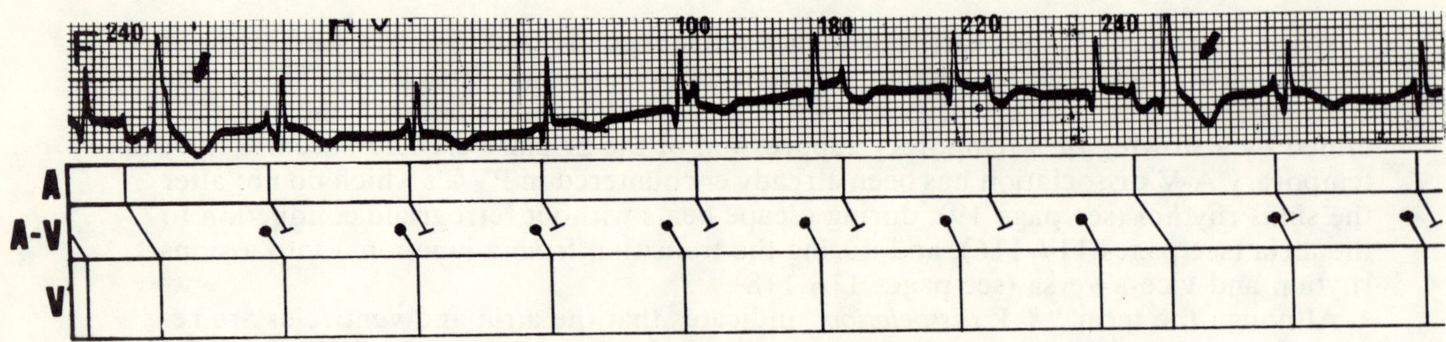

Fig. 61-A - A-V dissociation and escape capture beat. When the dissociated P waves follow the QRS complexes of an interval of 240 msecs., they cross the A-V junction and capture the ventricles.

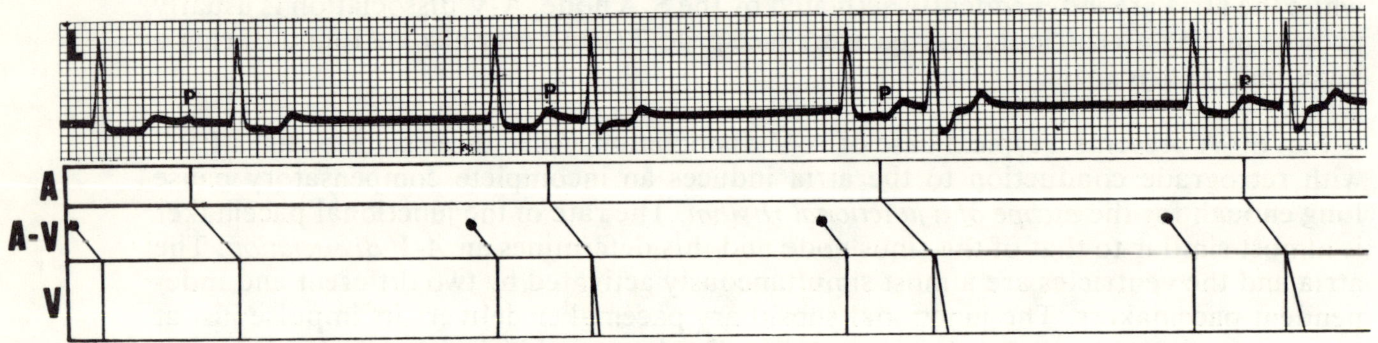

Fig. 61-B - A-V dissociation and escape capture bigeminy. Sinus P waves are "sandwiched" between two QRS's. Since they land far enough from the junctional QRS, they always capture the ventricles.

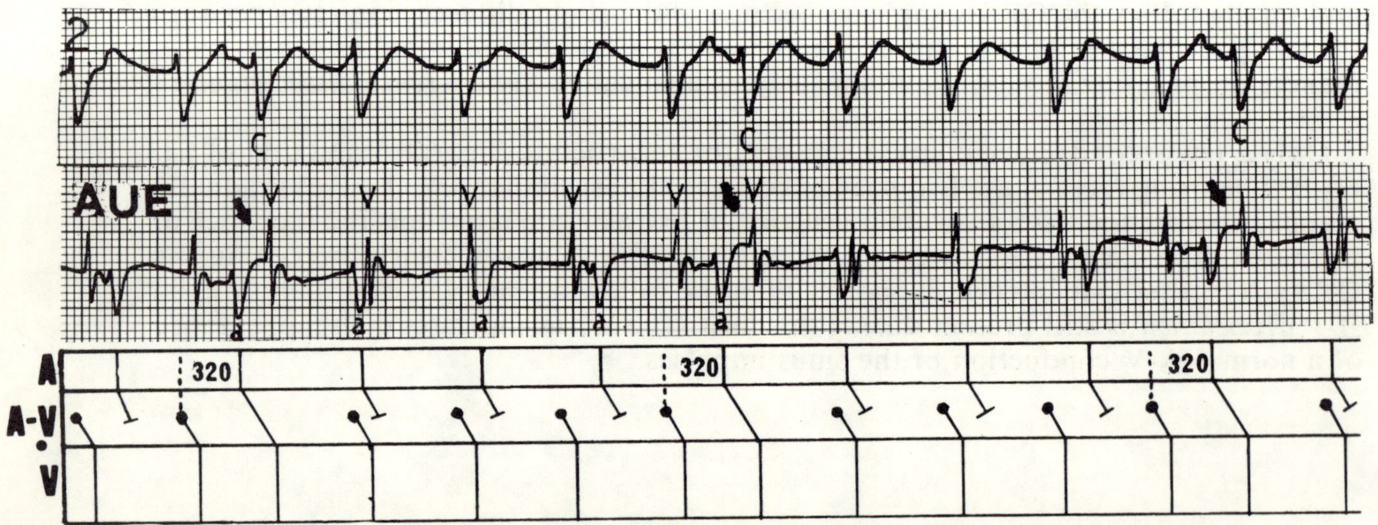

Fig. 61-C - A-V dissociation and ventricular capture beats. Capture beats are indicated with "C" on the surface ECG (L2). The mechanism of the arrhythmia is revealed by the unipolar atrial electrogram (UAE). This shows atrial waves (A) dissociated from ventricular waves (V), and ventricular capture beats (arrows).

A-V DISSOCIATION

During episodes of A-V dissociation, the sinus rate is often slower than that of the junctional pacemaker. Therefore, the sinus impulses will appear with an always greater delay over the junctional impulses and P waves may precede, be buried within or follow the QRS complexes. There will be a moment in which the atrial impulses will reach the A-V junction with such a delay from the preceding QRS, that they may find it no more refractory and completely repolarized. These impulses may conduct through the A-V junction and depolarize the ventricles before the formation and propagation of the next junctional impulse. This fact will determine an asystolic interval similar to an incomplete compensatory pause *(ventricular escape-capture beats)*. If the automaticity of the two foci remains unchanged after the escape-capture beats, the A-V dissociation continues and the sequence may repeat.

Fig. 61-A shows an A-V dissociation; the P waves first precede, are then buried and finally follow the QRS complexes. The second and tenth beats are premature when compared to other QRS's. In both instances, when the QRS-P interval is equal to 240 msec., the sinus impulses are able to penetrate the A-V junction, which is now fully repolarized, and are conducted to the ventricles *(escape-capture beats)*. It appears obvious how escape-capture beats may simulate PAC's or PVC's, especially when P waves are not clearly visible on the surface ECG.

Fig. 61-B shows an interesting, although uncommon, situation. At a rapid glance of the tracing, it appears immediately evident that the QRS complexes are grouped in "couplets" separated by long pauses. The first thing that comes to mind is some sort of bigeminal extrasystolic rhythm. However, a more careful observation reveals that, while the first QRS of each couplet is not preceded by a P wave, the second one has always a P wave sandwiched between the two QRS's. Furthermore, it may also be noted that the second QRS of the last three couplets shows a progressively increasing ventricular aberration. The ladder diagram explains the mysterious mechanism of the arrhythmia. The basic rhythm is a junctional escape mechanism dissociated from a markedly bradycardic sinus rhythm (or from a sinus rhythm with a 2:1 S-A block). The sinus P waves land always far enough from the preceding junctional QRS's and are able to cross the A-V junction and capture the ventricles. Therefore, the second QRS of each couplet is an *escape-capture beat*. Since the sinus rate is not perfectly regular, the P wave which falls too close to a junctional QRS captures the ventricles with a progressive ventricular aberration. The sequence in which a dissociated junctional beat is followed by an escape-capture beat has been descriptively named *"A-V dissociation with escape-capture bigeminy."*

Again, in fig. 61-C the beat indicated with "C" (L2) may be interpreted as an atrial premature beat or, since P waves are not clearly evident, the rhythm may be mistaken for an atrial fibrillation. The atrial unipolar electrogram (AUE), which is not recorded simultaneously, shows the A-V dissociation between a sinus and a junctional pacemaker and clearly reveals the ventricular capture beats (arrow). When the P wave falls 320 msecs. after a QRS it penetrates the A-V junction and is conducted to the ventricles (escape-capture beats).

Some authors use the term "interference dissociation" in describing a) ventricular escape-capture beats or b) an atrial rhythm that occasionally interferes with an otherwise regular junctional rhythm. Therefore, the term "interference dissociation" is used in a completely opposite fashion by different schools and it has been gradually changed into a simpler and less compromising classification of *A-V dissociation with or without escape-capture beats*. Other schools, finally, divide A-V dissociation into an *incomplete*, when escape-capture beats are present, and complete, when they are absent.

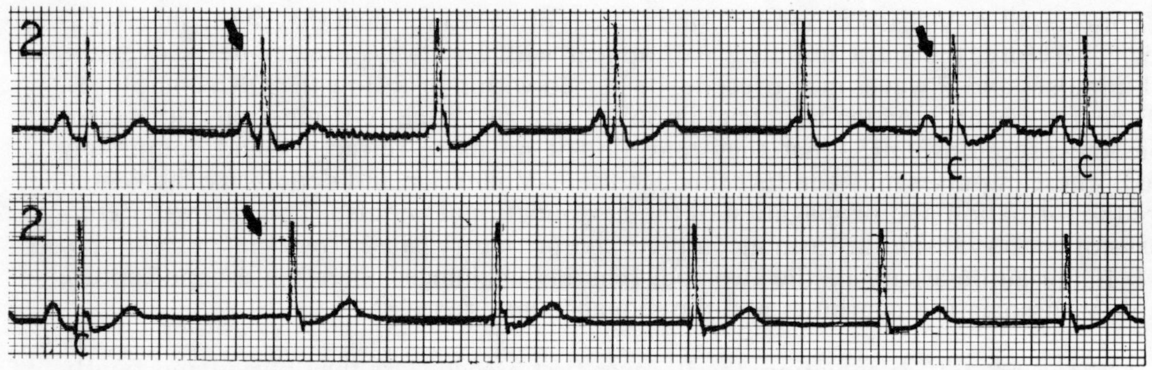

Fig. 62-A - A-V dissociation. Junctional beats appear during the phasic slowing of a sinus arrhythmia. The sinus impulses are conducted to the ventricle during expiration (C).

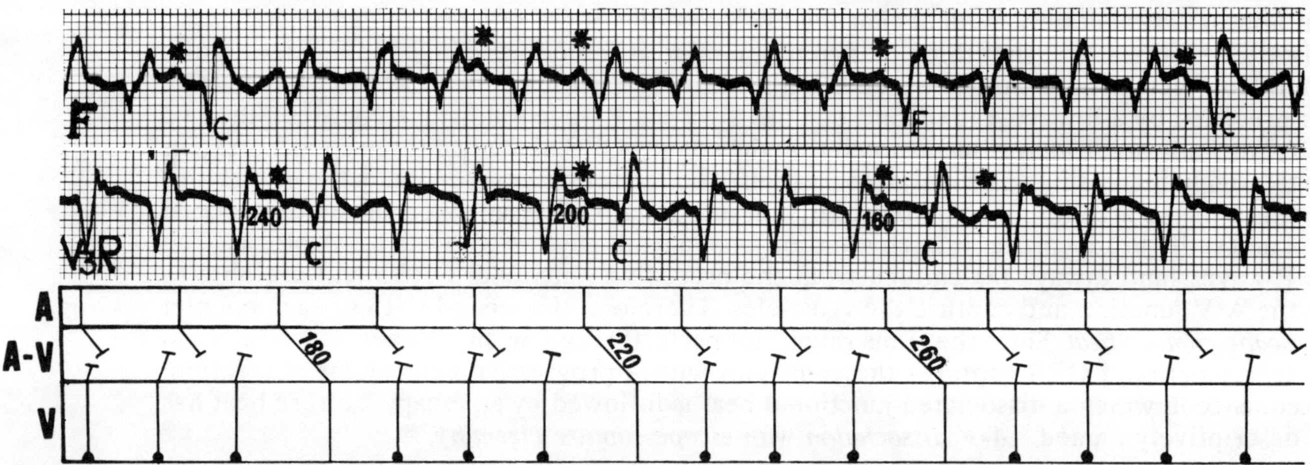

Fig. 62-B - A-V dissociation. This is present during a double tachycardia, atrial and ventricular. Ventricular capture beats (C) and fusion beats (F) are present. The length of the P-R interval of the capture beats has a reverse relationship with the preceding R-P¹ interval.

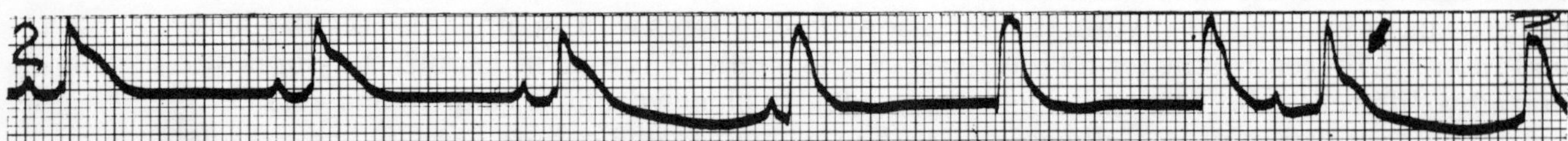

Fig. 62-C - A-V dissociation. The tracing was obtained during an acute myocardial infarction. The arrow indicates an escape capture beat.

An A-V dissociation may be initiated by the phasic slowing of a sinus arrhythmia. Fig. 62-A presents a respiratory sinus arrhythmia. At the slowing down of the sinus rate, a junctional rhythm emerges and induces an A-V dissociation for four consecutive beats. P waves approach and are then buried within the QRS's, but never surpass them. When the sinus node accelerates, it controls the cardiac rhythm (ventricular escape-capture beats = C). The R-R intervals of the escape-capture beats are shorter than those of the junctional rhythm. After the third sinus beat with ventricular capture (C) there is a pause without sinus activity. This determines, again, the reappearance of a "mid-junctional rhythm" which controls both atria and ventricles.

Although an A-V dissociation is usually determined by a slowing down of the sinus rate, it is possible to find it during a double atrial (or sinus) and ventricular tachycardia. Fig. 62-B shows a case of double tachycardia with A-V dissociation and ventricular escape-capture beats. The atrial rate is equal to 115/min. and the ventricular rate is 180/min. and some of the QRS's, which show a morphology totally different than others, are preceded by P[1] waves with variable P[1]-R intervals (C). P[1] waves are recognizable and indicated by the asterisks. The two rhythms are clearly dissociated. The *ventricular escape-capture beats* (C), therefore, confirm the diagnosis of a *double atrial and ventricular tachycardia with A-V dissociation*. Only the P[1] waves which fall far enough from the QRS's of the ventricular tachycardia capture the ventricles. The P[1]-R interval of the escape-capture beats is inversely proportional to the R-P[1] interval. Therefore, there is a reciprocal relation between R-P[1] and P[1]-R intervals in the cardiac cycles terminating with escape-capture beats. For example, in the second tracing of fig. 62-B, the P[1]-R intervals of the three capture beats are respectively 180, 220, 260 msec., while the distance between the P[1] waves and the preceding QRS's (R-P[1] intervals) are in order: 240, 200, 160 msec. Again, this indicates that the length of the P-R or P[1]-R intervals depends on both the state of function of the A-V junction and the position of the P or P[1] waves within the cardiac cycle. In fact, the more premature the P or P[1] wave with respect to the preceding beat (in this case the ventricular ectopic beats with retrograde penetration to the atria), the higher the possibility that it finds a refractory A-V junction during its trip to the ventricles.

Fig. 62-C shows a short episode of A-V dissociation in a patient with an acute myocardial infraction. After the third beat, the slower sinus rhythm dissociates from a fast junctional mechanism. The seventh beat is an *escape-capture beat* (C).

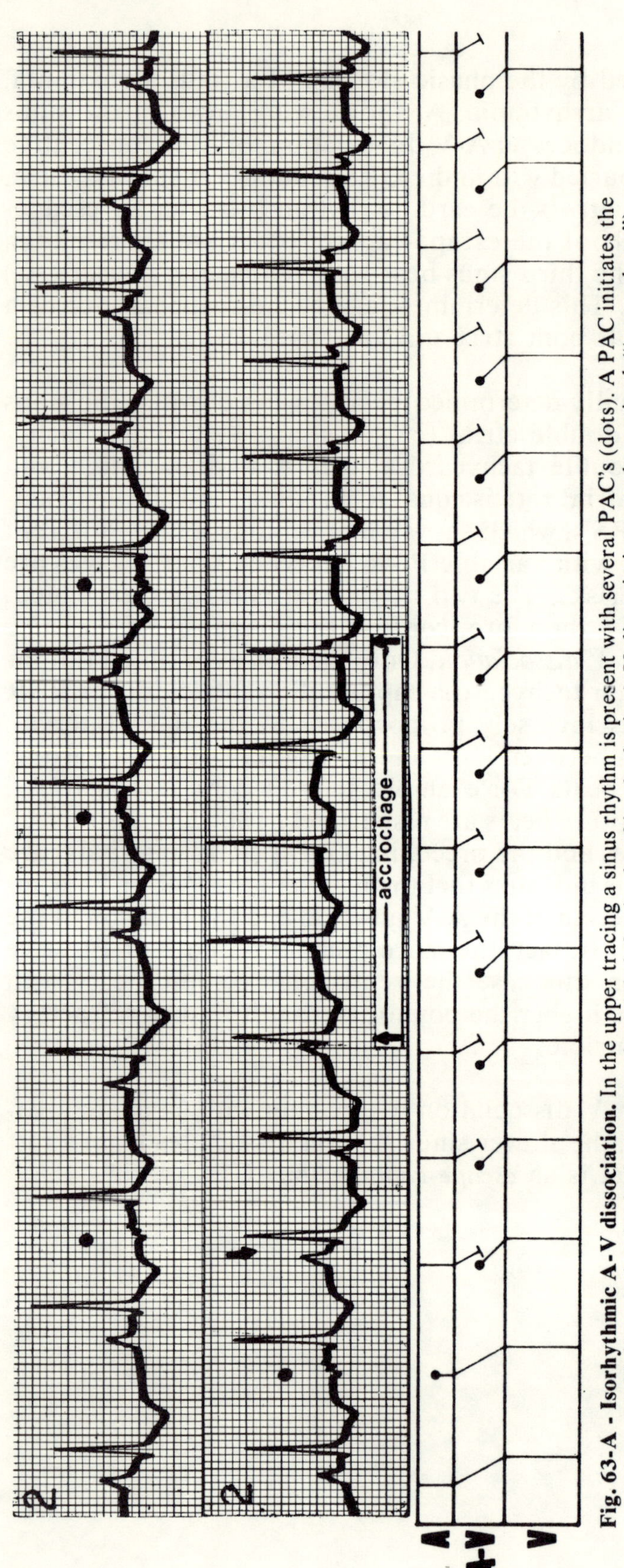

Fig. 63-A - Isorhythmic A-V dissociation. In the upper tracing a sinus rhythm is present with several PAC's (dots). A PAC initiates the A-V dissociation in the bottom tracing. A brief episode of isorhythmic A-V dissociation may be noticed ("accrochage").

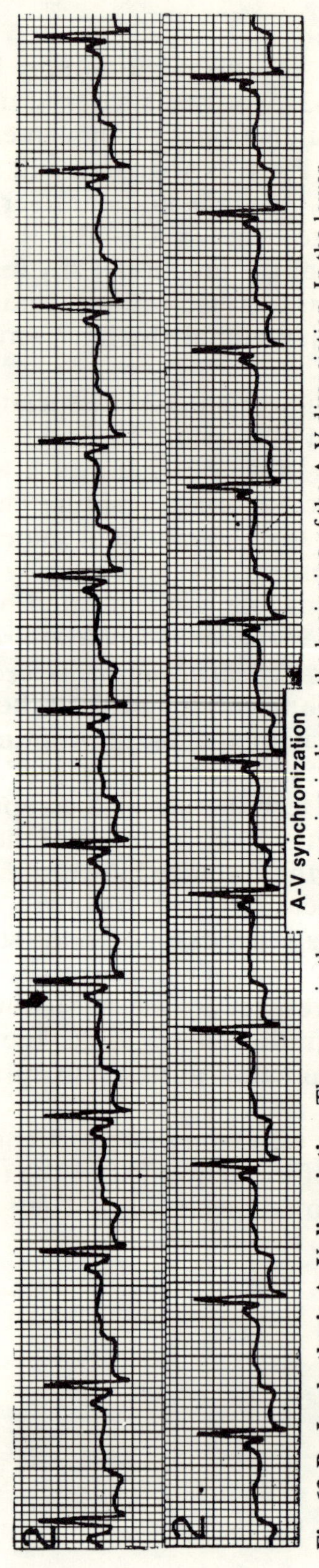

Fig. 63-B - Isorhythmic A-V dissociation. The arrow in the upper tracing indicates the beginning of the A-V dissociation. In the lower tracing, the atria and ventricles beat almost simultaneously ("A-V synchronization").

ISORHYTHMIC A-V DISSOCIATION

During an episode of A-V dissociation the rates of the two pacemakers, which separately control the atria and ventricles, is usually very similar. Since a junctional pacemaker does not show the phasic variations of a sinus arrhythmia, P waves may precede, be buried within, or follow the QRS complexes.

Fig. 63-A shows a sinus rhythm interrupted by atrial premature beats (dots). In the bottom tracing a PAC is followed by an episode of A-V dissociation between the S-A node and the A-V junction. The pacemaker's rates are almost similar and both are quite fast (110/min.). The atria and ventricles beat simultaneously for a period of four beats. This is known as *isorhythmic A-V dissociation* (beats included between the two arrows). However, an isorhythmic A-V dissociation may last for several seconds (as in the case of fig. 63-B where the dissociated atria and ventricles beat almost simultaneously). In the presence of these findings, a hypothesis has been formulated which holds that, during the A-V dissociation, the simultaneous formation of impulses in the two pacemakers would not occur by mere coincidence, but it would be determined by a state of electrical attraction between the two pacemakers. Therefore, the impulses delivered by the two pacemakers would synchronize, for variable periods of time.

During an A-V dissociation, brief episodes of simultaneous atrial and ventricular beating are commonly called "accrochage". Longer periods are called "A-V synchronization".

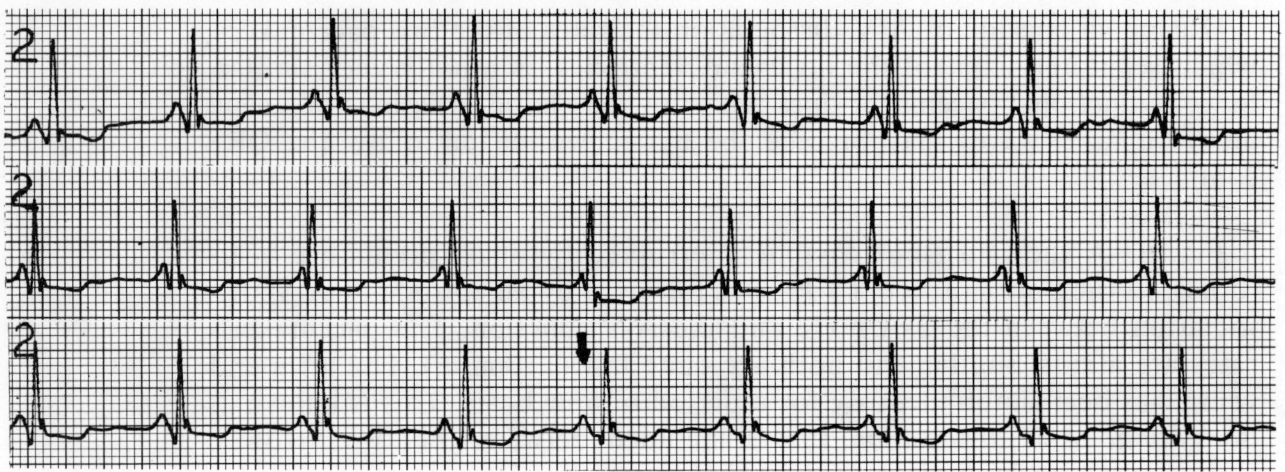

Fig. 64-A - Isorhythmic A-V dissociation.

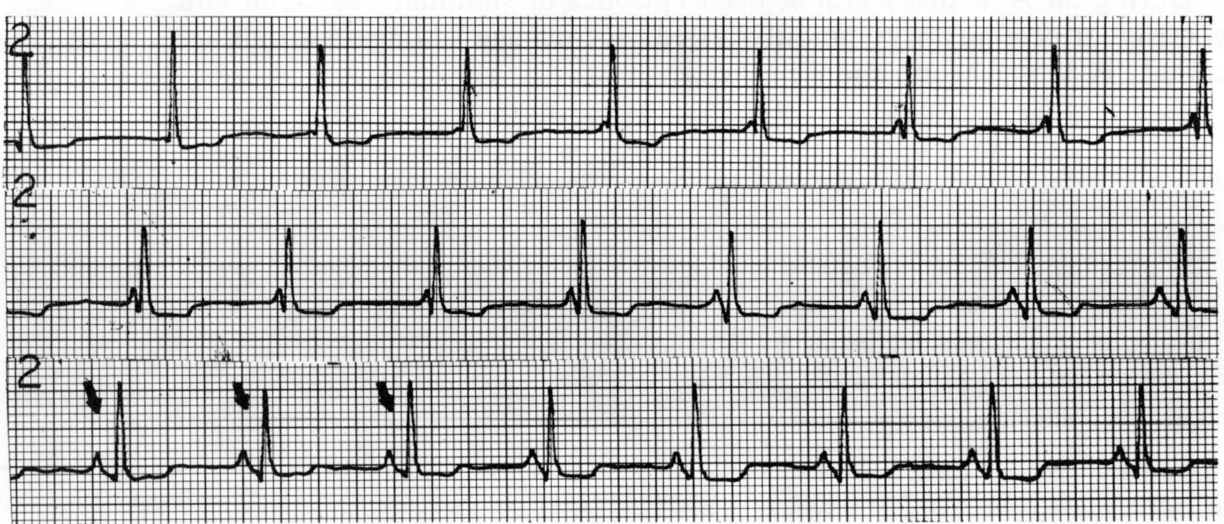

Fig. 64-B - Isorhythmic A-V dissociation.

ISORHYTHMIC A-V DISSOCIATION

Two examples of *isorhythmic A-V dissociation with periods of synchronization* are presented in fig. 64-A and 64-B. Obviously, during moments of isorhythmic A-V dissociation giant "a" waves will appear in the jugular veins because the atria contract against closed A-V valves. On auscultation, the first sound will be constant in intensity (differently from what happens in complete A-V block).

In fig. 64-A, thirteen seconds elapse with the atria and ventricle beating simultaneously, before the P wave is definitely re-established before the QRS.

Again in fig. 64-B, P waves gradually move across the QRS complexes for several beats in the presence of an isorhythmic A-V dissociation.

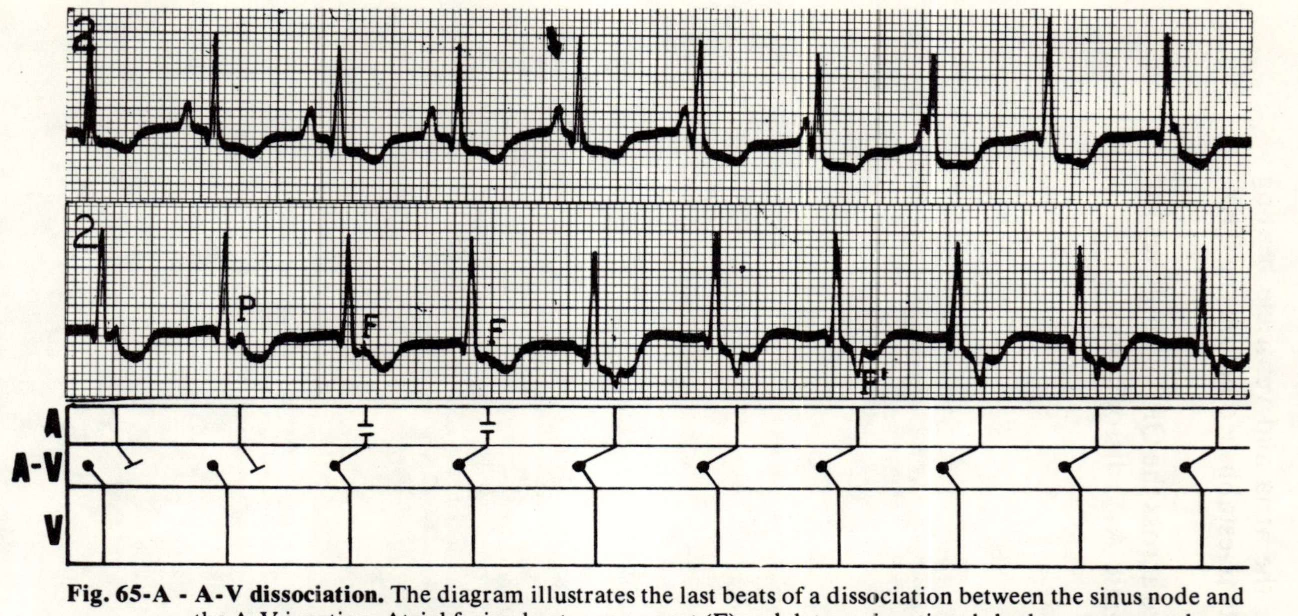

Fig. 65-A - A-V dissociation. The diagram illustrates the last beats of a dissociation between the sinus node and the A-V junction. Atrial fusion beats are present (F) and, later, a junctional rhythm appears and controls both atria and ventricles.

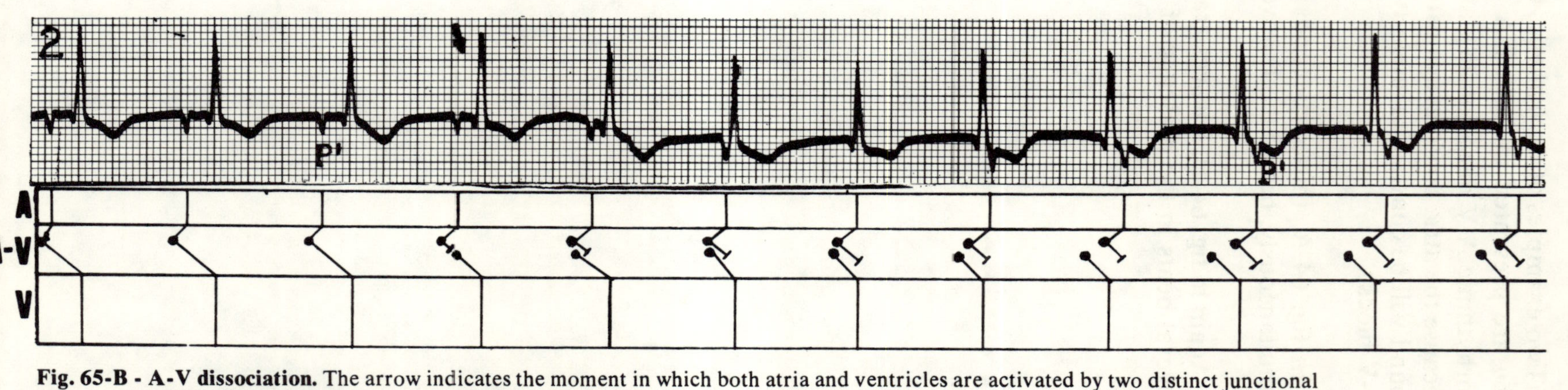

Fig. 65-B - A-V dissociation. The arrow indicates the moment in which both atria and ventricles are activated by two distinct junctional pacemakers (infra-junctional A-V dissociation).

When the firing rate of the junctional pacemaker, which induces an A-V dissociation, is slightly faster than the sinus rate, the atria could be depolarized in a retrograde fashion by the junctional impulses. For this not to happen it is necessary that a retrograde A-V block is present and protects the atria from the junctional control. Tracings 61-A-B-C, 62-B and 63-A show sinus P waves that are buried within or follow the QRS complexes, and only occasionally capture the ventricles. A retrograde block in the A-V junction must be present in these cases, otherwise the junctional impulses would have time enough to travel to and depolarize the atria before sinus impulses. When a retrograde block is not present, situations similar to that of fig. 65-A may be found. The sinus rhythm begins to dissociate from a junctional rhythm (fifth beat of the upper tracing) when the P-R interval becomes suddenly shortened (arrow). Because of the slower sinus node the P waves first approach, are then buried into, and finally follow the QRS complexes.

During the A-V dissociation, when the P wave falls far enough from the preceding QRS, the retrograde conduction to the atria of the junctional impulses starts to appear, first with atrial fusion beats (F) and later with clearly inverted P[1] waves. Therefore, in this case, the rhythm goes, in a matter of seconds, from a sinus rhythm dissociated from a junctional pacemaker, to a junctional rhythm which controls both the atria and the ventricles.

Occasionally, one may encounter extravagant arrhythmias as that presented in fig. 65-B, which belongs to the same patient of fig. 65-A. The tracing shows a dissociation between two pacemakers, both localized into the A-V junction *("infra-junctional A-V dissociation")*.

The first three beats originate from a high junctional rhythm (or a coronary rhythm) with clearly inverted P[1] waves. The P[1]-R interval becomes suddenly shortened at the fourth beat (arrow) and the P[1] wave is first buried within, and then reappears after the QRS complex. While the atria are always depolarized by the same pacemaker, the ventricular depolarization is controlled by a new junctional pacemaker.

An alternative to this explanation is that a retrograde (V-A) Wenckebach mechanism is operating into the junction, with a progressive delay of the conduction to the atria of the impulses originating from the same junctional pacemaker (see page 179).

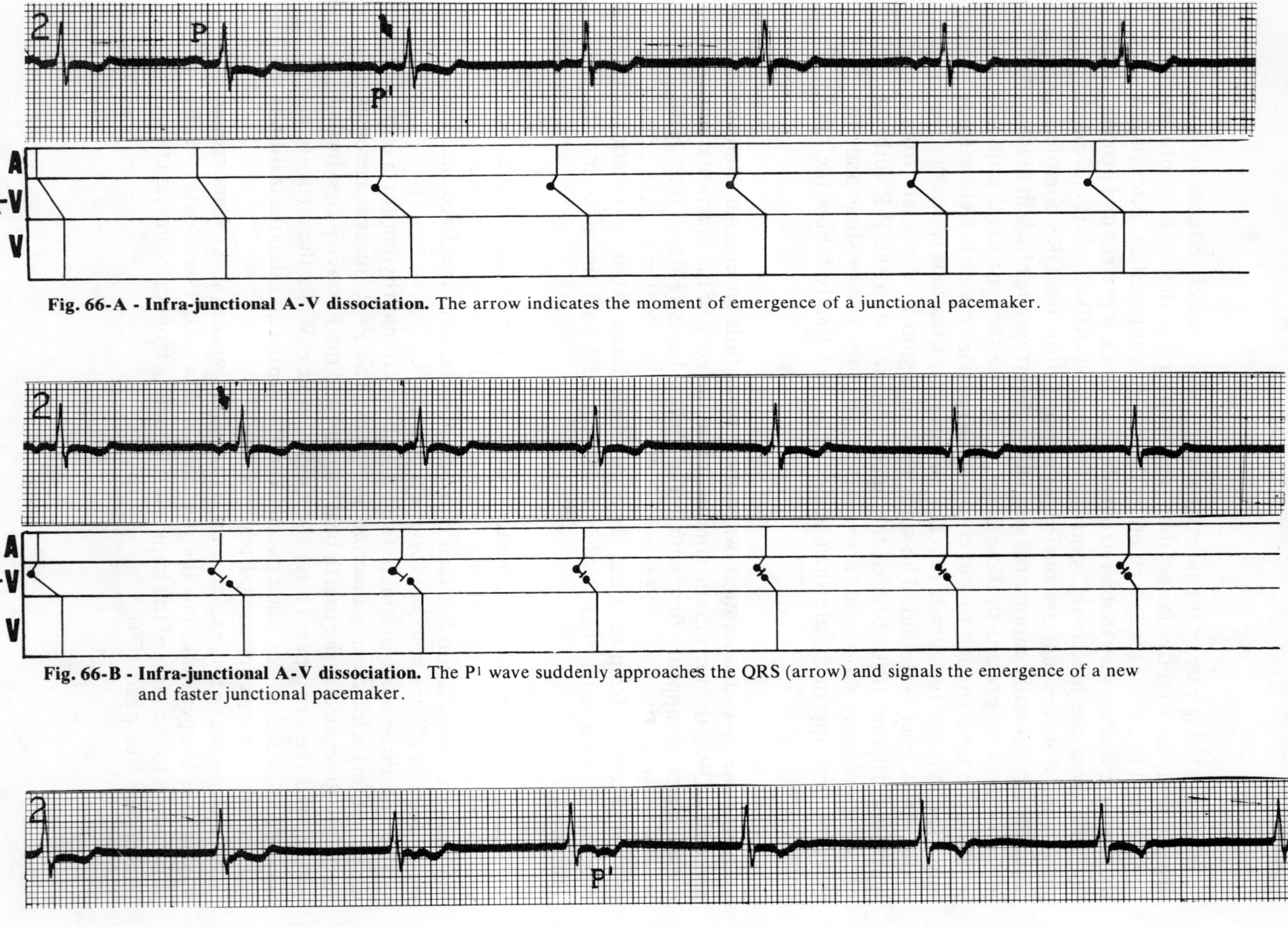

Fig. 66-A - **Infra-junctional A-V dissociation.** The arrow indicates the moment of emergence of a junctional pacemaker.

Fig. 66-B - **Infra-junctional A-V dissociation.** The P¹ wave suddenly approaches the QRS (arrow) and signals the emergence of a new and faster junctional pacemaker.

Fig. 66-C - **Infra-junctional A-V dissociation.** P¹ waves are first buried within and then follow the QRS complexes.

A-V DISSOCIATION

Tracings of fig. 66-A, 66-B and 66-C are continuous. The first two beats of fig. 66-A are of sinus origin. A brief period of a "high" junctional rhythm (or of coronary sinus rhythm) follows, and this controls both atrial and ventricular depolarization (a P[1] wave precedes each QRS complex).

In the tracing of fig. 66-B, the P[1] wave suddenly approaches the QRS (arrow) and then gradually disappears within the following QRS's. Therefore, atrial and ventricular activation are dissociated. The diagram illustrates a possible explanation of this phenomenon: the emergence of a second junctional pacemaker, more distal than the first one, which controls the ventricles while the atria are activated by the first junctional pacemaker (infrajunctional A-V dissociation). Therefore, a collision of impulses, delivered almost simultaneously, is present in the A-V junction and this determines the *A-V dissociation*. Since the rate of the new pacemaker is slightly faster than the first one, the QRS complexes move always closer to the P[1] waves until they fuse with them.

In tracing of fig. 66-C, the P[1] wave reappears after the QRS. The diagnosis is "infra-junctional A-V dissociation." An alternative explanation is possible in this case and calls upon the presence of a retrograde Wenckebach phenomenon in the conduction of the impulses to the atria (see page 179). Therefore, the impulses would originate always from the same junctional pacemaker, but, while the conduction to the ventricles remains constant, the retrograde conduction to the atria is progressively delayed. This fact would determine different P[1]-QRS ratios. While the surface ECG may leave doubts, the His bundle potentials recording has recently shown that both possibilities are valid.

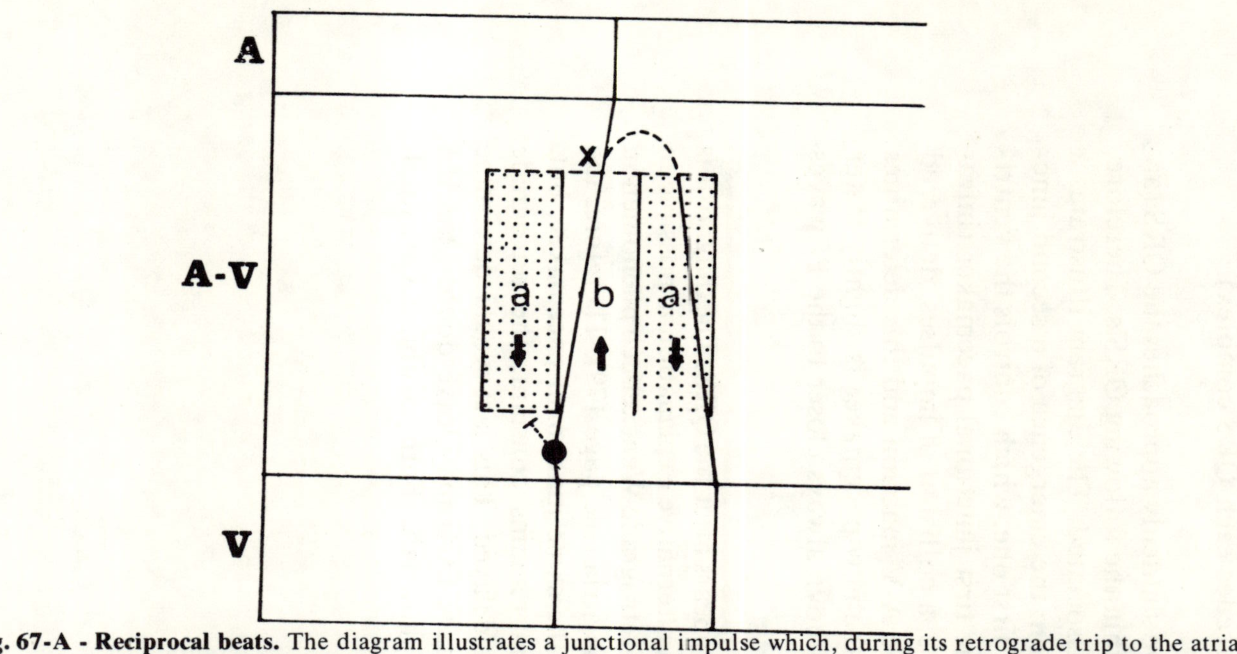

Fig. 67-A - Reciprocal beats. The diagram illustrates a junctional impulse which, during its retrograde trip to the atria, is reflected to the ventricles. a = conduction pathway with undirectional block; b = alternate A-V conduction pathway; x = reflection level.

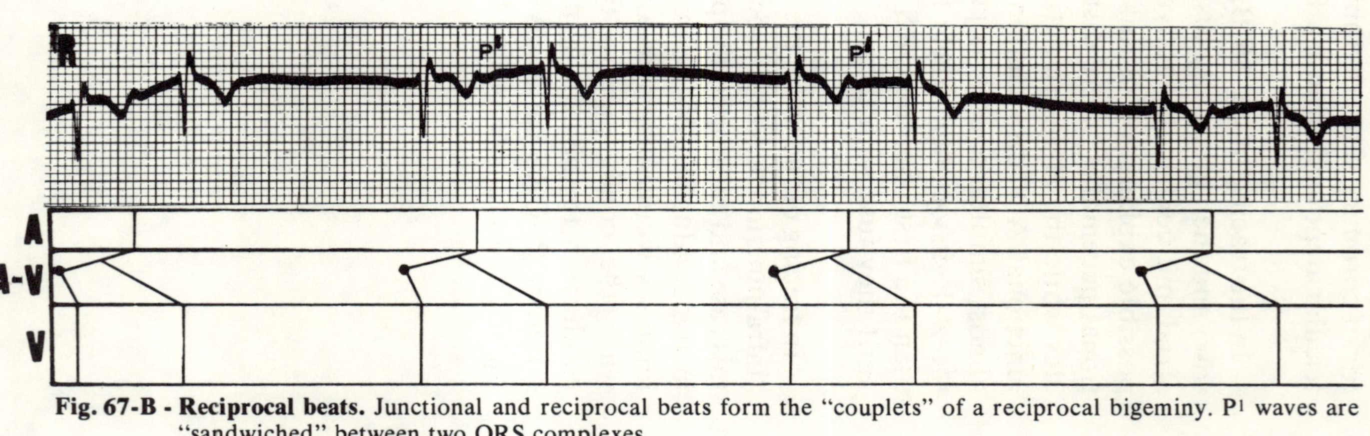

Fig. 67-B - Reciprocal beats. Junctional and reciprocal beats form the "couplets" of a reciprocal bigeminy. P¹ waves are "sandwiched" between two QRS complexes.

RECIPROCAL BEATS ("Echo beats")

When a junctional rhythm shows a delay in the retrograde conduction to the atria, it may give rise to *reciprocal beats*. Electrophysiologically this phenomenon is based upon the presence, in the A-V junction, of at least two conduction pathways, one of which has a "unindirectional block". The impulse originating in the A-V junction propagates distally to the ventricles and proximally to the atria. During its trip to the atria, it finds a totally refractory pathway (a) and, therefore, it proceeds toward the atria through an alternate conduction path (b) (fig. 67-A). When the impulse reaches the higher portions of the A-V junction, it may find an area in which path "a" is no longer refractory and, while still traveling to the atria, the impulse *reflects* and invades path "a", thereby returning to the ventricles and re-depolarizing them.

Naturally, the *reflection* and re-entry of impulses to the ventricles are favored by a delayed retrograde conduction through path "b". This offers to path "a" the necessary time to repolarize.

Heart beats coming from retrograde junctional impulses, which re-enter and re-excite the ventricles through anterograde conduction pathways, are called *reciprocal beats* or, more colorfully, *"echo beats"*. The rhythm which originates from these beats is called *reciprocal rhythm*. The level to which the impulses reflect within the A-V junction, and come back to the ventricles, is called *reflection level*.

More often a reciprocal rhythm presents itself in a form of "couplets" formed by a junctional beat and reciprocal beat, as is demonstrated in fig. 67-B. Such a rhythm is called *reciprocal bigeminy*. The P[1] wave is sandwiched between a QRS of junctional origin and a reciprocal one. The sequence is, in such a case, QRS-P[1]-QRS and it must not be confused with a sequence of an "A-V dissociation with escape capture" to which it has an extraordinary resemblance (see page 123). In the tracing of fig. 67-B the P[1] waves are easily traceable and present a constant interval with the QRS of the preceding junctional beats.

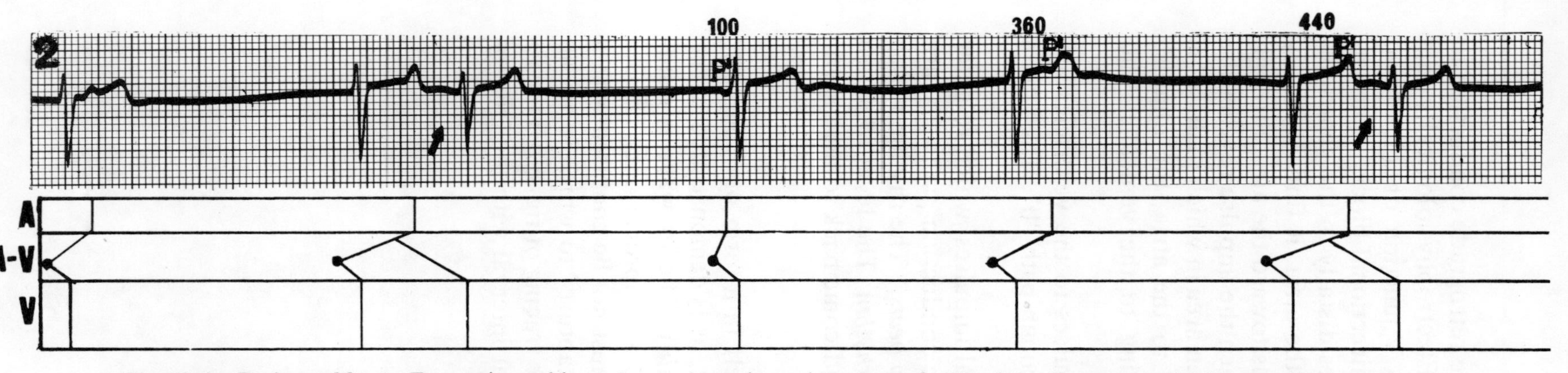

Fig. 68-A - **Reciprocal beats.** Two reciprocal beats (arrows) terminate the retrograde Wenckebach sequences. In the second sequence the P^1 wave first precedes the QRS, (100 msec.), then it follows it (360 msec.) and, finally, it becomes so prolonged (440 msec.) to allow for the reflection of the impulse to the ventricles (reciprocal beat).

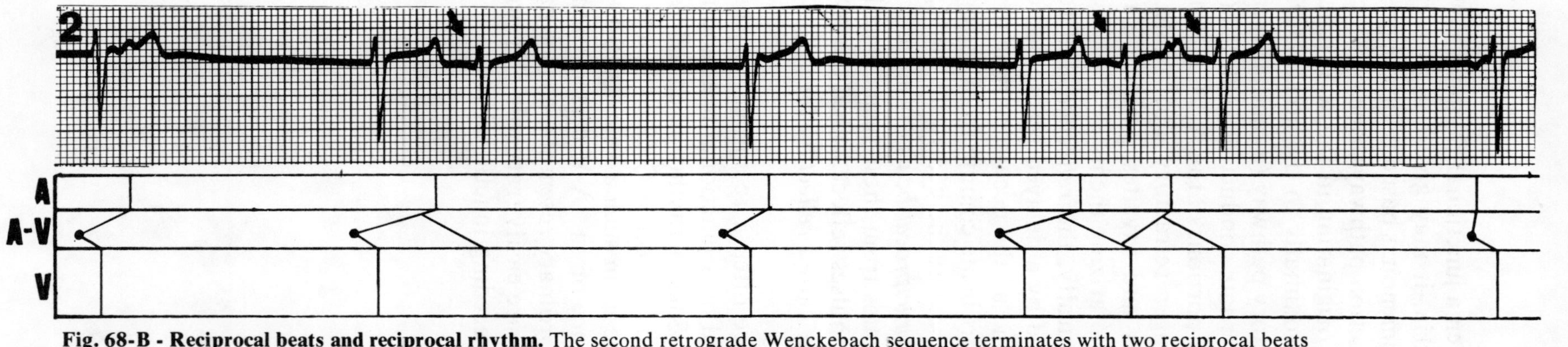

Fig. 68-B - **Reciprocal beats and reciprocal rhythm.** The second retrograde Wenckebach sequence terminates with two reciprocal beats (reciprocal rhythm). This is due to a double reflection of the junctional impulse toward the atria and ventricles.

Not unusually, a reciprocal beat may terminate a sequence of a *retrograde V-A Wenckebach phenomenon* (see page 179).

Fig. 68-A presents a "low" junctional rhythm, with a progressively slower retrograde conduction to the atria. There is a point in which the R-P^1 interval becomes so prolonged to allow for the "reflection" of the retrograde impulse and its re-entry into the ventricles. The reciprocal beats present in fig. 68-A are indicated by the arrows. The P^1 wave first precedes the QRS of 100 msec., then follows it with a progressively delayed R-P^1 interval (360 msec. to 440 msec.), and finally it induces a ventricular re-entry and a reciprocal beat.

Two sequences of a retrograde V-A Wenckebach are again presented in fig. 68-B. The second sequence is terminated not by one, but by two reciprocal beats. A sequence of several reciprocal beats deserves to be called a *reciprocal rhythm*. A reciprocal rhythm suggests the presence of two different levels of reflection within the A-V junction, one proximal and one distal. The retrograde junctional impulse is "reflected" and re-enters to the ventricles, and back again to the atria and then again to the ventricles and so on, with a pendulum type of motion of the excitation wave between atria and ventricles.

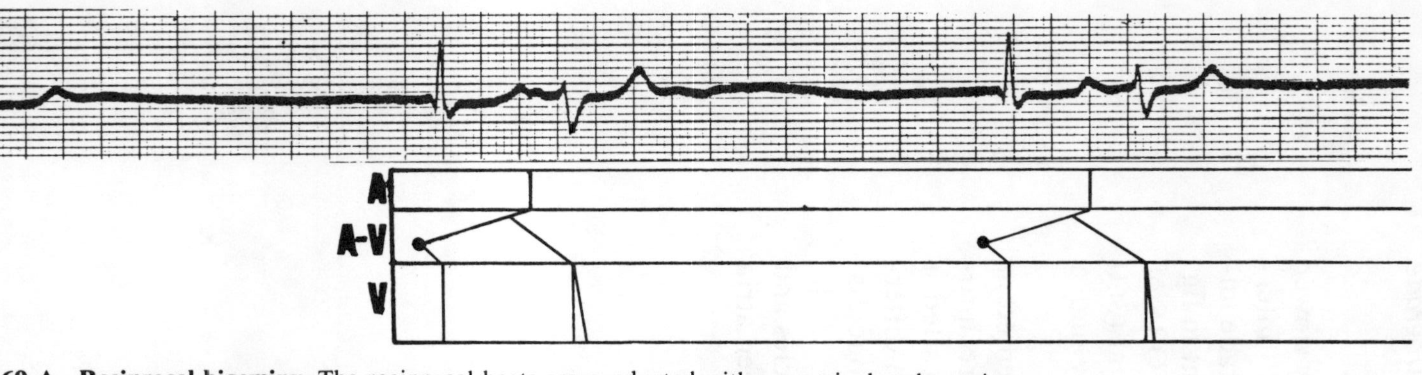

Fig. 69-A - **Reciprocal bigeminy.** The reciprocal beats are conducted with a ventricular aberration.

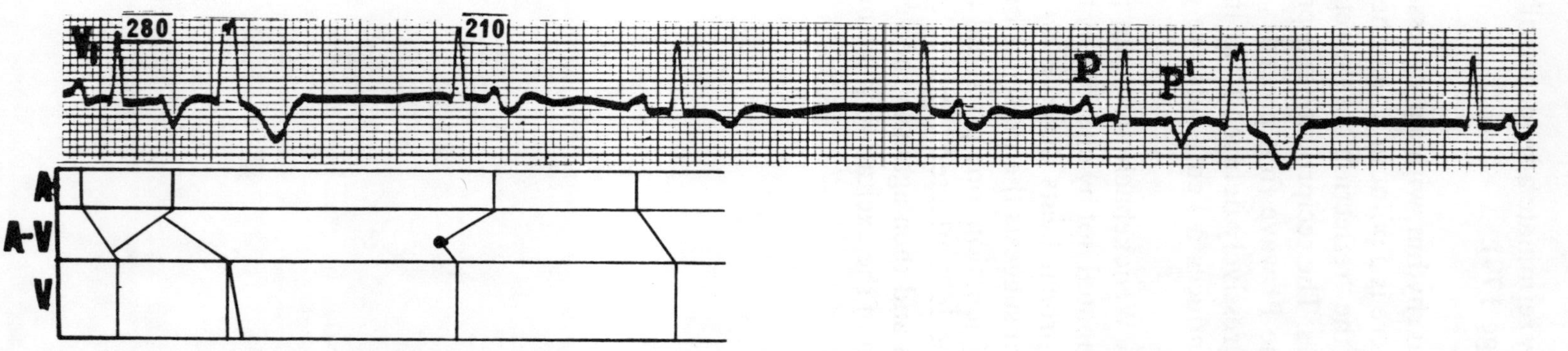

Fig. 69-B - **Inverse reciprocal beats.** The reciprocal sequence is initiated by a sinus impulse which, during its trip to the ventricles, is "reflected" and return to the atria and, again, to the ventricles with aberrant conduction.

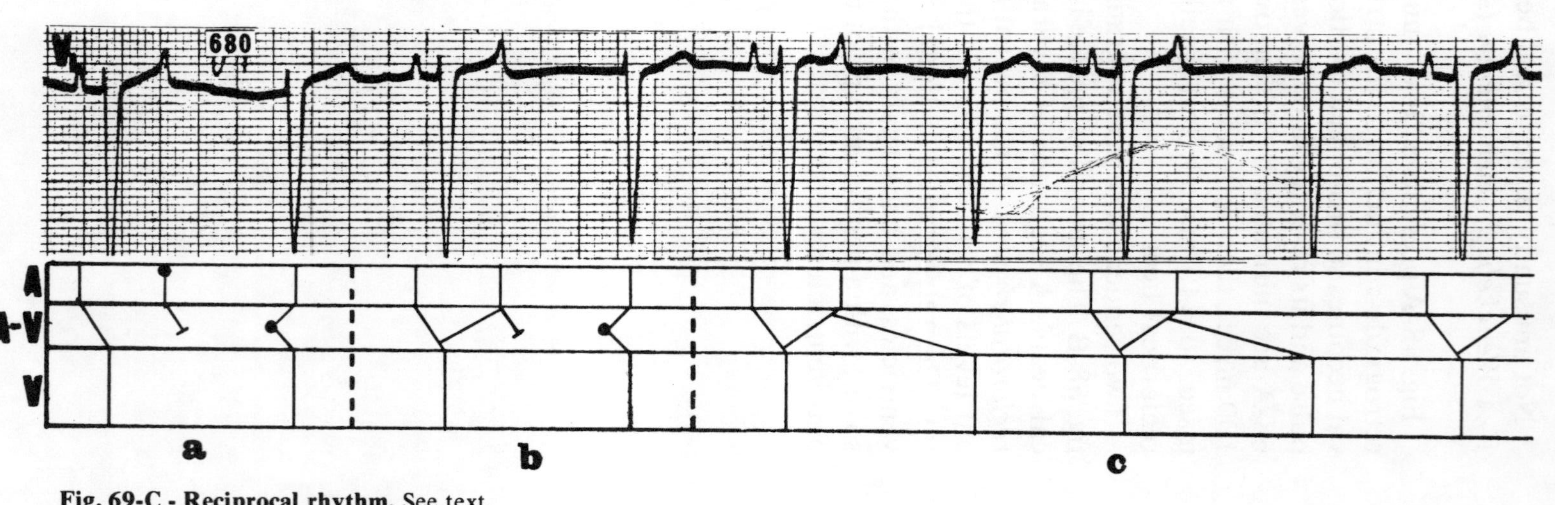

Fig. 69-C - **Reciprocal rhythm.** See text.

Fig. 69-A presents a *reciprocal bigeminy* with aberrant conduction of the reciprocal beats. An atrial P^1 wave is inscribed between two ventricular complexes. The surface ECG records the following sequence; normal QRS-P^1-aberrant QRS.

Occasionally, the impulse which initiates a reciprocal sequence originates from the S-A node and, while traveling to the ventricles, it reflects and returns to the atria. If the R-P^1 interval is long enough, the impulse can again reach the ventricles and originate a so-called *inverse reciprocal beat*. The resulting rhythm will be called *inverse reciprocal rhythm*.

In fig. 69-B, a sinus beat is followed by a reflected P^1 wave and by an aberrant QRS which terminates a reciprocal sequence. The following asystolic pause is followed by a junctional beat with retrograde conduction to the atria. This impulse does not induce a "ventricular echo beat", probably because the R-P^1 interval (210 msec.) is not long enough to determine the reciprocity. An *inverse reciprocal sequence* is again present at the end of the tracing.

Fig. 69-C presents a complex rhythm which may have three different and all valid explanations:
a) sinus rhythm interrupted by a blocked atrial extrasystole which is followed by a junctional escape beat;
b) sinus rhythm followed by an inverse reciprocal beat, which is blocked during its reflected descent, and which is followed by a junctional escape beat;
c) sinus rhythm and an inverse reciprocal rhythm with marked prolongation of the P^1-R interval of the reflected beat to the ventricles.

Since the phenomenon shows a regularity and a persistence of the same P^1-R interval (680 msec.), the third explanation is the most acceptable. Therefore, the sequence of the inverse reciprocal rhythm would be the following: P-QRS-P^1-QRS.

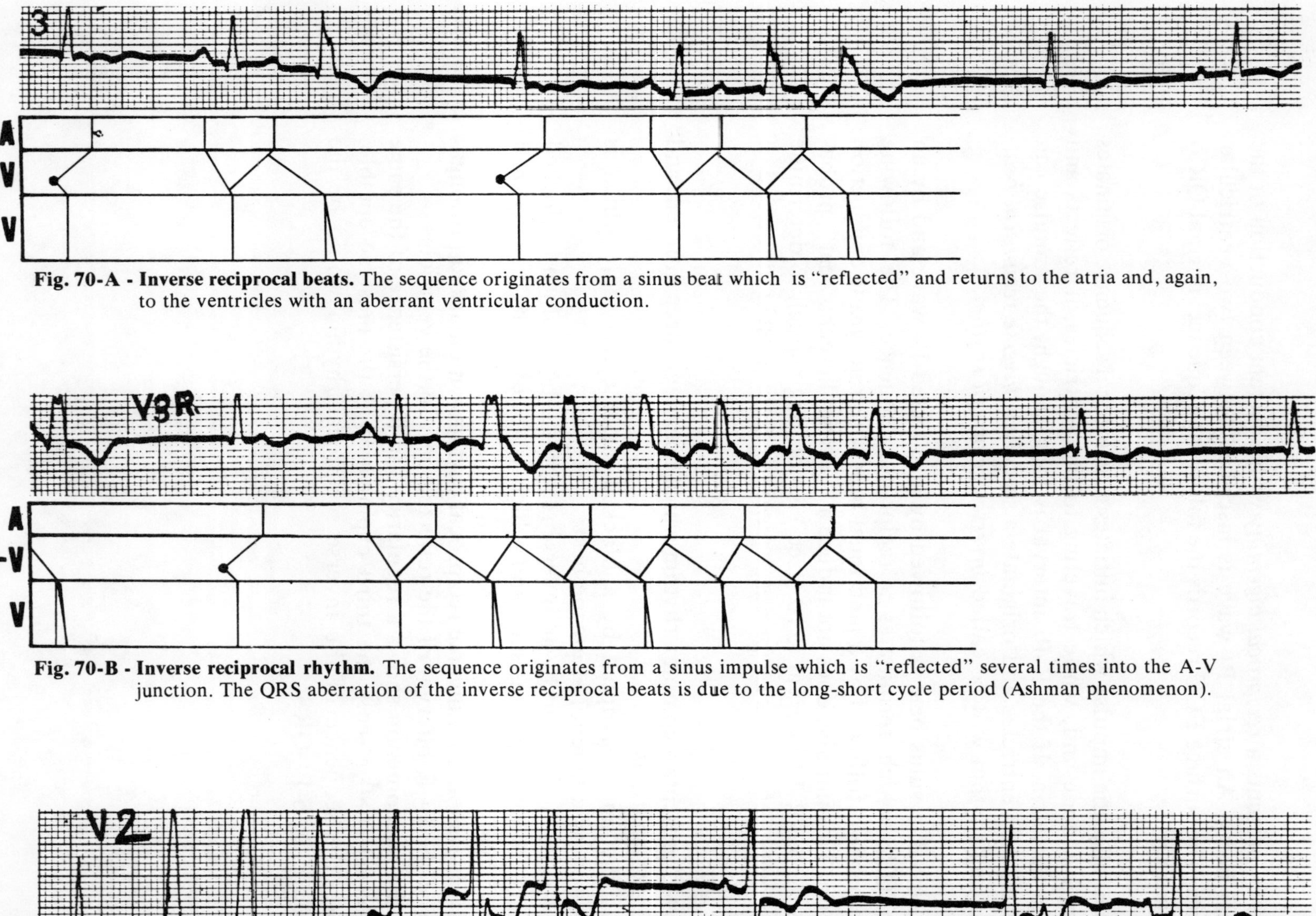

Fig. 70-A - **Inverse reciprocal beats.** The sequence originates from a sinus beat which is "reflected" and returns to the atria and, again, to the ventricles with an aberrant ventricular conduction.

Fig. 70-B - **Inverse reciprocal rhythm.** The sequence originates from a sinus impulse which is "reflected" several times into the A-V junction. The QRS aberration of the inverse reciprocal beats is due to the long-short cycle period (Ashman phenomenon).

Fig. 70-C - **Inverse reciprocal rhythm.** Another interesting example of junctional gymnastic with ventricular aberration in "diminuendo".

RECIPROCAL BEATS

Other examples of *inverse reciprocal rhythms* are presented in the next three figures. In fig. 70-A junctional beats, with retrograde activation of the atria, are followed by a sinus beat, a P^1 wave and a reciprocal aberrant QRS. Later in the tracing, another inverse reciprocal sequence, with two aberrant QRS's, can be observed.

A paroxysm of an *inverse reciprocal rhythm* is presented in fig. 70-B. The atrial re-entry of the first inverse reciprocal impulse originates an interesting sequence of junctional gymnastic. This is made by a reciprocal beat which is directed first to the atria, and then again to the ventricle with aberrant conduction. The ventricular aberration of the first QRS which follows the sinus beat of the reciprocal sequence is at a maximum, and progressively decreases in the following beats. This sequence may simulate a ventricular tachycardia.

A similar sequence is presented in fig. 70-C. Once again, the first QRS following the sinus beat is clearly aberrant, while the following QRS's gradually approach a normal morphology. The explanation of the ventricular aberration in "diminuendo" must be searched in the so-called *Ashman phenomenon* (see page 187) which may operate also during reciprocal rhythms. Note that the first of the inverse reciprocal beats always closes a short cardiac cycle after a longer one.

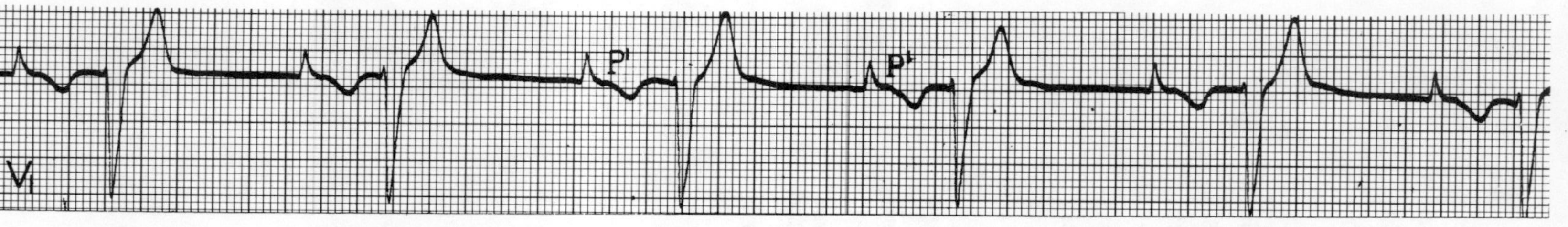

Fig. 71-A - **"Low" junctional rhythm.** The atrial activation is delayed (P') and the ventricular extrasystoles have a fixed coupling interval and a bigeminal pattern.

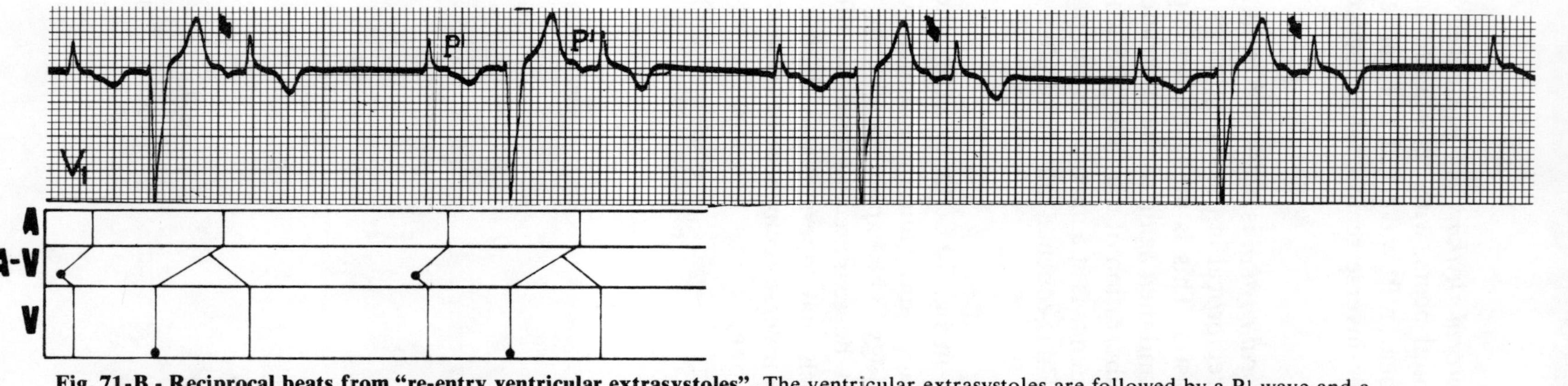

Fig. 71-B - **Reciprocal beats from "re-entry ventricular extrasystoles".** The ventricular extrasystoles are followed by a P' wave and a reciprocal QRS complex.

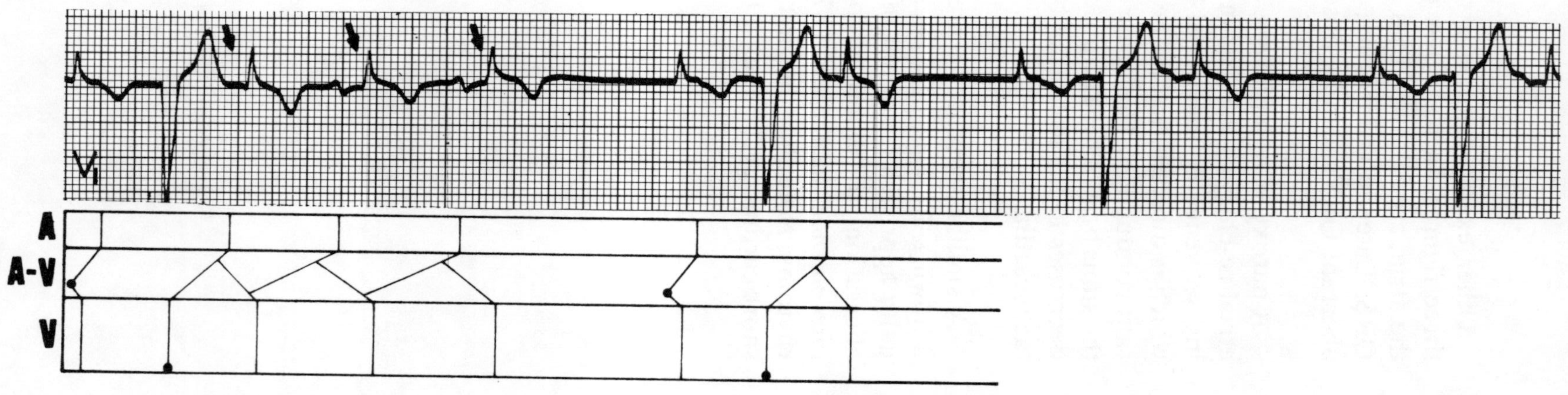

Fig. 71-C - **Reciprocal beats from "re-entry ventricular extrasystoles".** A brief reciprocal rhythm is initiated by a re-entry extrasystole.

RECIPROCAL BEATS

A variant of reciprocal beat may originate from ventricular extrasystoles with a retrograde conduction to the atria. This type of beat is also called *re-entry extrasystole*.

Fig. 71-A presents the tracing of a young patient after a surgical correction of a congenital abnormality (anamalous pulmonary venous drainage). The recording is made in V_1 and the morphology of the QRS complexes suggest the presence of right ventricular hypertrophy. A "low" junctional rhythm is present, with a delayed retrograde activation of the atria (P¹), and each QRS is followed by a ventricular extrasystole with fixed coupling (ventricular bigeminy).

Fig. 71-B is recorded from the same patient and presents new findings; the impulse of the ventricular extrasystole penetrates into the atria (P¹) and, during its retrograde trip, re-enters into the ventricles and originates "echo beats". The *reciprocal beats* are due to impulses which originate in the ventricles and the *reciprocal sequences* are formed by *extrasystole-P¹-reciprocal QRS*.

Naturally, for this to happen it is necessary that the retrograde conduction to the atria is slow enough to allow for the complete repolarization of the A-V junction and of the ventricles. In fact, many cases of interpolated ventricular extrasystoles may be *extrasystoles with ventricular re-entry*. In such a case, what seems to be a sinus beat following the extrasystole, is nothing else than an *"echo beat"*.

Fig. 71-C is again recorded from the same patient and shows a reciprocal rhythm with re-entry extrasystoles as the basic rhythm. However, the first sequence is followed by two beats with negative P¹ waves and with P¹-R intervals of 190 msec. Therefore, the rhythm is a brief *reciprocal rhythm* initiated by a ventricular extrasystole and lasting for three beats. This rhythm is caused by the reflection of the impulses which re-enter sequentially to the atria and ventricles.

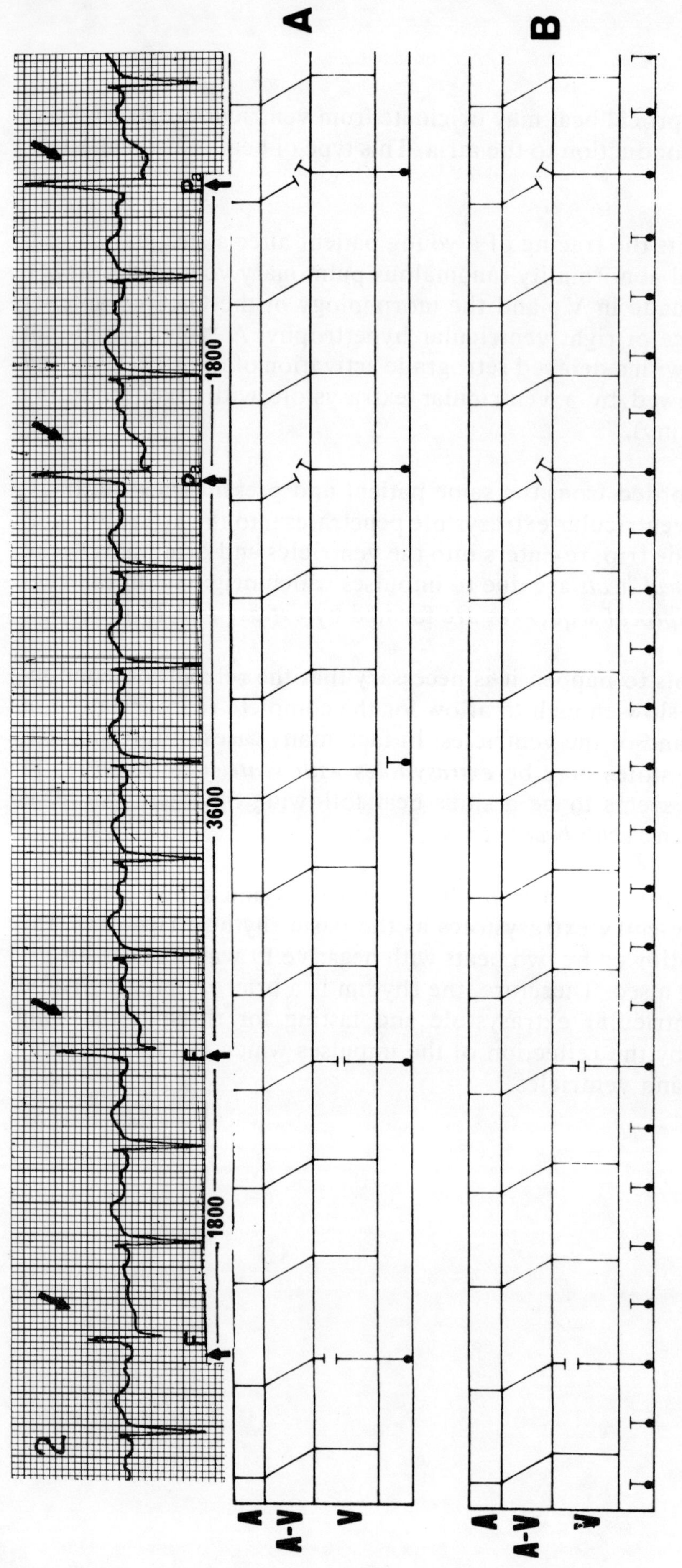

Fig. 72.-A - Ventricular parasystole. Pa = parasystolic impulses with complete ventricular capture. F = fusion beats between a sinus and a ventricular ectopic impulse. The common denominator interectopic interval is equal to 1800 msec. The firing rate of the parasystolic focus may be the one represented in diagram A (36/min.) or that of a potential ventricular tachycardia (180/min.) with a "5:1 exit block" (as represented in diagram B).

PARASYSTOLE

The *parasystole* is a strange phenomenon of electrical symbiosis for which an ectopic focus, independent and protected, co-exists and competes with a normal sinus pacemaker. In order for the *symbiosis* to exist, it is necessary that one of the two natural pacemakers be immune to the penetration of the other. The parasystolic focus, which operates by the side (from the Greek = para) of the primary cardiac pacemaker, is surrounded by a mechanism of protection which makes it impenetrable to the invasion of sinus impulses. Although it may show slight variations, the regular firing rate of a parasystolic focus is usually superior even to that of the sinus node. The rates most commonly found fluctuate between 34 and 60 impulses per minute. Parasystolic foci may be present in the atria, in the A-V junction and in the ventricles. The parasystole most commonly encountered and most easily recognized is the *ventricular parasystole*.

VENTRICULAR PARASYSTOLE

In the ventricular parasystole a ventricular ectopic focus delivers impulses in a regular and rhythmic fashion, undisturbed by the impulses coming from the sinus node. A classic example of ventricular parasystole is presented in the tracing of fig. 72-A. The cardinal criteria for the recognition of this arrhythmia are:
   a) the ventricular premature beats have a *variable coupling interval* (see page 25).
   b) the shortest *interectopic interval* (interval between two extrasystoles) must be a *common denominator* and, therefore, must divide easily the longer interectopic intervals.
   c) presence of *fusion beats.* These are not essential for the diagnosis but, if present, strongly suggest the presence of a parasystolic focus.

In fig. 72-A, a parasystolic focus with a rate of 36/min., co-exists with sinus impulses with a rate of 100/min. The coupling interval of the extrasystoles is variable, suggesting an independent mechanism. This also indicates that the extrasystoles do not have a cause-effect-relationship with the preceding sinus beats. The mathematic relation of the interectopic intervals is present, with a common denominator of 1800 msec. The longest interectopic interval is twice (3600 msec.) the basic one. This suggests the presence of a protective mechanism or "entrance block" which prevents the interruption of the parasystolic rhythm. Fusion beats (F) are clearly recognized. They are "hybrid" beats and their morphology appear as something in between that of sinus and that of parasystolic beats (Pa).

Therefore, the protective mechanism is the basic element of a parasystole and is called *"entrance block"* or *"protective block"* (diagram A). The nature of this protective mechanism is not clear. The most commonly accepted theory is that there is an area of a unidirectional block within the myocardial tissue surrounding the ectopic focus which enables the exit of impulses from the ectopic focus but not for its penetration by impulses coming from outside. Recently, other researchers have suggested that the parasystolic foci have an automaticity and a rate much faster than the one recorded on the surface ECG. In other words, parasystolic foci would conceal potential ventricular tachycardias. Therefore, the fast depolarization and repolarization of the myocardial tissue surrounding the parasystolic focus would at the same time determine a trench of physiologic refractoriness (entrance block) toward stimuli coming from outside and an *exit block* (see page 191) which results in a low parasystolic rate (30-60/min.). In other words, the automaticity of the parasystolic focus of fig. 72-A could be equal to 180/min., and this would determine the protective mechanism (or entrance block), while a simultaneous exit block of 5:1 would produce a parasystolic rate of 36/min. (diagram B).

The latter theory is interesting because it suggests an electrophysiologic explanation of the entrance block. It also coincides with the almost universally recognized fact that ventricular parasystoles often degenerate into repetitive phenomena, salvos of PVC's, and ventricular tachycardias (see page 83).

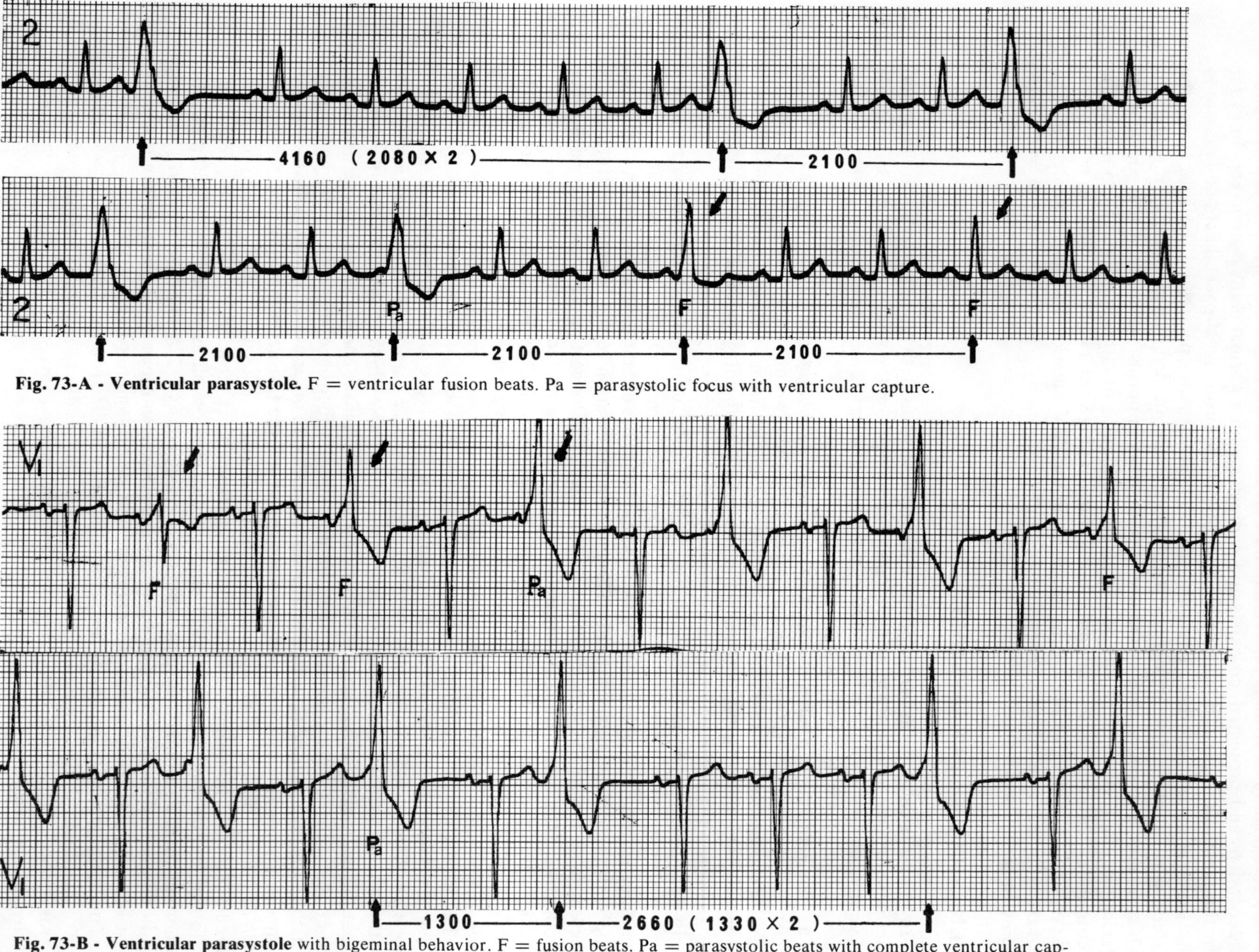

Fig. 73-A - **Ventricular parasystole.** F = ventricular fusion beats. Pa = parasystolic focus with ventricular capture.

Fig. 73-B - **Ventricular parasystole** with bigeminal behavior. F = fusion beats. Pa = parasystolic beats with complete ventricular capture.

VENTRICULAR PARASYSTOLE

Two examples of ventricular parasystole are presented on the opposite page. Fig. 73-A is the continuous recording of a tracing which shows numerous ventricular extrasystoles with variable coupling intervals. When the coupling interval becomes long enough, the extrasystole falling immediately after a sinus P wave presents a QRS complex very similar to that of a sinus beat (last two PVC's of the lower tracing). These beats are *fusion beats* (F) between the parasystolic focus and the sinus node. The *interectopic interval common denominator* is about 2100 msec. and the longest interectopic interval (upper tracing) is twice the basic one. Therefore, all the criteria for the diagnosis of a *ventricular parasystole* are present in this tracing.

Fig. 73-B presents a ventricular parasystole which results in a ventricular bigeminal rhythm. The coupling interval of the premature beats varies markedly and produces different morphologies of the parasystolic QRS's.

Since the impulses of a parasystolic focus are regular, once the basic interectopic interval is localized, one can accurately predict when the next parasystolic impulse should appear on the tracing. The parasystolic impulse may fall at any point of the sinus cycle. Some of them fall within the absolute ventricular refractory phase following a sinus beat. Therefore, they do not depolarize the ventricles and do not appear on the surface ECG. This determines an *interectopic interval multiple of a common denominator*. Other parasystolic impulses may slightly precede the sinus beat and activate only a portion of the ventricular myocardium, while the rest is normally depolarized by the sinus impulse. This determines the appearance of *fusion beats*. The sharing of the ventricular activation may be in favor of one or the other pacemaker, and this will determine several morphological combinations of fusion beats. (Notice the different configuration of the first and second fusion beat of fig. 73-B).

If the parasystolic impulse emerges far enough from the preceding sinus beat and finds the myocardium excitable, the ventricular activation will be entirely controlled by the parasystolic focus. The QRS morphology will be that typical of a ventricular extrasystole. (The parasystolic beats are indicated with Pa.)

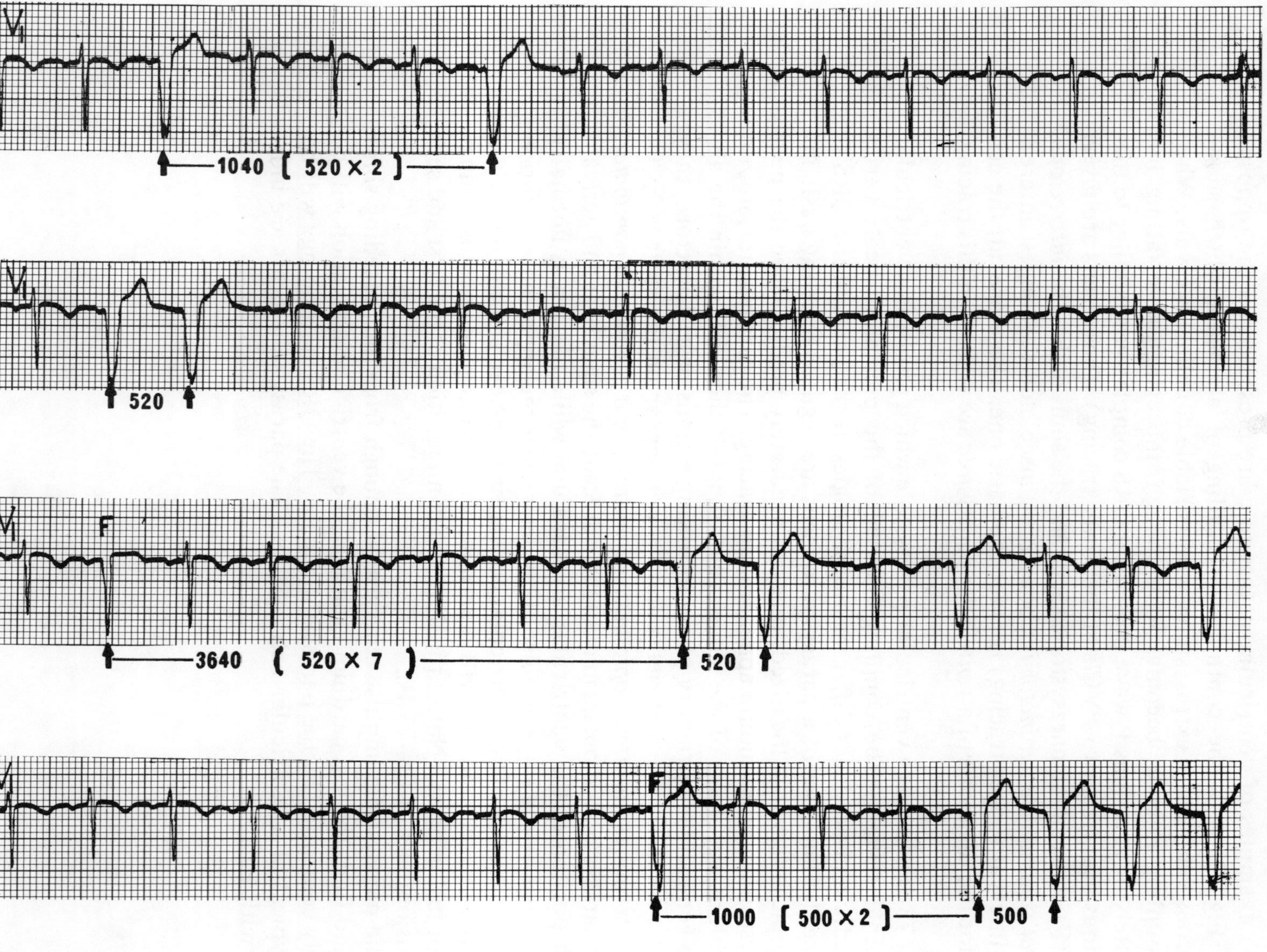

Fig. 74-A - Ventricular parasystole. The parasystolic focus hides a ventricular tachycardia. This is manifested by the repetitive ectopic beats (second and third tracing) and by a salvo of ventricular tachycardia (end of the bottom tracing).

VENTRICULAR PARASYSTOLE

Fig. 74-A illustrates a sinus rhythm counterpointed by numerous ventricular extrasystoles. The coupling interval between the premature beats and the preceding sinus QRS's is variable, and the various interectopic intervals are multiples of a common denominator of 500-520 msec. Fusion beats are recognizable (F) at the beginning of the third and in the last tracing. In two occasions (second and third tracing) the extrasystoles are repetitive and this suggests the presence of an underlying ventricular tachycardia.

The last tracing ends with a series of beats originating from the same ventricular parasystolic focus and in the form of a ventricular tachycardia. The rate of the *parasystolic ventricular tachycardia* indicates the real automaticity of the parasystolic focus (which is equal to 140/min.)

This example shows that a parasystole has a tendency to temporarily suppress the surrounding "exit block" (see page 145) and to compete with the sinus rhythm.

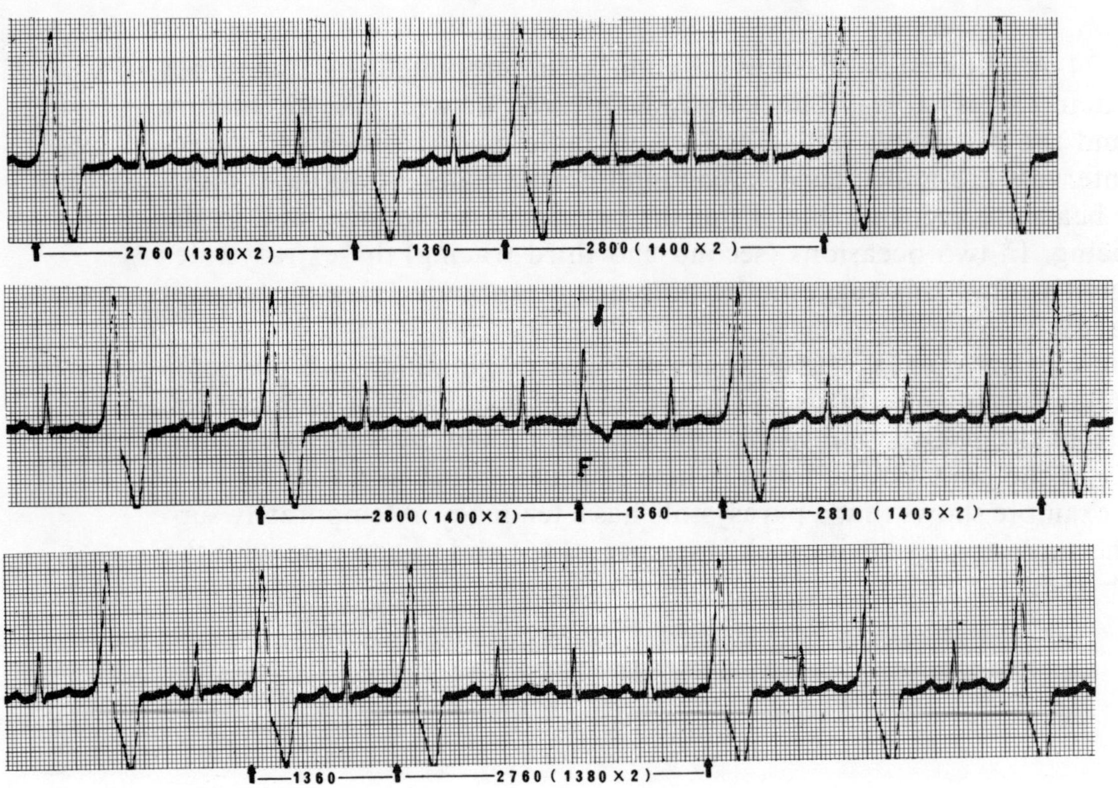

Fig. 75-A - Ventricular parasystole. The ectopic beats show a tendency toward a ventricular bigeminy. The interectopic interval common denominator is between 1360 and 1405 msecs. "F" is a fusion beat.

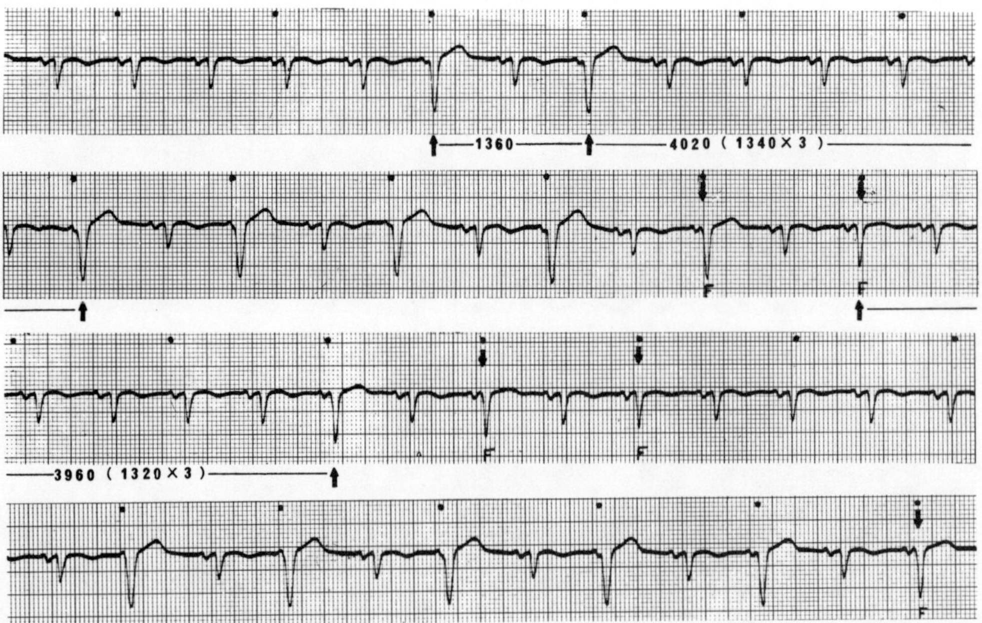

Fig. 75-B - Ventricular parasystole. Dots indicate the firing rate of the parasystolic focus. F = fusion beats.

VENTRICULAR PARASYSTOLE

A ventricular parasystole is a more common finding than is usually believed. It is usually misinterpreted as a common ventricular extrasystole and its recognition is greatly limited by the necessity of obtaining long ECG recordings. Since the advent of the dynamic Holter monitors and of ECG monitoring in the Intensive and Coronary Care Units, it has been possible to observe this type of arrhythmia which once was thought to be a rare finding. Parasystoles, and in particular ventricular parasystole, have become some of the most common, though not the most innocent, of the cardiac arrhythmias noted in long term monitoring of cardiac rhythms.

Two examples of ventricular parasystolic rhythms are presented in fig. 75-A and 75-B. In the case of fig. 75-A, the interectopic interval common denominator fluctuates between 1360-1405 msec.; a fusion beat (F) is present in the middle tracing and the rhythm has a tendency to have a bigeminal behavior.

A similar situation is that of fig. 75-B where numerous fusion beats are present (F) and the interectopic intervals are, at times, multiples of the basic interval of 1320-1360 msec. It must be kept in mind that, in both cases the real parasystolic rate is much faster than what is measured from the interectopic intervals. For example, the actual rate of the parasystolic foci could be twice, or four times, that determined from the surface ECG, and an exit block of 4:1 or 2:1 would determine the parasystolic rate which appears on the surface ECG.

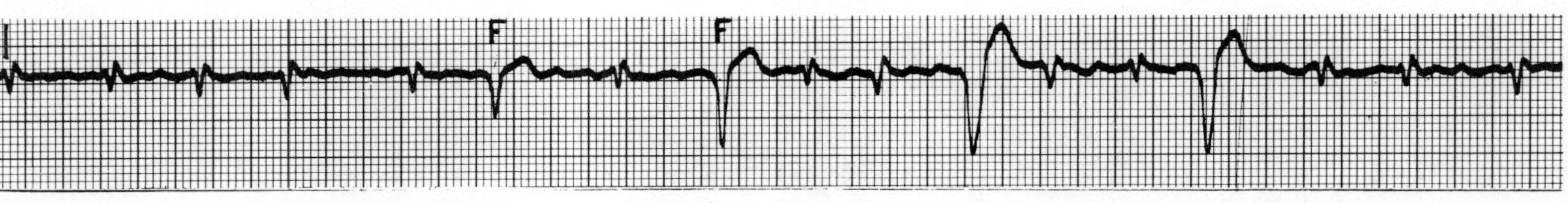

Fig. 76-A - **Ventricular parasystole and atrial fibrillation.** The parasystolic focus emerges among the irregular QRS complexes of an atrial fibrillation. Two fusion beats are present (F).

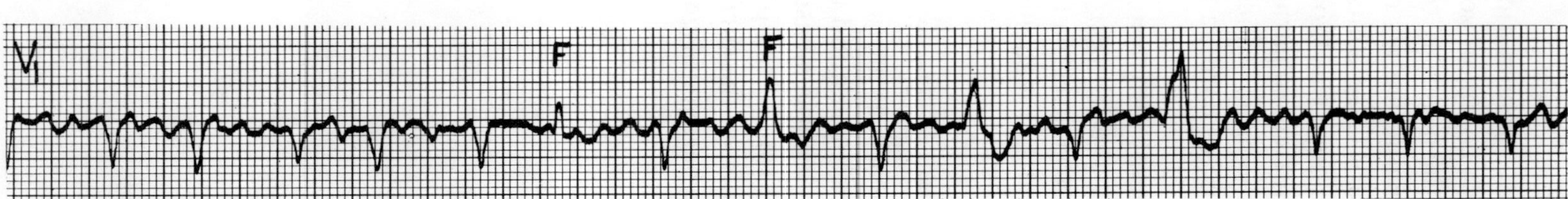

Fig. 76-B - **Ventricular parasystole and atrial fibrillation.** F = fusion beats.

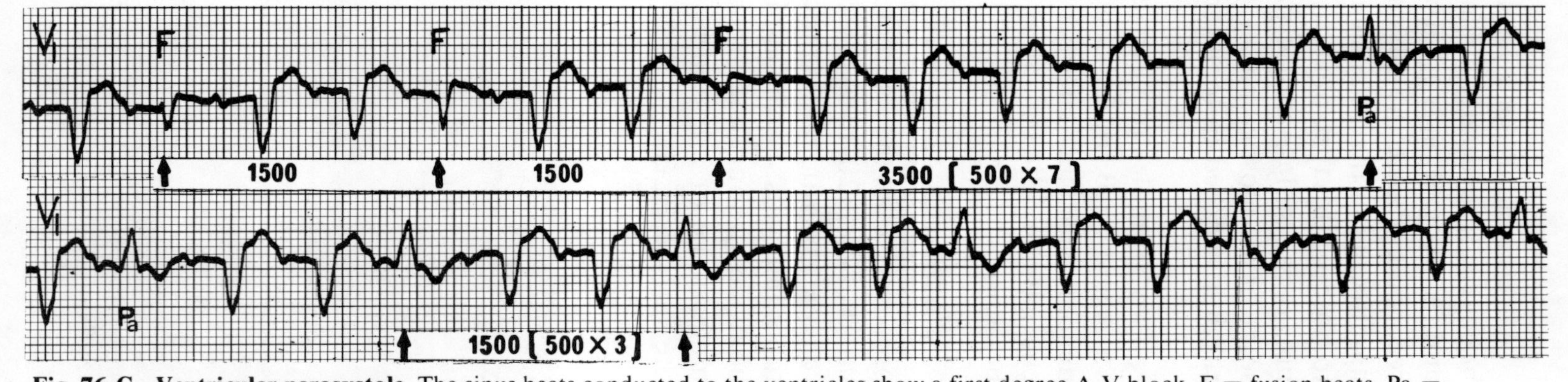

Fig. 76-C - **Ventricular parasystole.** The sinus beats conducted to the ventricles show a first degree A-V block. F = fusion beats. Pa = parasystolic impulses with complete ventricular capture. The common denominator interectopic interval is equal to 1500 msec., but it could also be shorter (for ex. 500 msec.) and associated to a 3:1 block.

VENTRICULAR PARASYSTOLE

Ventricular parasystolic rhythms may manifest themselves within the contest of an atrial fibrillation. Fig. 76-A presents an atrial fibrillation punctuated by four QRS complexes of a clear ventricular origin. (Notice the fine undulation of the baseline and the irregular ventricular response). The interectopic interval is constant and the first two premature beats show a QRS complex with a shorter duration and a morphology in between that of atrial fibrillation and that of ventricular extrasystoles (fusion beats = F). Therefore, the ventricular parasystolic focus is competing for ventricular capture with impulses coming from the atria.

A similar situation is that of fig. 76-B. In this case the atrial fibrillatory waves are coarse and easily recognized; the ventricular ectopic beats have a polarity opposite to that of supraventricular beats. Once again two fusion beats are recognized (F). Within the contest of an atrial fibrillation, fusion beats are not always easily recognized. Because of the irregular ventricular rate, one is never sure when the next supraventricular beat would appear on the tracing (see page 183). Therefore, the recognition of fusion beats relies entirely upon their intermediate morphology, which is in between that of a supraventricular and of a ventricular beat.

A sinus tachycardia, with a first degree A-V block, and a ventricular parasystolic focus are presented in fig. 76-C. The interectopic interval common denominator is equal to 1500 msec. However, note that it may also be equal to 500 msec. and may be associated to an exit block of 3:1 (see page 145). Several fusion beats are present (F) and the QRS complex is gradually widened until it indicates a complete ventricular capture by the parasystolic focus (Pa).

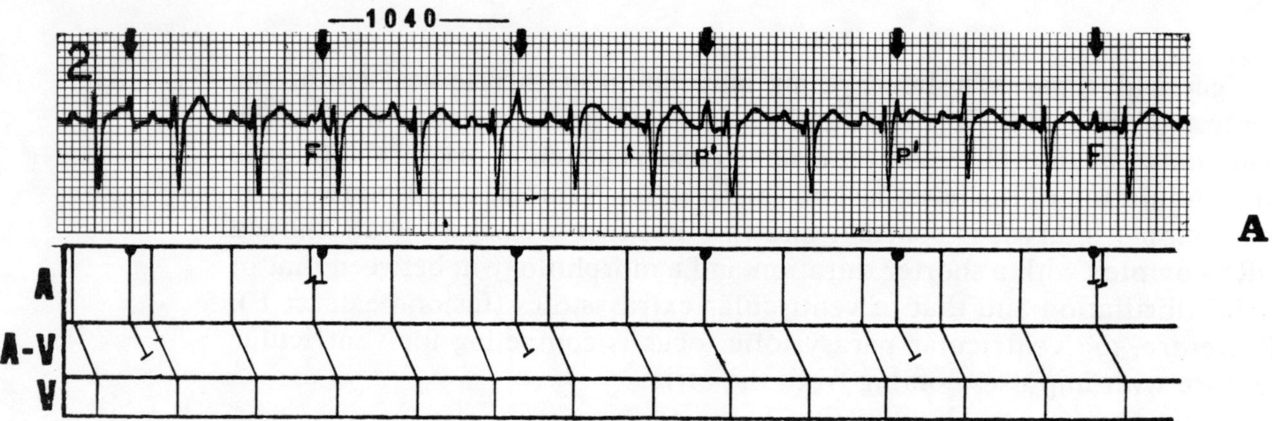

Fig. 77-A - Atrial parasystole. The arrows indicate P¹ waves of the atrial parasystolic focus. The common denominator interectopic interval is 1040 msec. F = atrial fusion beats.

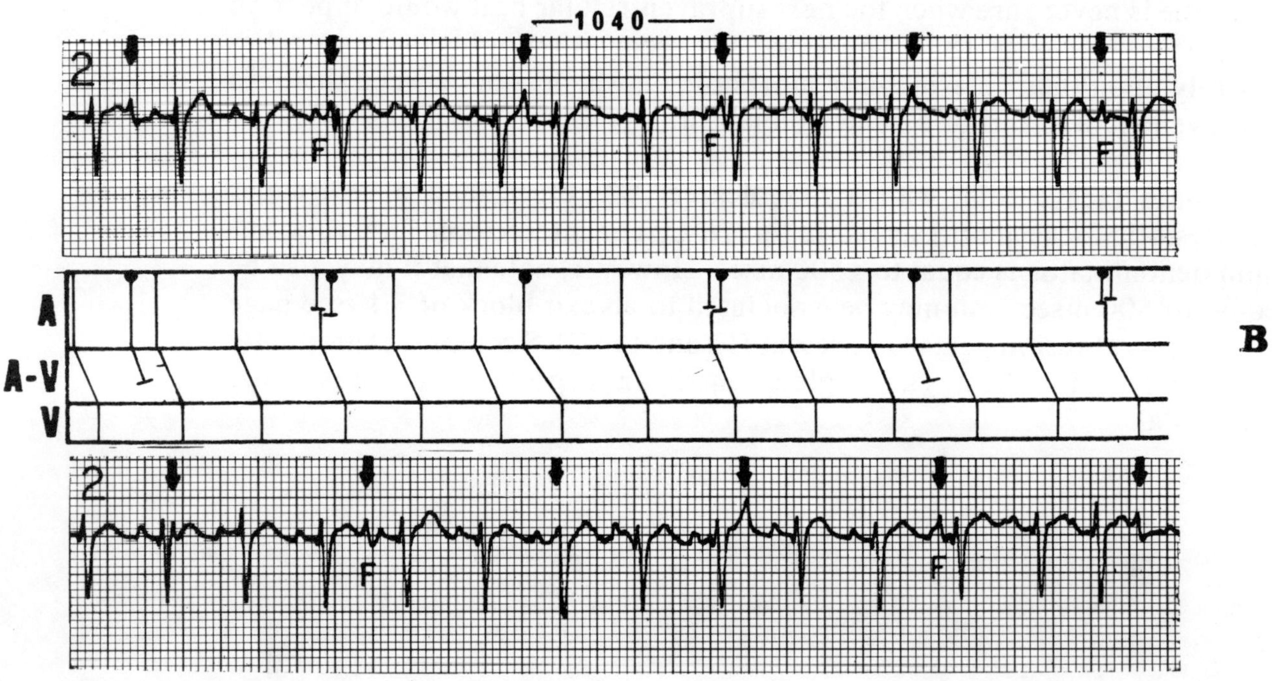

Fig. 77-B - Atrial parasystole (see text).

ATRIAL PARASYSTOLE

Atrial parasystoles are not as common as the ventricular and are not so easily recognized. Usually they are interpreted as atrial extrasystoles or chaotic atrial tachycardias.

All the diagnostic criteria that are valid for a ventricular parasystole are also applicable to an atrial parasystole, and therefore:

a)   the *atrial premature beat must have a variable coupling interval* (variable P^1-P^1 interval);

b)   the *interectopic interval* must be fixed and be a *common denominator* of longer intervals;

c)   *atrial fusion beats* may be present.

Examples of atrial parasystoles are presented in fig. 77-A and 77-B (the tracings are continuous). The sinus rate is 140/min., and the parasystolic rate is 58/min. Some of the parasystolic atrial impulses conduct prematurely to the ventricles and behave just as atrial extrasystoles. Other impulses are blocked because they fall too prematurely and during the repolarization of the A-V junction. Finally, some parasystolic impulses fuse with sinus beats and conduct to the ventricles without disturbing the ventricular rate *(atrial fusion beats)*.

The atrial waves originating from the atrial parasystolic focus are indicated by the arrows (P^1). Atrial fusion beats (F) have an intermediate morphology between that of sinus P waves and P^1 waves from the parasystolic focus. The interectopic interval is equal to 1040 msec.

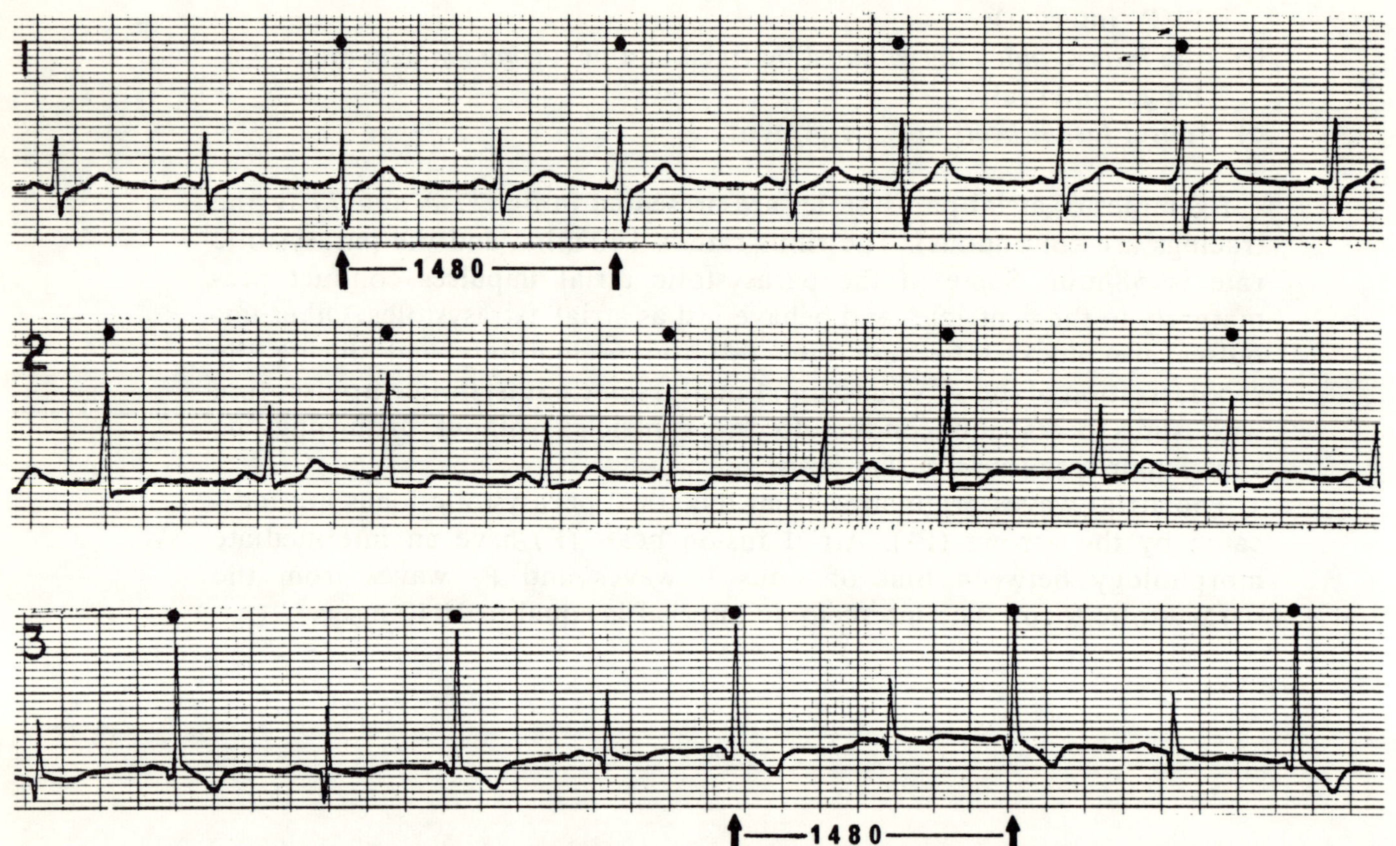

Fig. 78-A - Junctional parasystole. Dots indicate parasystolic beats. The coupling interval with the preceding sinus beat is variable. The interectopic interval is 1480 msec. The parasystolic QRS's are similar to those of sinus beats.

JUNCTIONAL PARASYSTOLE

A *junctional parasystole* may originate anywhere within the A-V junction and above the His bundle. The criteria for the diagnosis of a junctional parasystole are the same used for other type of parasystoles, atrial and ventricular, except for the absence of fusion beats on the surface ECG. Although there is a possibility that a sinus beat originates simultaneously to a junctional ectopic beat, the ventricular depolarization will not be affected; this is because the fusion of the two impulses occurs in that period electrocardiographically silent which is the P-R interval. It must be noted, however, that the junctional parasystolic impulses may be conducted to the ventricles with aberration, simulating the presence of fusion beats of a ventricular parasystole.

Fig. 78-A presents a typical case of a junctional parasystole. Junctional ectopic beats are present (dots). The coupling interval with the sinus beat is variable, while the interectopic interval is fixed (1480 msec.).

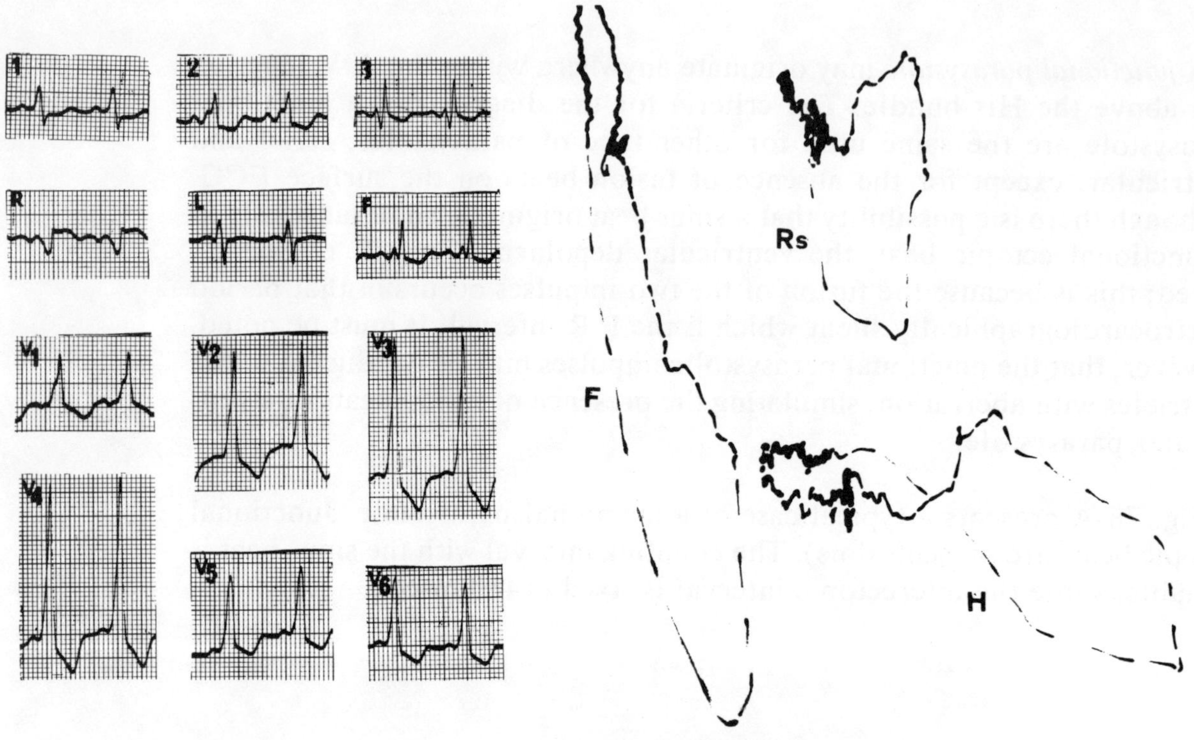

Fig. 79-A - Wolff-Parkinson-White syndrome, type A. ECG and VCG.

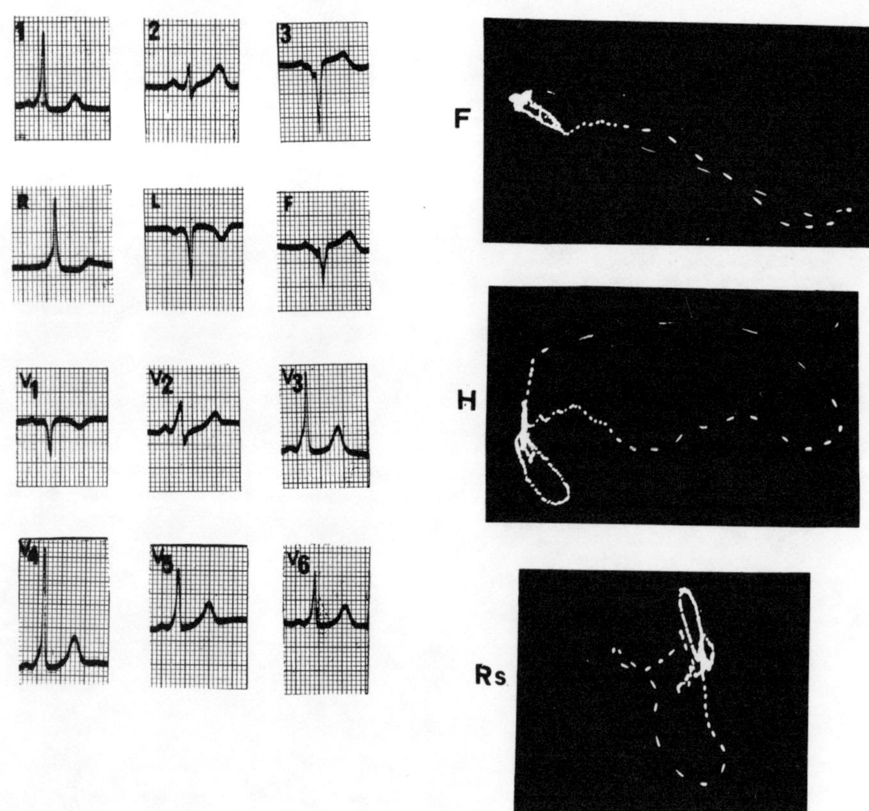

Fig. 79-B - Wolff-Parkinson-White syndrome, type B.

WOLFF-PARKINSON-WHITE SYNDROME (W-P-W)

This is a fascinating, although not very common, electrocardiographic finding. It may be easily confused with a bundle branch block or, when present in a intermittent form, with endiastolic ventricular extrasystoles or intermittent bundle branch blocks.

Patients with electrocardiographic findings of W-P-W have a high incidence of cardiac arrhythmias. Among the most common are paroxysmal supraventricular and ventricular tachycardias. One of the most accepted theories is that a W-P-W syndrome is caused by the congenital presence in the conduction system of specific fibers which bypass the normal A-V conduction pathways and allow for a faster transmission of atrial impulses to the ventricles. Therefore, part of the right or of the left ventricular musculature is prematurely depolarized, while the remaining is activated in a conventional fashion. This explains why this syndrome is also known as *"pre-excitatory syndrome"* and why the presence of the classical *delta waves* is pathognomonic of W-P-W. Delta waves are slowly inscribed at the beginning of the QRS complex, which is altered in such a way as to simulate a bundle branch block. Furthermore, the P-R interval is also shortened in such a way that the abnormal QRS's simulate endiastolic ventricular extrasystoles.

The W-P-W syndrome has been separated electrocardiographically and vectocardiographically in two different types:

TYPE A: the ventricular pre-excitation initiates in the epicardium of the posterior basal area of the left ventricle and it is directed anteriorly. The delta wave vector is directed anteriorly and slightly to the left; the QRS loop is usually inscribed in a counterclockwise fashion. On the surface ECG delta waves appear positive in all the precordial leads (fig. 79-A).

TYPE B: the ventricular pre-excitation initiates in the epicardium of the posterior basal wall of the right ventricle and the impulse propagates from right to left. The delta wave vector appears negative in V1 but is positive in the remaining precordial leads (fig. 79-B).

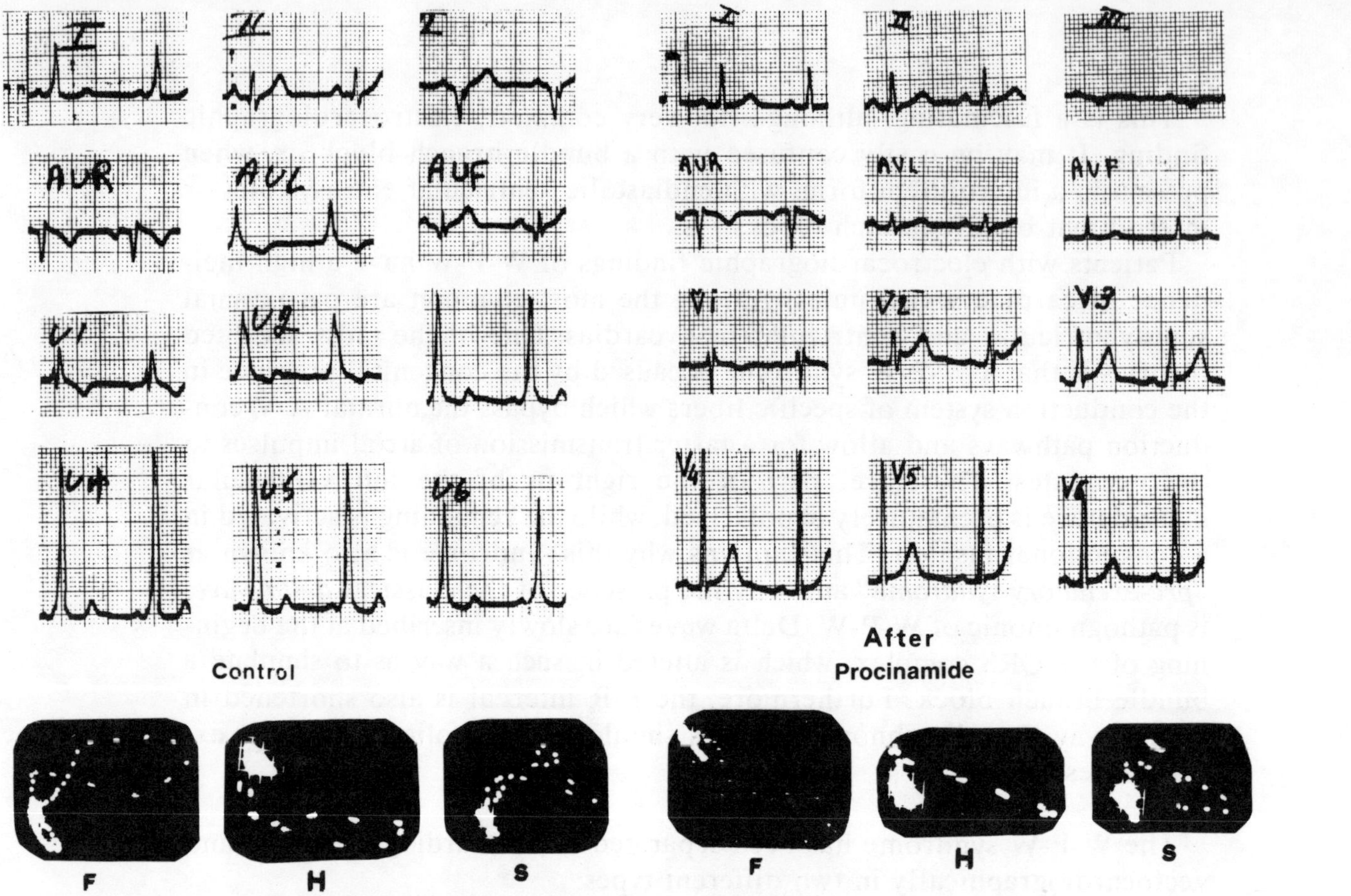

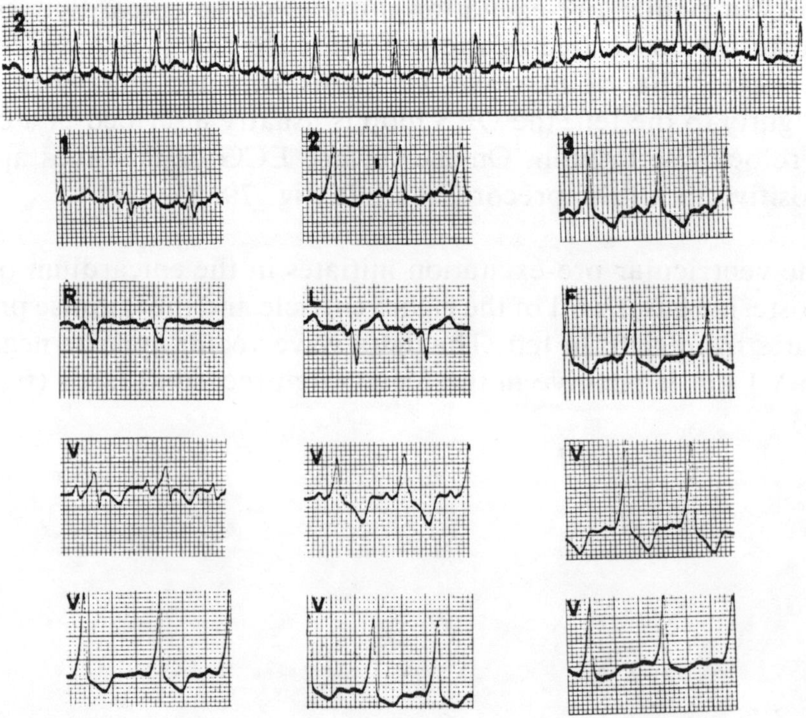

Fig. 80-A - Wolff-Parkinson-White syndrome, before and after IV Pronestyl.

Fig. 80-B - Wolff-Parkinson-White syndrome. Twelve leads ECG recorded at the end of a
paroxysmal atrial tachycardia (upper tracing).

Fig. 80-A presents a patient with a Wolff-Parkinson-White syndrome of type A, before and after the administration of Pronestyl I.V. The drug depresses the conduction of the anomalous bundle and re-establishes a normal A-V conduction. The control tracing clearly shows the *delta waves*. They are directed anteriorly and are positive in V1. The P-R interval is markedly shortened. The vectorcardiogram confirms the diagnosis of a Wolff-Parkinson-White type A. After the administration of Pronestyl I.V., both the A-V conduction and the ventricular activation returns within normal limits. The P-R interval becomes 0.20 seconds and delta waves are no longer present.

The upper tracing of fig. 80-B shows a patient during an episode of paroxysmal supraventricular tachycardia with a rate of 180/min. After the cessation of the arrhythmia, a control 12 leads ECG clearly reveals positive delta waves in L1, and the QRS complexes resemble those of a right bundle branch block. Therefore, the SVT was occuring in a patient with a Wolff-Parkinson-White syndrome type A.

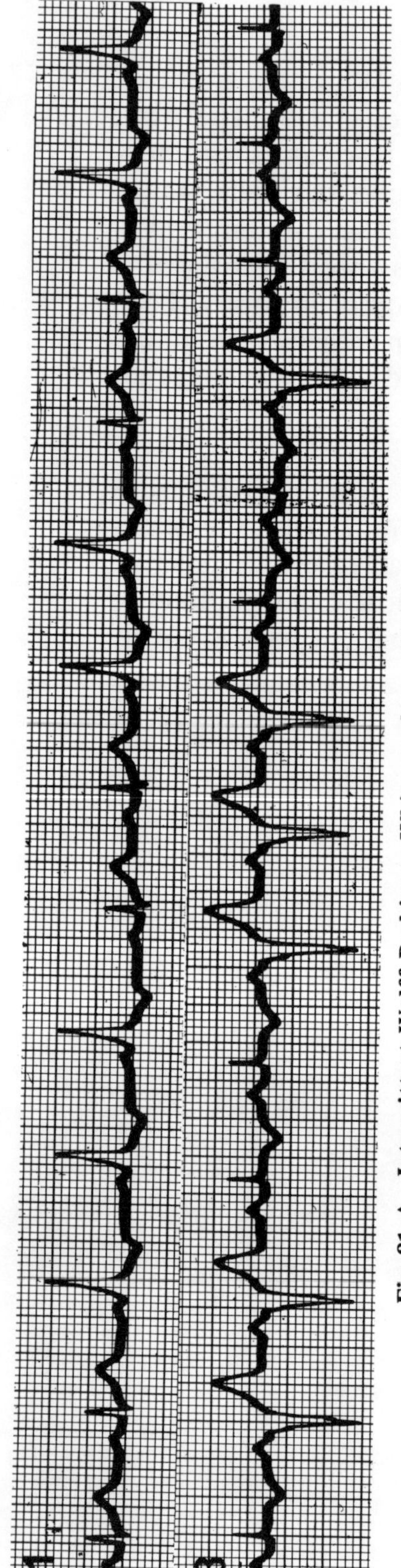

Fig. 81-A - **Intermittent Wolff-Parkinson-White syndrome.** The beats are aberrant for the presence of "delta waves" and simulate ventricular extrasystoles.

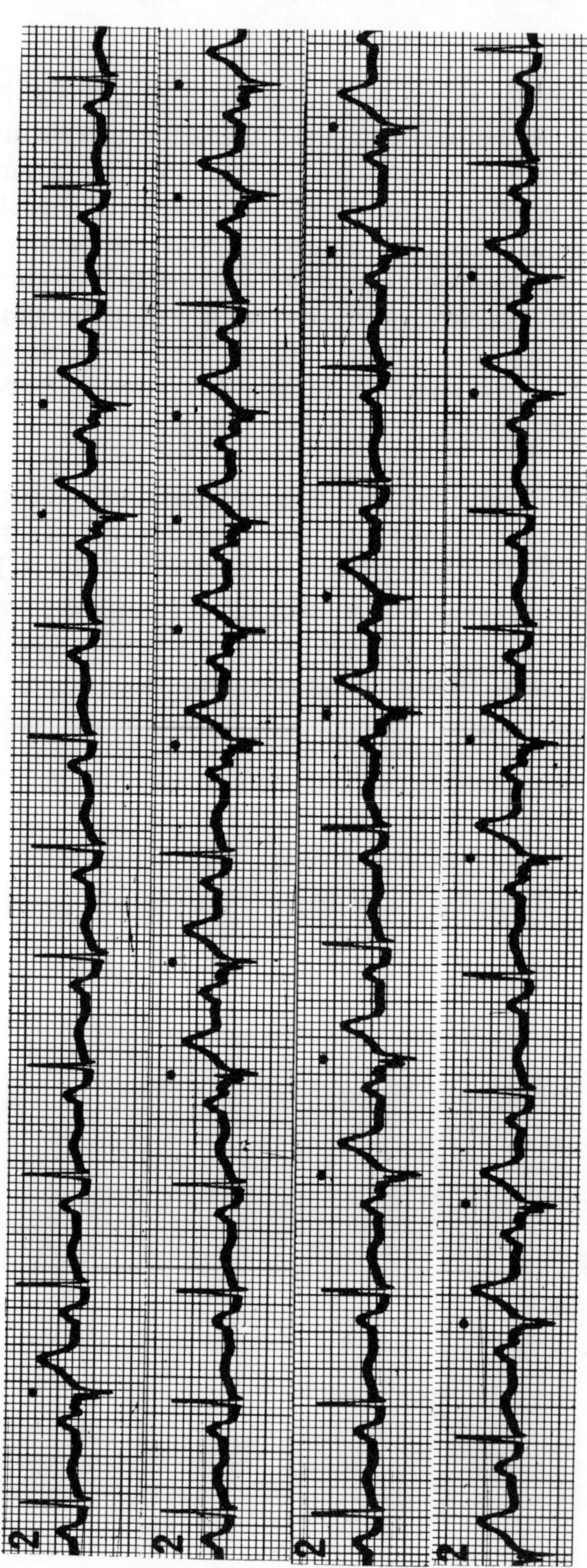

Fig. 81-B - **Intermittent Wolff-Parkinson-White syndrome.** The anomalous beats of the "pre-excitation syndrome" are indicated by dots. The tracing belongs to the same patient of fig. 81-A.

WOLFF-PARKINSON-WHITE SYNDROME

The tracings of fig. 81-A and 81-B are recorded from an airplane pilot who is asymptomatic and who has an otherwise normal heart. Several bizarre and widened QRS complexes punctuate the sinus rhythm of L1 and L2 of fig. 81-A. They are preceded by P waves with P-R intervals of 0.12 sec. and they are separated by a interectopic interval common denominator. Therefore, at a superficial examination of the tracing, the abnormal beats suggest the presence of endiastolic ventricular extrasystoles or of a ventricular parasystolic focus.

Fig. 81-B is a continuous recording of L2 of the same patient. The anomalous beats are indicated by a dot. A careful examination of the three standard leads (fig. 81-A and B) reveals that the longer duration of the QRS complexes and the shortening of the P-R intervals of the anomalous beats, is due to the presence of slow and aberrant initial forces which are typical of a Wolff-Parkinson-White syndrome. This is not an uncommon form of W-P-W, and is the *intermittent type,* and usually offers a great diagnostic challenge to the arrhythmologist. Furthermore, observe that the delta waves and the R-S vectors determine, in L3 of the surface ECG, QRS complexes which falsely suggest the presence of an inferior wall infarction. This error may occur especially when it is not possible to compare abnormal and normal QRS complexes in a same tracing (for ex. with a stable W-P.W. syndrome).

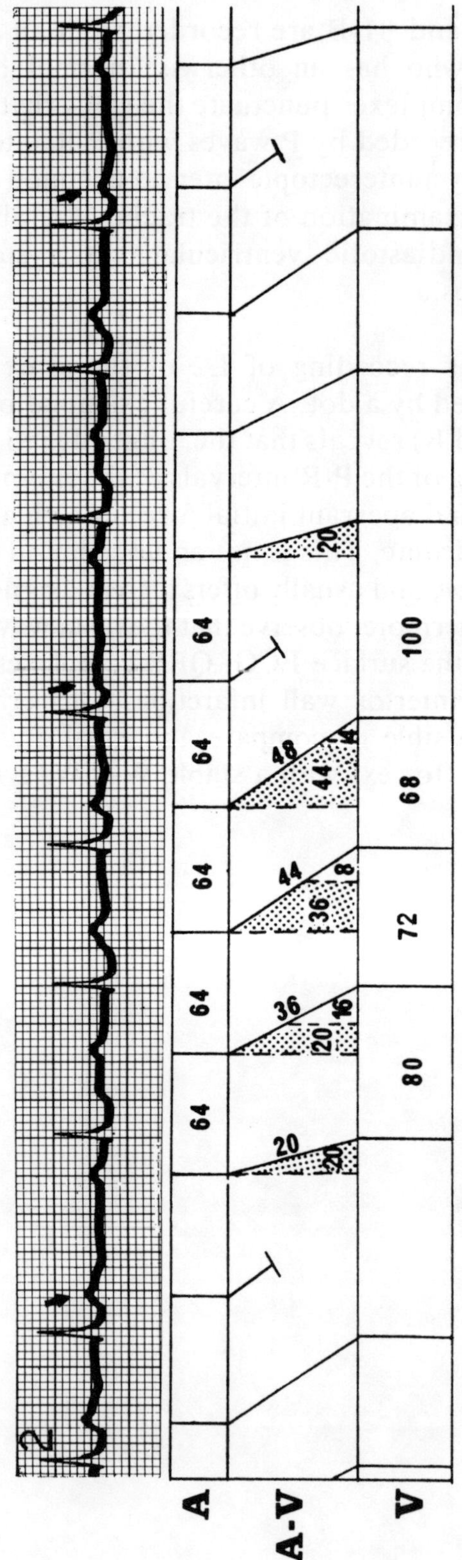

Fig. 82-A - A-V Wenckebach phenomenon. At least two entire sequences are recorded (a 5:4 Wenckebach period followed by a 4: Wenckebach). The blocked P waves are indicated by the arrows. Notice that the maximal prolongation of the P-R interval is always present on the second beat of the sequence. The following P-R increments are always of a smaller degree (16-8-4). This determines a progressive shortening of the R-R intervals (90-72-68), until a pause induced by the blocked P wave, is reached.

THE WENCKEBACH PHENOMENON

A-V WENCKEBACH

The A-V Wenckebach is recognized on a surface ECG by the presence of progressively longer P-R intervals until a P wave is blocked in the A-V junction. The beat following the non-conducted P wave has the shortest P-R interval of the sequence. The P-R interval may start to lengthen again and the sequence is repeated. The entire sequence is also known as a *Wenckebach period.*

Fig. 82-A presents a typical case of A-V Wenckebach phenomenon and enables one to observe at least two entire *periods.* The P-R interval is progressively prolonged from 20 to 48 (the numbers indicate hundredths of a second; ex: 20 = 0.20 sec.) until a P wave is blocked in the A-V junction. The P-R interval of the following beat is again equal to 20 and the sequence repeats itself. The first of the two sequences is a Wenckebach period of 5:4 (of five P waves only four are conducted to the ventricles), while the second is a period of 4:3.

In the classic A-V Wenckebach, the greatest lengthening of the P-R interval occurs between the first and the second beat of the sequence (ex: from 20 to 36); the P-R interval continues to lengthen, but with an always smaller increment with respect to the first P-R (16, 8, 4). This determines a visibly parodoxical effect on the rate of the cardiac chambers distal to the block, and is represented by a *progressive shortening of the R-R intervals* (80, 72, 68). Therefore, the pause, which is determined by the blocked P wave and which includes the shorter P-R interval of the sequence, is always non compensatory.

Hence, the presence of an A-V Wenckebach phenomenon leaves two important prints on the surface ECG tracing:

a) *a progressive lengthening of the P-R interval, which ends in a blocked P wave; the cycle then restarts with the shortest P-R interval;*
b) *a progressive shortening of the R-R interval and, therefore, a progressive acceleration of the ventricular rate, which ends in an asystolic pause.*

The second of these two elements is very important because it allows one to recognize a Wenckebach type of conduction even when P waves are not easily recognizable, or when this phenomenon occurs in areas different than in the A-V junction (see page 176 and 178).

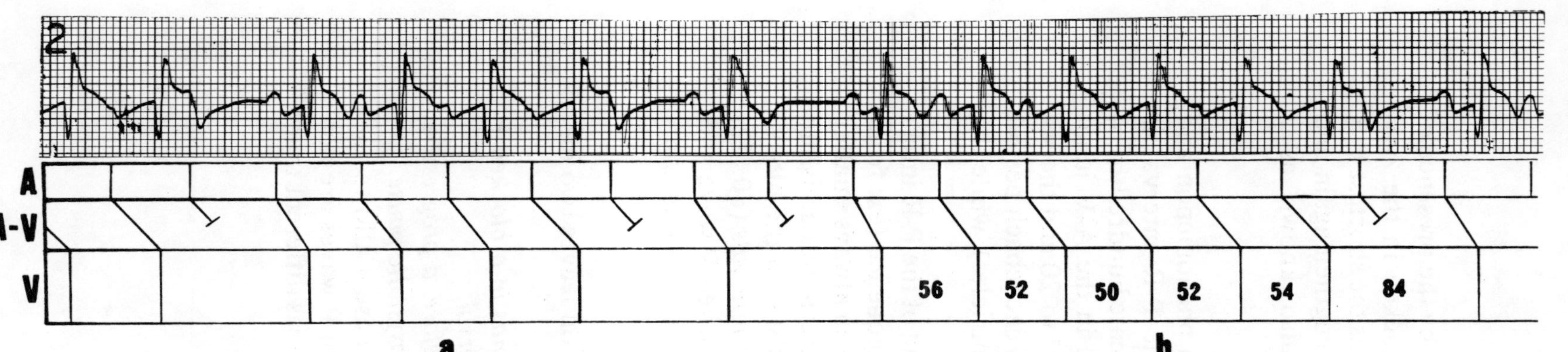

Fig. 83-A - A-V Wenckebach phenomenon. Sequence "a" is a classical 5:4 Wenckebach period. Instead of a progressive shortening, sequence "b" shows a sudden prolongation of the last two R-R intervals. This is called "paradoxycal prolongation" and is due to a lack of regularity of the sinus rate.

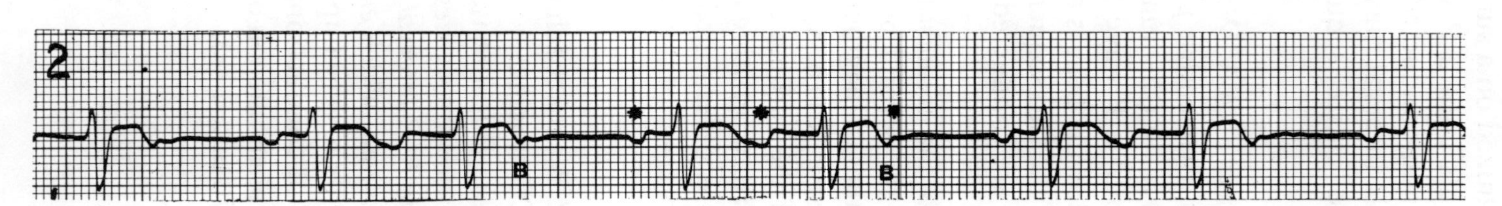

Fig. 83-B - A-V Wenckebach phenomenon. The bigeminal rhythm is due to a 3:2 Wenckebach. The asterisks indicate the sinus P waves. B = blocked P waves.

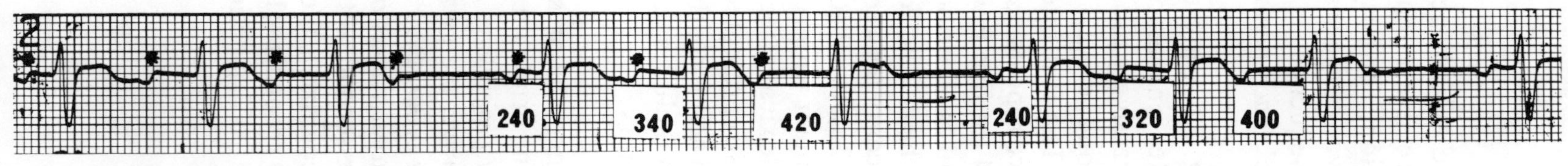

Fig. 83-C - A-V Wenckebach phenomenon. Same patient of fig. 83-B with A-V Wenckebach periods of 4:3 type which determines a ventricular bigeminy.

THE WENCKEBACH PHENOMENON

A-V WENCKEBACH

The typical ECG findings of an A-V Wenckebach phenomenon are not the rule. They may often be altered by a sinus arrhythmia and by a sudden lengthening of the P-R intervals.

Fig. 83-A shows at least two entire A-V Wenckebach periods. The first is a 5:4 period (a); this is followed by a conducted sinus beat and one blocked in the A-V junction. The second (b), however, is a Wenckebach period of 7:6.

It may be observed that the second of the two Wenckebach periods shows a progressive shortening of the first three R-R intervals. However, the last two R-R intervals, immediately preceding the pause, instead of a shortening they present a sudden increase in their length (50-52-54). This phenomenon is called *paradoxical lengthening* of the R-R interval and is due to a sudden and marked increment of the R-R interval *(inverse increment)* caused by a sinus arrhythmia.

Fig. 83-B shows the classic QRS couplets of a bigeminal rhythm. With a careful examination of the tracing P waves may be recognized (*) and they reveal the mechanism of the arrhythmia. The rhythm is sinus with A-V Wenckebach periods of 3:2. Every third P wave is blocked in the A-V junction and determines the QRS couplets.

The same patient is presented again in fig. 83-C. A-V Wenckebach periods of 4:3 determine the QRS triplets and a ventricular trigeminy.

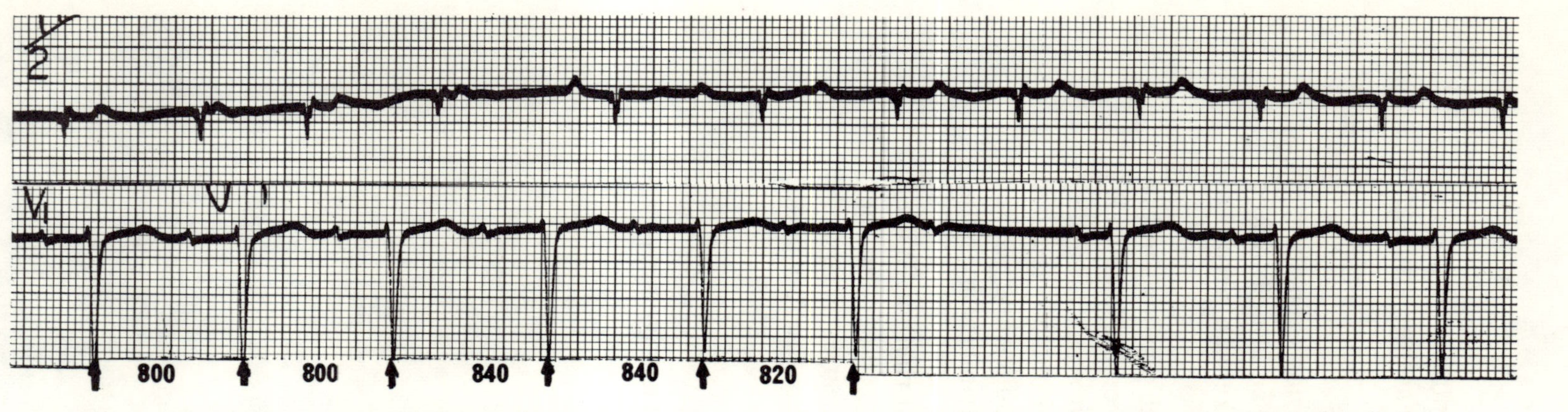

Fig. 84-A - A-V Wenckebach phenomenon. In the bottom tracing, two cycles (840 msec.) show a paroxysmal prolongation of the R-R intervals. This is secondary to a sudden increase of the P-R interval (inverse increment). The R-R interval preceding the blocked P waves is again shortened (820 msec.).

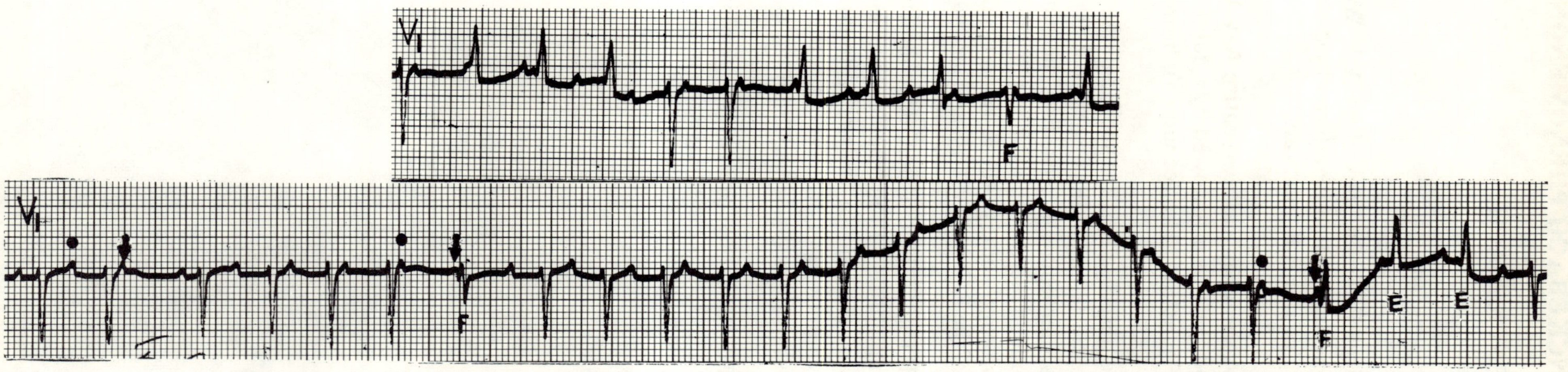

Fig. 84-B - A-V Wenckebach phenomenon. An atrial tachycardia, with long Wenckebach periods (periods of 6:5 and 15:14 are present in the lower tracing), alternate with a ventricular tachycardia (V) when the P-R interval becomes markedly prolonged (P waves indicated by dots). Arrows indicate blocked P waves. F = fusion beats.

THE WENCKEBACH PHENOMENON

A-V WENCKEBACH

Fig. 84-A presents another example of A-V Wenckebach with *paradoxical lengthening* of some of the R-R intervals. The pheonomenon is present in both tracings, but it is better observed in V1. While the P-R interval of the first three beats lengthens gradually and progressively, that of the following beats becomes excessively long (inverse increment) and this determines a lengthening, instead of a gradual shortening, of the R-R interval (from 800 to 840 msec.). The R-R interval preceding the blocked P wave is agan shortened (820 msec.), in relation to a further and gradual increase of the P-R interval.

Fig. 84-B presents two tracings obtained a few seconds apart. The upper tracing may create some confusion in the mind of the interpreter. The T waves seem dissociated from the QRS's, which show at least two different morphologies: one with a positive and one with a negative R wave. The rate of the positive-R wave-beats is 135/min., while that of the negative-R-wave beats is 160/min. Beat "F" has a morphology which is something in between that of the two opposite QRS's. The lower tracing clarifies the mechanism of this complex arrhythmia. It is an *atrial tachycardia with a second degree A-V block Mobitz type I*. At least two entire A-V Wenckebach periods are recognizable, one of 6:5 and the other of 15:14. The Wenckebach periods permit a separation of the QRS complexes of supraventricular origin (those with a faster rate and negative R waves) from the other QRS's. The latter are *ventricular escape beats*, which emerge when the P-R interval is so long as to enable their ventricular escape. Furthermore, fusion beats definitely sanction the presence of two almost simultaneous pacemakers, and localize in the ventricles the origin of the escape beats.

The blocked sinus P waves are indicated with an arrow. The P waves which show a critical lengthening of the P-R interval, allowing for the appearance of the escape beats, are indicated with a dot.

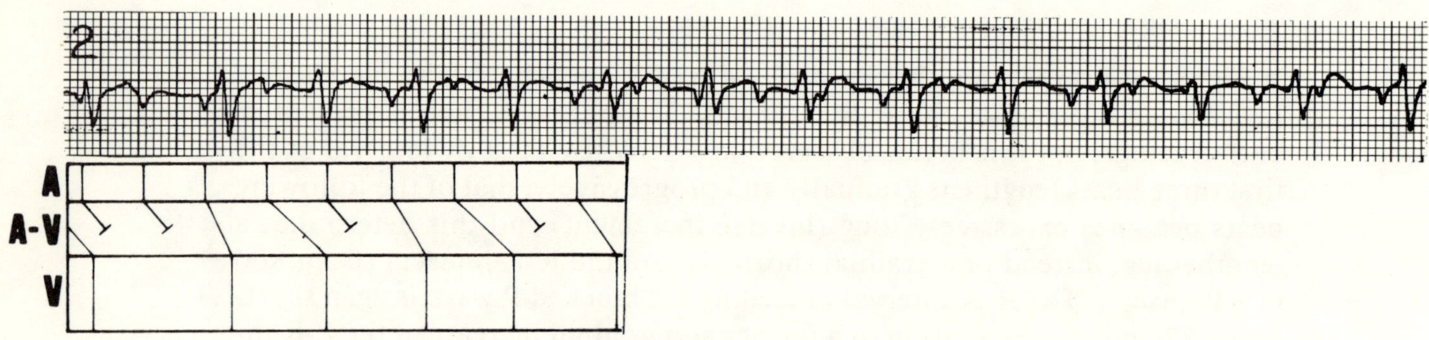

Fig. 85-A - Atrial tachycardia and A-V Wenckebach phenomenon. Every third P¹ wave is blocked in the A-V junction, after a progressive prolongation of the P¹-R interval.

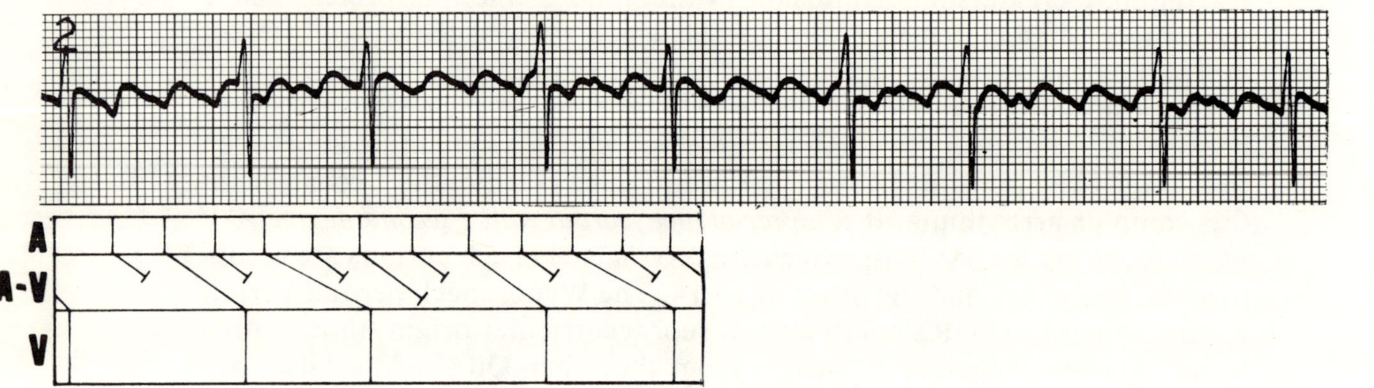

Fig. 85-B - Atrial flutter and A-V Wenckebach phenomenon. The A-V ratio varies between 4:1 and 2:1. A stable 2:1 A-V block is present in the proximal areas of the A-V junction while a Wenckebach mechanism is acting distally.

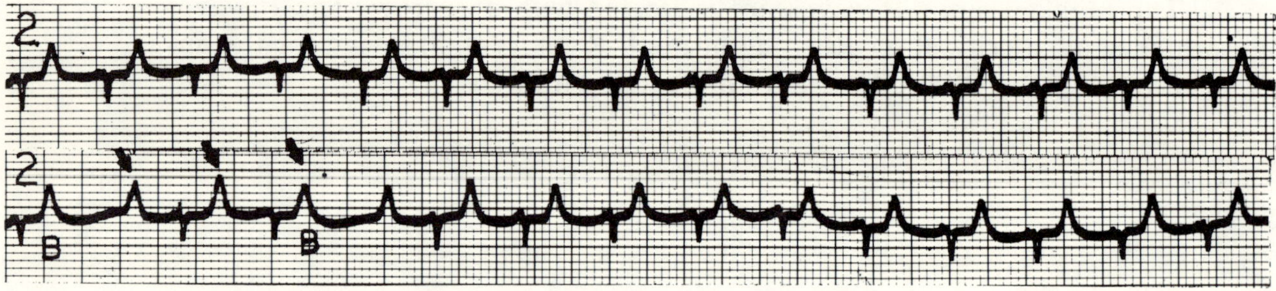

Fig. 85-C - A-V Wenckebach phenomenon. A first degree A-V block (upper tracing) heralds more advanced conduction abnormalities. A second degree A-V block, Mobitz type I, is present in the bottom tracing (Wenckebach periods of 3:2).

THE WENCKEBACH PHENOMENON

A-V WENCKEBACH

An A-V Wenckebach is often present during supraventricular tachycardias and occasionally during junctional or ventricular tachycardias.

Fig. 85-A shows an atrial tachycardia (atrial rate = 200/min.) with a slightly irregular ventricular rate and without a fixed A-V ratio. With a careful examination of the tracing, it appears evident that brief episodes of A-V Wenckebach conduction are present (3:2 periods). The conduction of the atrial impulses to the ventricle is irregular and the *A-V Wenckebach* determines a reduction in the ventricular rate.

A similar situation is that of the atrial flutter in fig. 85-B, in which the A-V ratio changes from 4:1 to 3:1. Again, a Wenckebach mechanism is operating in the distal portions of the A-V junction while, at the same time, a constant 2:1 A-V block is present in the more proximal areas. Every other F wave presents a progressively longer F-R interval, until an F wave is blocked in the distal part of the A-V junction (see page 51).

A sinus tachycardia with a first degree A-V block is presented in the upper tracing of fig. 85-C. Often, a first degree A-V block announces more serious conduction defects. The lower tracing shows a brief *A-V Wenckebach period of 3:2* (arrows). After a blocked P wave, a sinus rhythm reappears, with a slight but progressive lengthening of the P-R intervals.

WENCKEBACH PHENOMENON

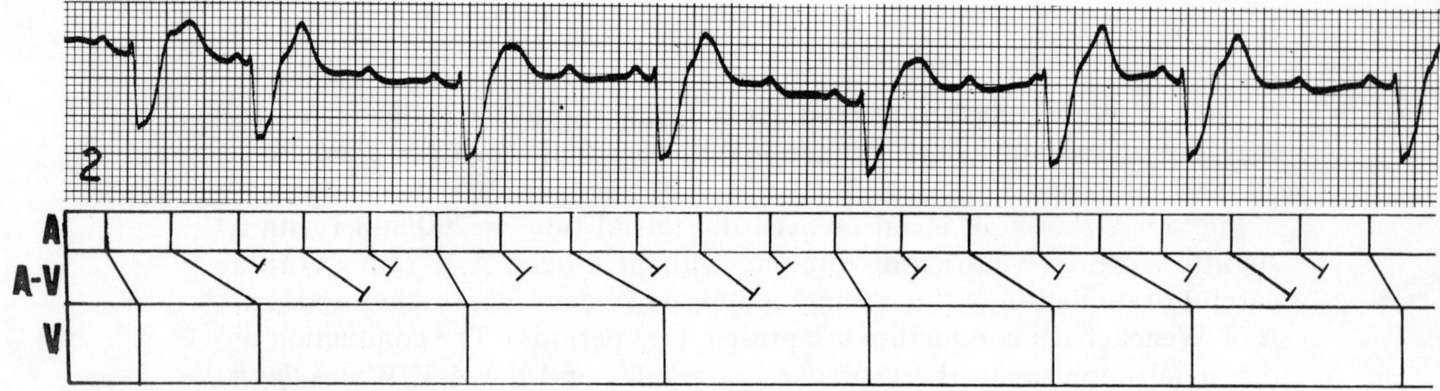

Fig. 86-A - A-V Wenckebach phenomenon. The atrial tachycardia has a constant 2:1 A-V block in the proximal portion of the A-V junction while a Wenckebach mechanism is present in the more distal areas.

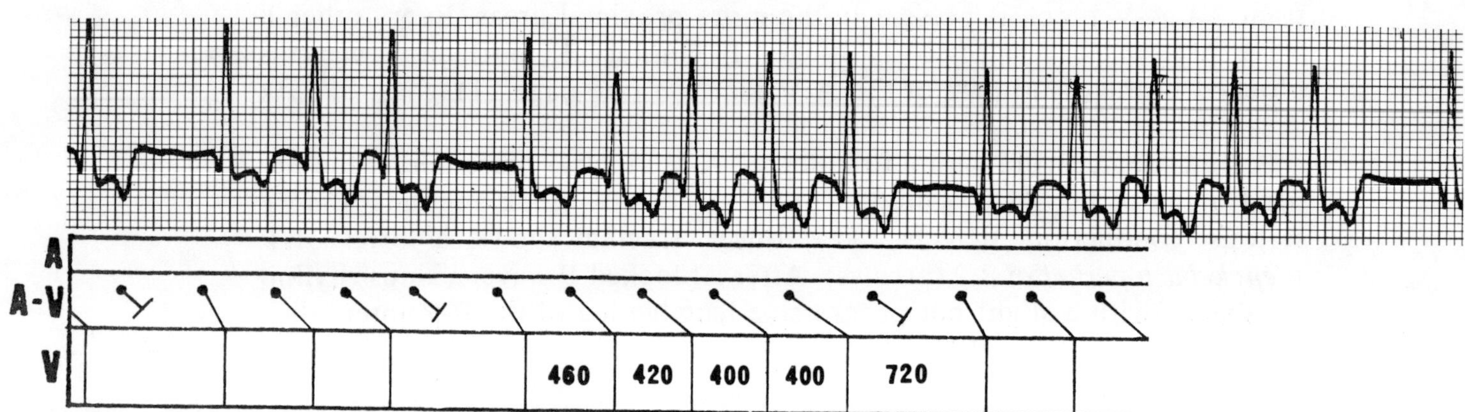

Fig. 86-B - A-V Wenckebach phenomenon. The irregular rhythm is probably due to a junctional tachycardia with an A-V Wenckebach mechanism. The flat baseline suggests a sinus arrest.

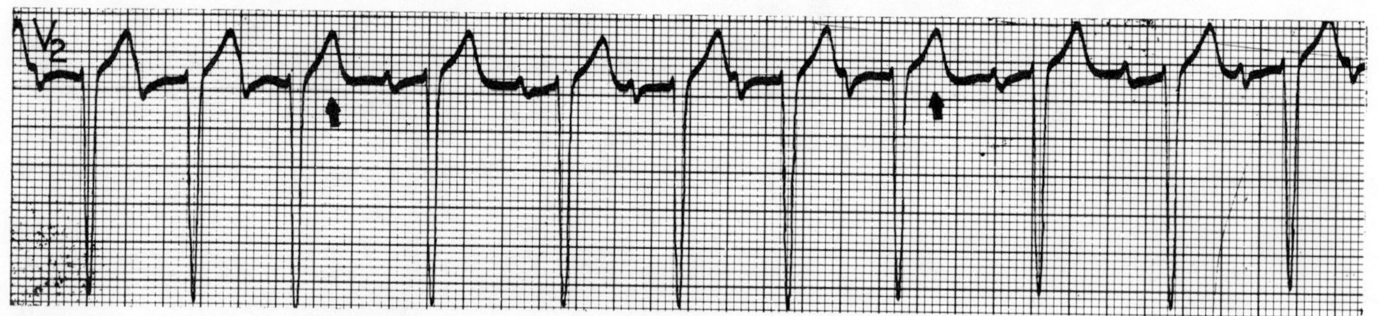

Fig. 86-C - A-V Wenckebach phenomenon. P waves are first gradually absorped and then completely buried in the preceding T waves.

THE WENCKEBACH PHENOMENON

A-V WENCKEBACH

Fig. 86-A shows a slow atrial tachycardia, with impulses conducted to the ventricle in an irregular fashion, and with a left bundle branch block type of aberration. The diagram below illustrates the reason of the irregular transmission of atrial impulses to the ventricles. The tracing starts with two atrial beats which are conducted to the ventricles with a progressive delay and with a lengthening of the P-R interval. Starting from the third atrial wave, an A-V Wenckebach conduction, similar to that of an atrial flutter with a variable A-V ratio, is established (see page 170). Therefore, while an A-V Wenckebach mechanism is present in the lower parts of the A-V junction, a 2:1 A-V block operates in the more proximal areas.

Fig. 86-B shows beats with progressively shorter R-R intervals, separated by longer, but constant, asystolic pauses (720 msec.). The behavior of the R-R intervals, and the presence of asystolic pauses, suggest that an A-V Wenckebach phenomenon is in action. Atrial activity (P waves) is not recognizable. The mechanism of this arrhythmia may have at least two explanations:
a)   sinus arrest and a junctional tachycardia with an A-V Wenckebach.
b)   atrial fibrillation with complete A-V block, escape junctional tachycardia with A-V Wenckebach conduction.

A sinus tachycardia with an A-V Wenckebach is present in fig. 86-C. Notice the gradual absorption of the sinus P wave by the preceding T wave. The blocked P wave is buried in the peak of a T wave (arrow).

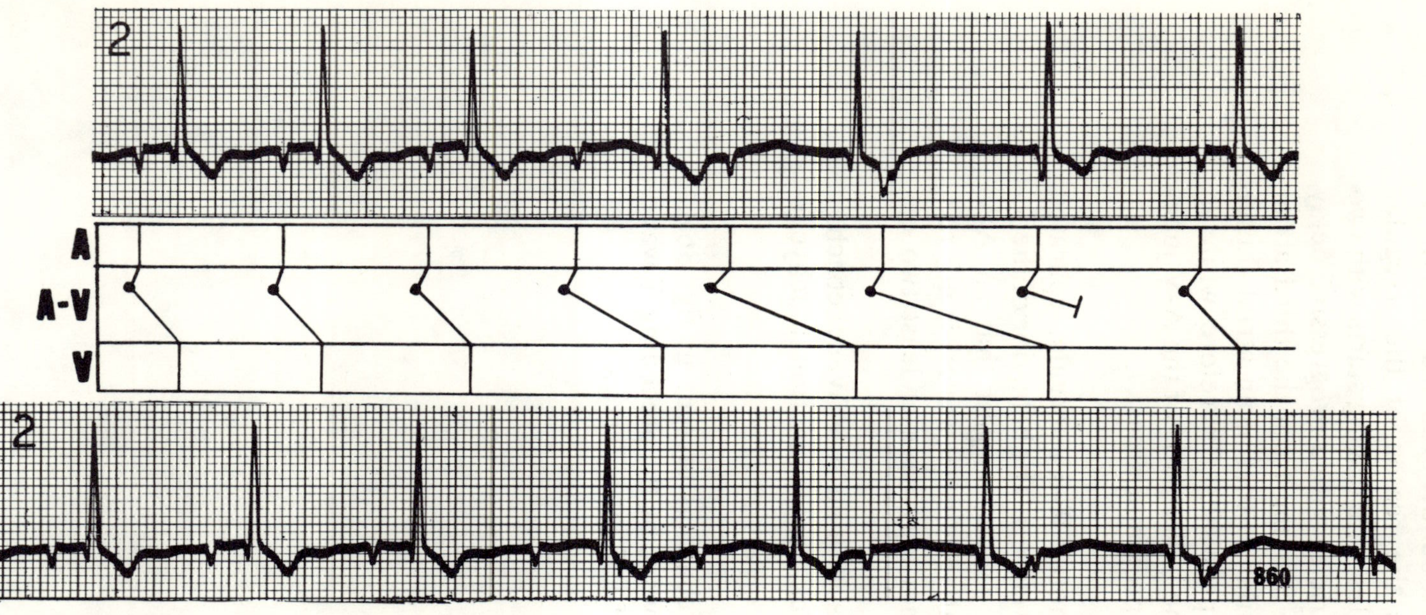

Fig. 87-A - "Infra-junctional" Wenckebach phenomenon. The pacemaker is localized in the A-V junction (or in the coronary sinus), as is indicated by the morphology of the P^1 waves. The blocked P^1 wave is preceded by a progressive prolongation of the P^1-R interval.

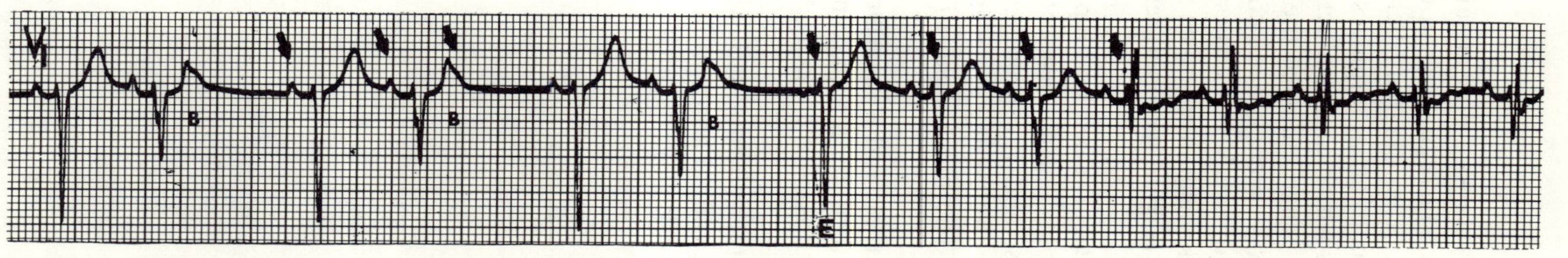

Fig. 87-B - Wenckebach phenomenon of the right bundle. The second QRS complex of the first three couplets shows a conduction delay in the right bundle. A PAC is blocked in the A-V junction. The following escape junctional beat (E) shows a progressive conduction delay in the right bundle until rsR^1 type complexes appear.

WENCKEBACH PHENOMENON

A-V WENCKEBACH

Fig. 87-A shows a particular form of A-V Wenckebach phenomenon during a "high" junctional rhythm (or a coronary sinus rhythm). The retrograde conduction to the atria is constant, while the anterograde conduction to the ventricles becomes progressively slower until an impulse is blocked. This example demonstrates that the P^1-R, or the R-P^1, ratio of a junctional rhythm (or a coronary sinus rhythm) is strictly dependent on the retrograde and anterograde conduction velocity of the impulses, and not on the anatomic location of the pacemaker.

The sequence of this *"infra-junctional Wenckebach"* is repeated in the second tracing of fig. 87-A where, among other things, it may also be noticed that the prolongation of the P^1-R interval of the last beat is of a remarkable degree (860 msec.). Everything happens within the A-V junction; the impulse originates in the A-V junction and there it is delayed during its trip to the ventricles.

Occasionally, a Wenckebach phenomenon has been found in the conduction of the impulses in the right or left bundle. A sinus rhythm is usually present, with a normal or prolonged P-R interval. The QRS complexes are progressively widened and show the characteristics, first of an incomplete and then of a complete left or right bundle branch block. The sequence may repeat itself and, usually, is favored by a slight acceleration of the sinus rate *(critical cardiac rate)* (see page 107).

An example of a *right bundle Wenckebach phenomenon* is presented in fig. 87-B. Three QRS couplets are present at the beginning of the tracing, and the sequence is formed by a sinus beat, followed by one with aberrant ventricular conduction, and by a blocked atrial extrasystole. (P waves are indicated with three arrows.) The third blocked PAC is followed by a junctional escape beat (E) which, however, shows a normal appearing QRS. A sinus rhythm follows, with progressively wider QRS complexes and with a delay in the inscription of terminal forces, until rsR^1 complexes are reached. The second set of arrows indicate QRS complexes which go from a normal morphology into one of a right bundle branch block type. Therefore, this sequence shows a progressive delay in the conduction of the right bundle until a complete block is reached. This type of sequence has been deservingly called *"right bundle Wenchebach phenomenon"* or *"Wenchebach of the right bundle"*.

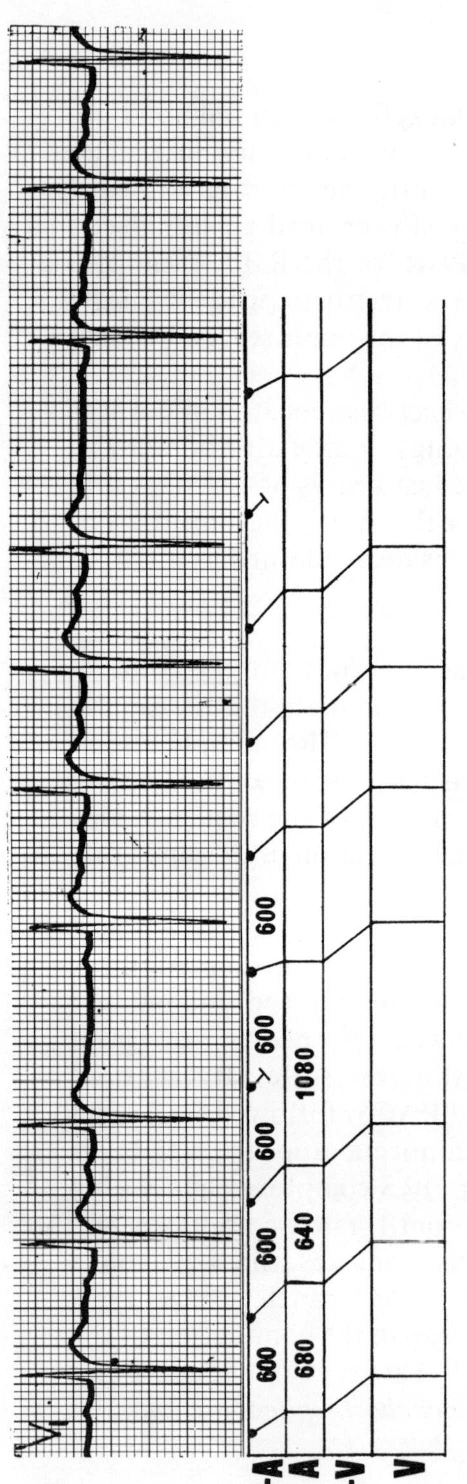

Fig. 88-A - Sino-Atrial (S-A) Wenckebach. The rate of formation of impulses in the sinus node is constant (600 msec.). The conduction in the S-A junction is progressively delayed until the impulse is blocked and does not reach the atria. This determines a progressive shortening of the P-P intervals until a pause is reached. The sequence repeats itself.

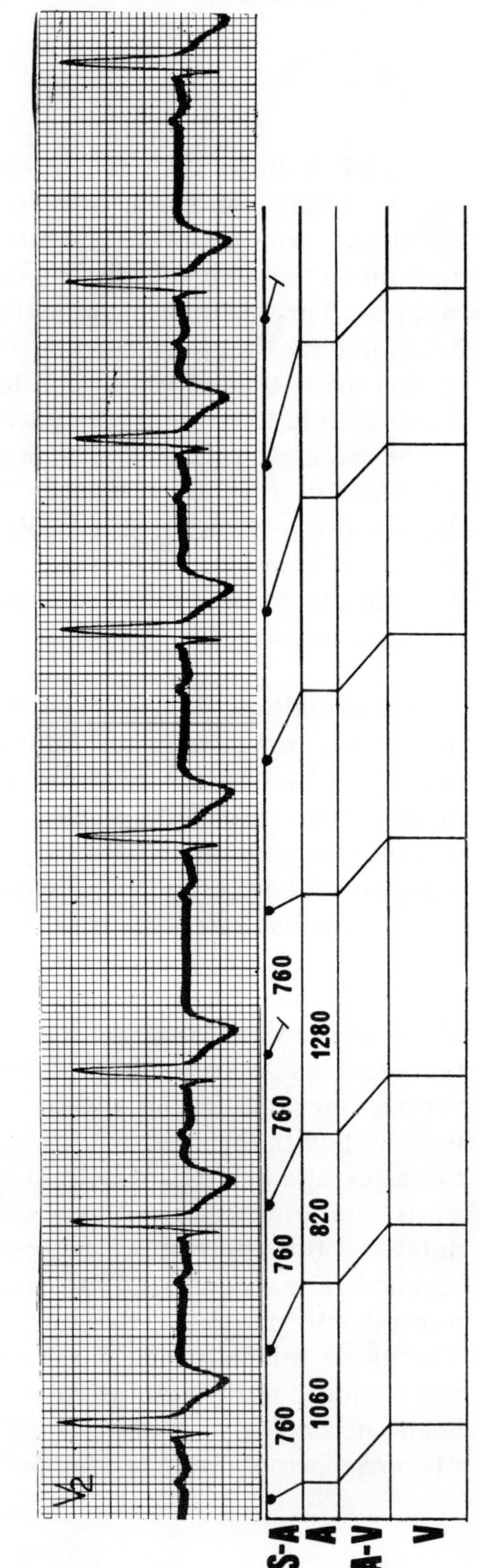

Fig. 88-B - Sino-Atrial (S-A) Wenckebach. The progressive shortening of the P-P intervals is evident; the conduction of the impulse into the atria and ventricles remains constant.

THE WENCKEBACH PHENOMENON

S-A WENCKEBACH

The impulses originating in the S-A node may be conducted with delay to the surrounding atrial tissue. The S-A conduction delay may be progressively longer until an impulse is blocked within the S-A junction. The next impulse is again conducted with a normal velocity and the sequence may repeat itself. This type of S-A conduction disturbance is known as *sino-atrial Wenckebach phenomenon*.

While the A-V conduction of a sinus impulse is represented on the surface ECG by the P-R interval, the conduction within the S-A junction is silent and may only be determined indirectly. It is possible to find a situation in which the P-P interval behaves in the same fashion as the R-R interval of the A-V Wenckebach phenomenon. *The P-P interval may become progressively shorter until a pause is reached*. The cardiac cycle then starts again with progressively shorter P-P intervals until a new pause is reached. (The asystolic pauses will never be equal to two complete cardiac cycles).

An example of S-A Wenckebach is presented in fig. 88-A. The diagram illustrates the sino-atrial and the distal conduction of the impulses. The P-P interval becomes progressively shorter and, after three beats, there is a pause; this is followed by another sequence of four beats, with progressively shorter P-P intervals, and again another pause. While the rate of impulse formation in the S-A node is constant (one impulse every 600 msec.), the impulse conduction between the S-A node and the surrounding atrial tissue shows a Wenckebach phenomenon.

Another example of *S-A Wenckebach* is that of fig. 88-B. Again, the rate of formation of impulses is regular (760 msec.) while the conduction in the S-A junction varies and determines a progressive shortening of the P-P intervals. Once the impulse crosses the S-A junction, the conduction through the atria, the A-V junction, and the ventricles occurs in a normal and constant fashion. Therefore, the asystolic pauses are due to a sinus impulse which does not reach the atria. The following impulse finds the S-A junction totally repolarized and is conducted to the atria with the maximum velocity.

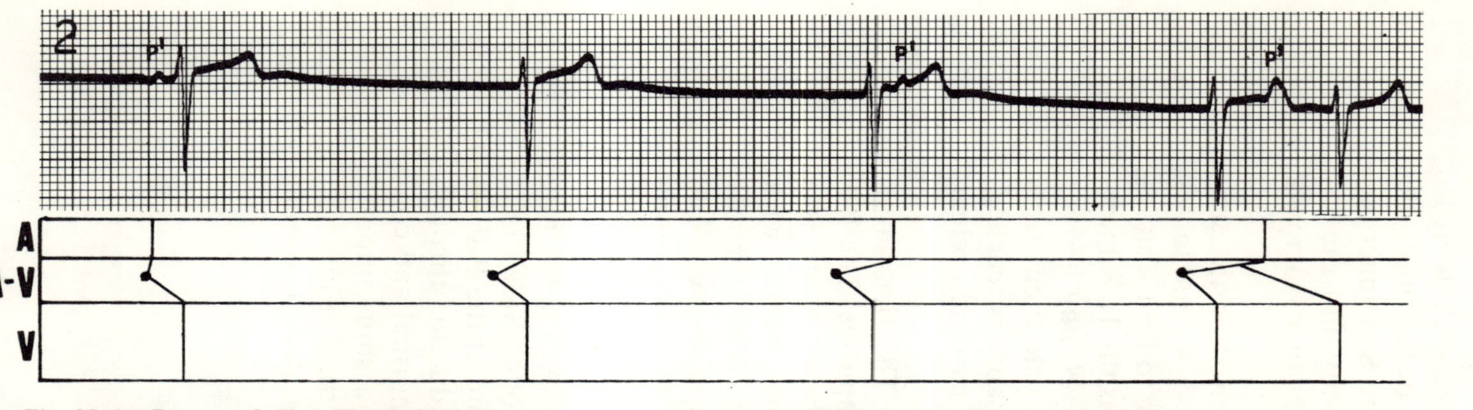

Fig. 89-A - **Retrograde V-A Wenckebach.** P¹ waves first precede and then follow the QRS complexes. The R-P¹ interval of the last beat is so prolonged that it allows for the "reflection" and the re-entry of the impulse into the ventricles (reciprocal beats).

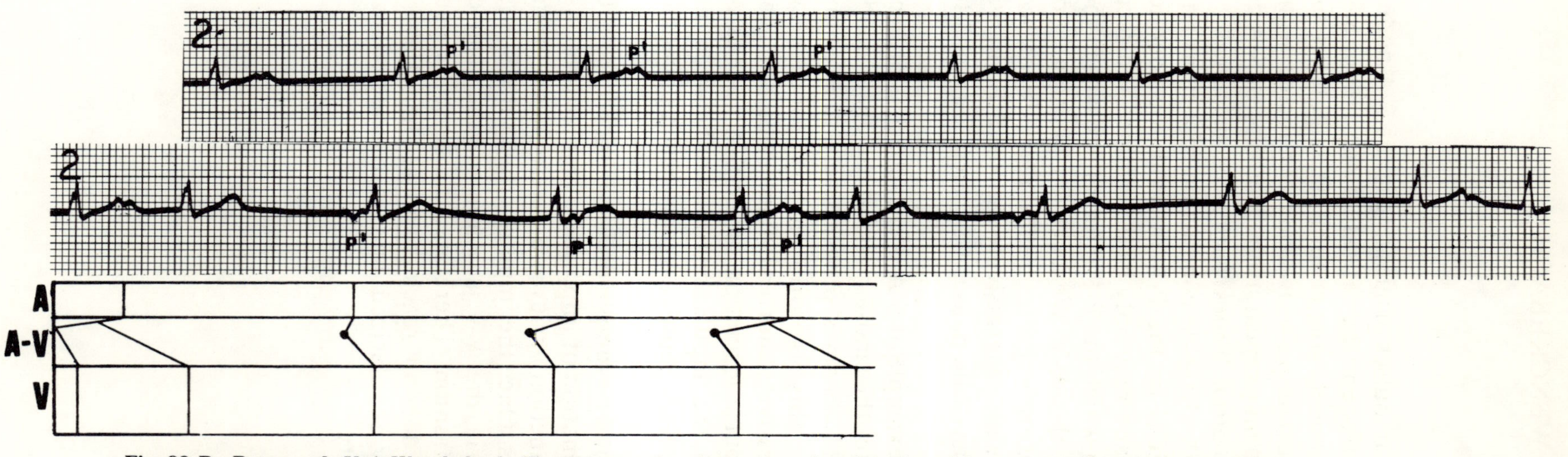

Fig. 89-B - **Retrograde V-A Wenckebach.** The upper tracing shows a junctional rhythm with a constant delay in the retrograde atrial activation (R-P¹ = 0.30 sec.). The lower tracing presents periods of a retrograde V-A Wenckebach which terminate with reciprical beats ("echo beats").

THE WENCKEBACH PHENOMENON

RETROGRADE V-A WENCKEBACH

The Wenckebach phenomenon may also appear when impulses cross the A-V junction in a retrograde fashion. Since, in these cases, the cardiac chambers distal to the block are the atria, a progressive prolongation of the R-P^1 interval will be present, and will be associated with a progressive shortening of the P^1-P^1 intervals.

Two examples of junctional rhythm with a normal anterograde conduction and a *retrograde V-A Wenckebach phenomenon* are presented in fig. 89-A and 89-B.

In fig. 89-A the retrograde atrial activation by a junctional pacemaker first precedes, is then simultaneous, and finally follows the ventricular depolarization, as can be observed in the first three beats. The last impulse is delayed so much in its trip to the atria that it reflects in the high portion of the A-V junction and returns to the ventricles *(reciprocal beat)*.

As is usually the case, in the *retrograde V-A Wenckebach* the blocked P^1 wave is not present because the sequence ends with a reciprocal beat. When the R-P^1 interval becomes long enough, the retrograde impulse reflects into the A-V junction and returns to the ventricles.

The upper tracing of fig. 89-B presents a junctional rhythm with P^1 waves following the QRS complex after a prolonged (0.32 seconds) but constant R-P^1 interval *(first degree V-A block)*. In the lower tracing, the conduction of the junctional impulse to the atria slows down progressively, until the R-P^1 interval is long enough to allow for a reciprocal beat ("echo beat"). Therefore, while the anterograde conduction to the ventricle is constant, the conduction to the atria shows a *retrograde V-A Wenckebach phenomenon*.

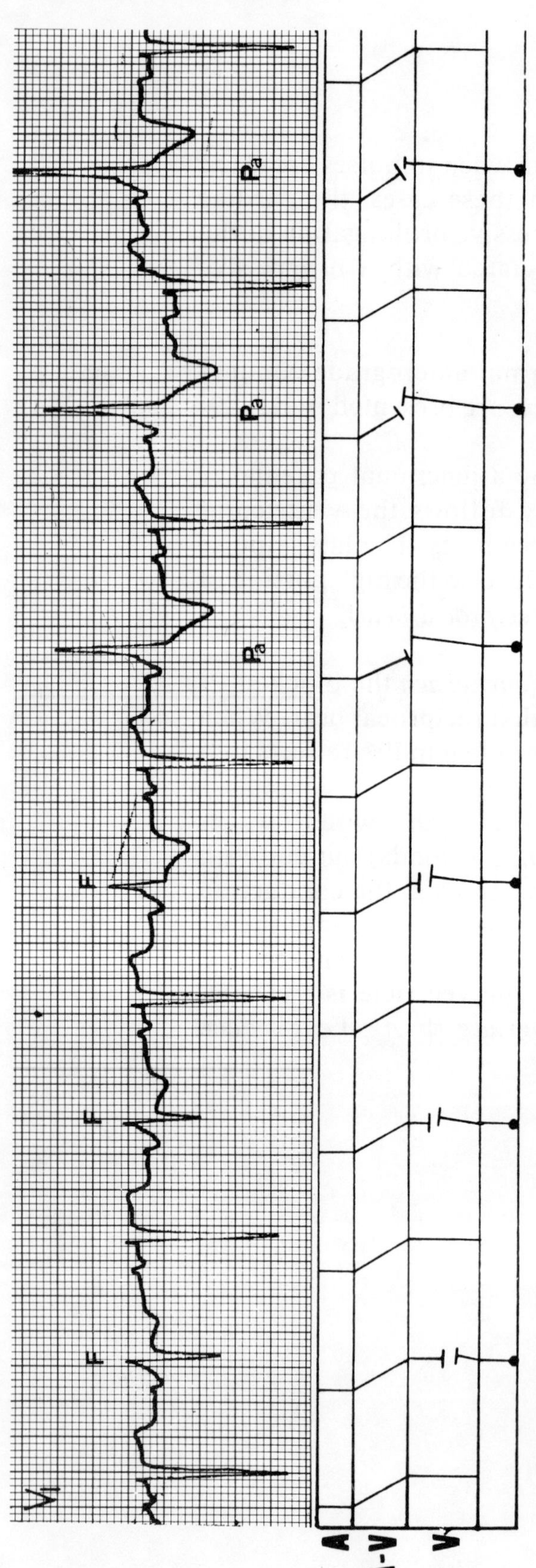

Fig. 90-A - Fusion beats. The first three anomalous beats are fusion beats (F). They are due to a ventricular depolarization which is partly due to the sinus impulse and partly to the parasystolic focus (Pa). A gradual shortening of the coupling interval of the ectopic beat determines a greater degree of aberration of the fusion beats. Pa indicates parasystolic impulses with complete ventricular capture.

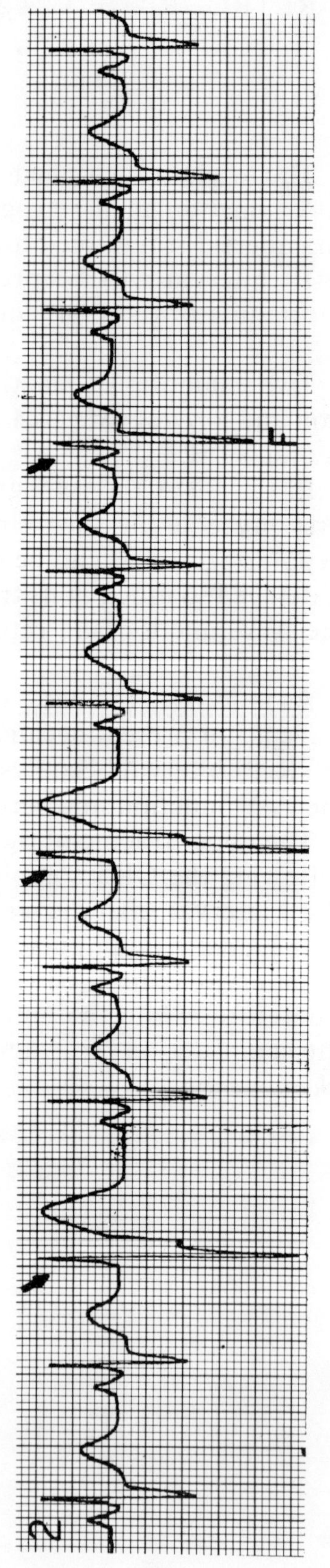

Fig. 90-B - Fusion beats. The last of the three premature beats is a fusion beat (F). The QRS complex follows a P wave and has an intermediate morphology between that of a sinus QRS and that of a PVC.

FUSION BEATS

There are two types of fusion:

a) *pseudofusion:* this is found everytime P waves and QRS complexes are overimposed on the surface ECG. It is caused by the almost simultaneous activation of both atria and ventricles (A-V dissociation, ventricular extrasystoles, etc.). In this case, the fusion is only an ECG recording ("pseudofusion") and does not indicate a fusion of two impulses within one of the cardiac chambers. Pseudofusion is the superimposition of two distinct phenomena (P waves and QRS complexes) which are independent but, in this case, almost simultaneous. It is amazing how often the beginner does not separate the pseudofusion from the true *fusion beats.*

b) *true fusion:* the activation of one of the cardiac chambers, atria or ventricles, is shared by the simultaneous propagation of impulses from two different foci. Therefore, the resulting QRS complex on the surface ECG is the vectorial summation of the myocardial areas activated by one and by the other pacemaker.

Atrial fusion beats (see page 91 and 155) are not very common and their recognition is difficult on the surface ECG. More common and significant are *ventricular fusion beats.* They are often a pathognomonic finding for the diagnosis of ventricular tachycardia (see page 75), for the recognition of parasystoles (see page 145), for the distinction between supraventricular tachycardia with aberrant conduction and ventricular tachycardia, and for the diagnosis of A-V dissociation between a sinus rhythm and an ectopic ventricular rhythm.

Fusion beats are usually a common finding in the presence of endiastolic extrasystoles and parasystolic foci. Fig. 90-A presents a sinus rhythm with a progressively different morphology due to a gradual shortening of the coupling interval between the extrasystoles and the preceeding sinus beats. The ectopic focus delivers impulses with a rate of 43/min., while the sinus rhythm has a rate of 90/min. (P-P interval = 680 msec.). The first extrasystole depolarizes only a small part of the ventricles, while the remaining ventricular myocardium is activated by the almost simultaneous sinus impulse. This determines a *fusion beat* with a morphology similar to that of sinus beats. Because of a slight but progressive shortening of the coupling interval, the second and the third extrasystoles capture an always greater area of ventricular myocardium while the one under sinus control decreases. Therefore, the resulting fusion beats show an increasingly bizarre and wider QRS. The fourth and following extrasystoles capture the entire ventricular myocardium (Pa). The presence of fusion beats, the variable coupling intervals, and the constant interectopic intervals clearly indicate a ventricular parasystolic focus.

Tracing of fig. 90-B presents three ventricular extrasystoles within the context of a sinus rhythm. The last extrasystole falls after a P wave and shows a configuration which is in between that of a sinus beat and that of a PVC. Therefore it is a *fusion beat* (F), resulting from the fusion of a sinus impulse and the almost simultaneous ventricular ectopic impulse.

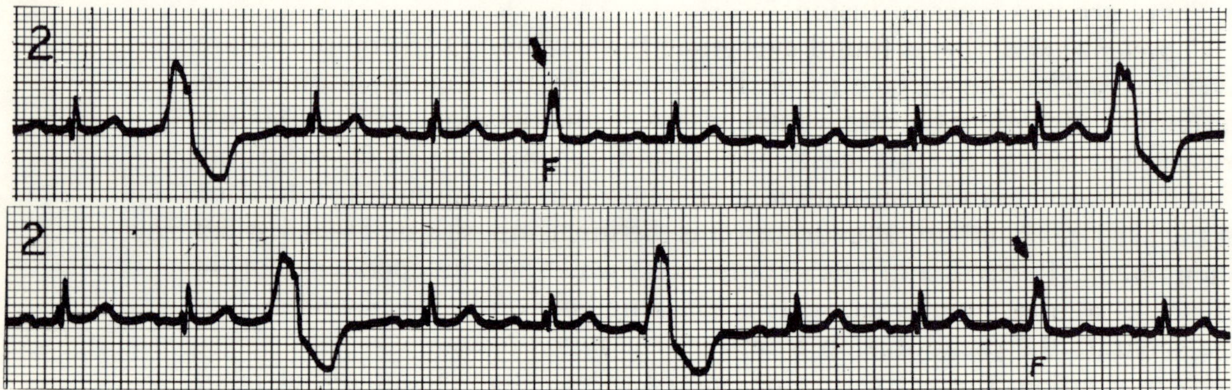

Fig. 91-A - Fusion beats. The morphology of fusion beats (F) is something in between that of a sinus beat and that of ventricular extrasystoles.

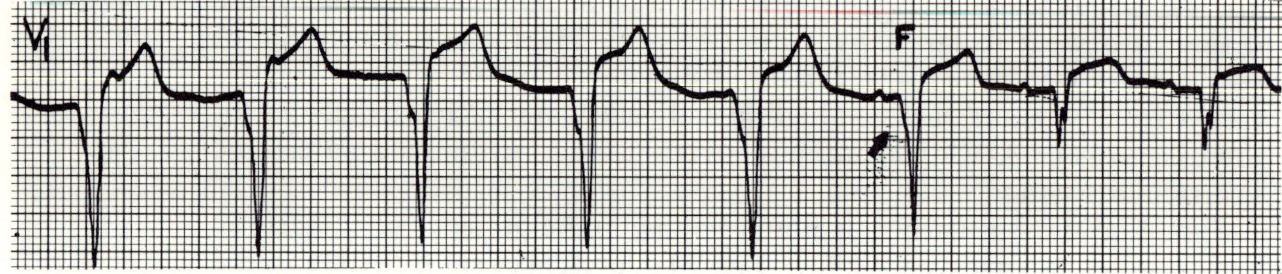

Fig. 91-B - Fusion beats. A fusion beat (F) signals the transition from a ventricular tachycardia into a sinus rhythm.

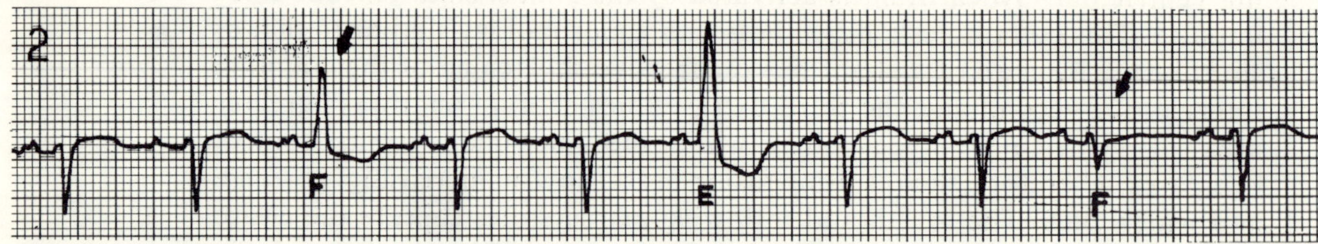

Fig. 91-C - Fusion beats. The coupling interval of the last fusion beat (F) is slightly longer than the first one. This determines a QRS morphology more similar to a sinus beat then to a ventricular extrasystole (E).

FUSION BEATS

Fig. 91-A presents a case of endiastolic ventricular extrasystoles with variable coupling intervals and fusion beats (F). Once again the morphology and duration of fusion beats is something in between that of ventricular extrasystoles and that of sinus beats. As a general rule, keep in mind that a fusion beat must appear in a moment in which, knowing the rate of the two competitive pacemakers, an almost simultaneous firing of both impulses would be expected. (This rule cannot apply for the irregular ventricular response of an atrial fibrillation.)

A *fusion beat* (F) is present also in the tracing of fig. 91-B. An *idioventricular rhythm,* with a rate of 70/min., controls the ventricles for the first five beats. A fusion beat (F) is recorded immediately before the last two sinus QRS's, which are preceded by a P wave and by a constant P-R interval. The fusion beat is also preceded by a P wave, but with a shorter P-R interval. Although sometimes it may be equal, the P-R interval of the fusion beat is usually shorter than that of a sinus beat. The *P-S interval* (from the beginning of a P wave to the end of the QRS) of a fusion beat is always longer than the P-R interval of a sinus beat.

Fig. 91-C presents two fusion beats (F) and endiastolic ventricular extrasystole (E). The configuration of the second fusion beat is almost similar to that of a sinus QRS, except for the inscription of the terminal forces. This is due to the fact that the coupling interval of the last premature beat is slightly longer than others.

While the initial vector may or may not be different, the terminal vector of a fusion beat is always different than that of a sinus beat. The initial forces will be determined by the one, of the two foci in competition which will initiate the ventricular depolarization.

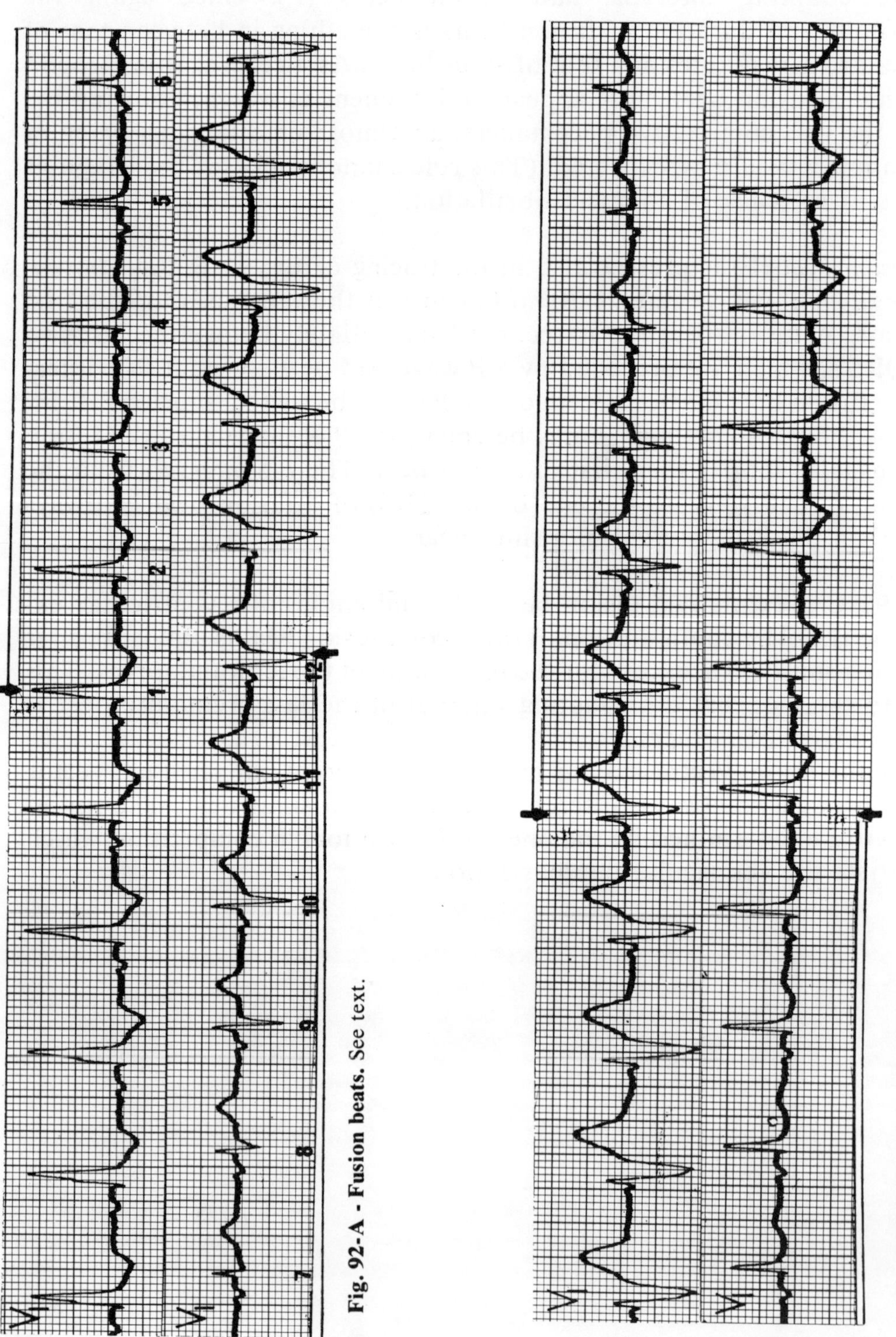

Fig. 92-A - Fusion beats. See text.

Fig. 92-B - Fusion beats. See text.

FUSION BEATS

It has been stated that, as a general criteria, a *fusion beat* has a morphology which is between that of a sinus beat and that of the competitive pacemaker. The QRS duration of a fusion beat is usually longer than that of a sinus beat. An exception to this rule is presented in the rare and fascinating tracings of fig. 92-A and 92-B.

The patient has a sinus rhythm with a complete right bundle branch block. The heart rate is 85/min. and the P-R interval is normal (fig. 92-A). Although the rhythm is practically unchanged throughout the tracing and the rate is similar to that of the first beats, it may be observed that, starting from the beat indicated by the arrow, the QRS complexes show a morphology and a duration which is gradually changing. From complexes of the qR type (1-6) with a maximal duration of 0.12 sec., the pattern changes first into complexes of the Rs type (7-8) and then of the rS type (8-12) with a shorter duration and, finally, into complexes of a clear left bundle branch block type (last 5 QRS's of the second tracing).

Notice that the P-R interval of the beats included between the two arrows becomes progressively shorter. Therefore, this continuous tracing shows the *transition from a sinus rhythm with a complete right bundle branch block into a slow ventricular tachycardia with a rate very similar to the sinus rate.* The left bundle branch block morphology of the idio-ventricular beats sharply contrasts with the right bundle branch block morphology of the sinus beats. This suggests that the ventricular ectopic focus must be situated in the right ventricle. The very similar firing rate of the sinus and idio- ventricular pacemakers determines the appearance of fusion beats with different morphology (12 beats between the two arrows) and a sharing of the ventricular depolarization. Furthermore, it may be observed that the fusion beats have a shorter duration than other QRS's and that their morphology approaches one vectorially normal for V1. The ninth and tenth beats have a "normal" duration and morphology for V1. This is explained as follows: (a) the ectopic focus is situated in that ventricle where the incoming sinus beats are blocked by the specific bundle branch (right ventricle); (b) the rate of the ectopic focus is very similar to the sinus rate.

Therefore, during a fusion beat, the right ventricle will be controlled more by the ventricular ectopic focus and less by the sinus impulse (which is delayed for the presence of a right bundle branch block). This will determine a progressively minor delay in the inscription of terminal forces (beat 1 through 5). During beats 6 through 8, the ventricular activation is shared between the two pacemakers, but only a very small portion of the right ventricle is activated by sinus beats. Beats 9 and 10 are "vectorially normal beats" for the V1 lead and they indicate an equal sharing of the ventricular activation between the two pacemakers. Therefore, the right ventricle will be entirely depolarized by the ectopic ventricular focus while the left ventricle is simultaneously being depolarized by the sinus impulse. The next beats (11, 12, etc.) show a configuration of left bundle branch block type, and indicate a total control of both ventricles by the ectopic ventricular focus.

A similar, but inverse, sequence is presented in the continous tracing of fig. 92-B, which is from the same patient of fig. 91-A. The rhythm goes from a ventricular tachycardia to a sinus rhythm, with a complete right bundle branch block, through several *fusion beats.* The fusion beats have shorter QRS's and some of them show a "normal morphology for the V1 lead.

ASHMAN PHENOMENON

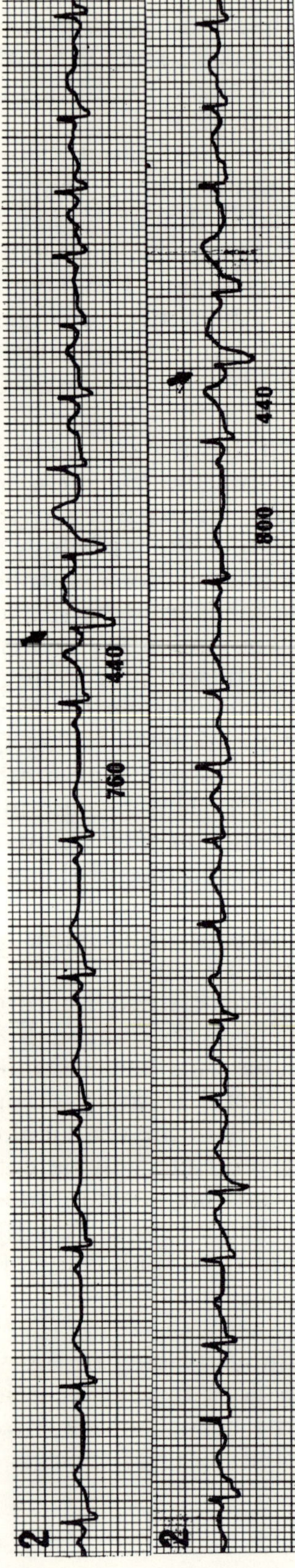

Fig. 93- A - Ashman phenomenon. The continuous tracing shows a sinus rhythm interrupted by two bursts of atrial fibrillation. The first two beats of the paroxysm show a ventricular aberration, of RBBB type, which terminate a short cardiac cycle (440 msec.) after a longer one (760-800 msec.).

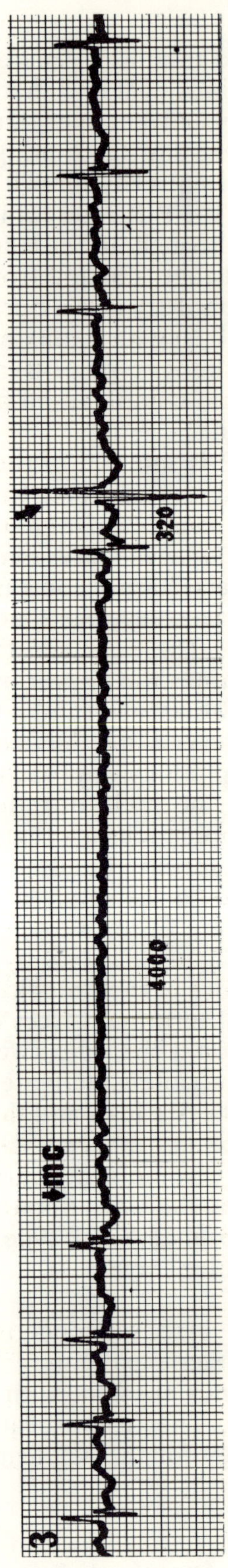

Fig. 93-B - Ashman phenomenon. The ventricular response of the atrial fibrillation is interrupted, for 4 msecs., by the application of a carotid sinus massage. The long pause is ended by two beats, one with a QRS complex similar to preceding beats, and one showing an aberrant ventricular conduction. The aberrant QRS closes a short cardiac cycle (320 msec.) after a long asystolic cycle (4000 msec.).

ASHMAN PHENOMENON

The aberrant ventricular conduction of a supraventricular beat may be secondary a) to the prematurity of the impulse within the cardiac cycles and b) to the fact that it terminates a shorter cardiac cycle after a longer one (see page 54, 68, 70).

The "long-short" sequence, with a ventricular aberration of the beats terminating the shorter cycle, is also known as the *Ashman phenomenon*. This phenomenon is so common, and causes so many diagnostic errors, that it requires further elaboration.

Fig. 93-A presents a continuous tracing where, in two different occasions, a paroxysmal atrial fibrillation interrupts a normal sinus rhythm. In both cases, the paroxysmal atrial fibrillation starts with more than one beat showing a right bundle branch block aberration, before the restoration of a normal intraventricular conduction. The beat initiating the paroxysm closes a shorter cardiac cycle following a longer sinus cycle *(Ashman phenomenon)*.

Therefore, the *Ashman phenomenon* indicates that, in a given cardiac cycle, the refractory period of the *intraventricular conduction is directly related to the length of the preceding cycle*. In other words, for a given beat, the *aberrant ventricular conduction* (which means that the impulse falls within the refractory period of the intraventricular conduction tissue) may be determined by:

a) *the impulse prematurity within the basic cardiac cycles;*
b) *a lengthening of the preceding cardiac cycles.*

Fig. 93-B shows an atrial fibrillation with a prolonged asystolic pause determined by the vagal stimulation of a carotid sinus massage (cm). The pause terminates with a normal looking QRS, followed by a complex with aberrant ventricular conduction (arrow). Again, the aberrant beat terminates a shorter cardiac cycle (320 msec.) after a longer one (4000 msec.). The assumption that a similar phenomenon could happen in proximal areas of the A-V junction (A-V node and His bundle) enables one to understand why, during the A-V Wenckebach, the longest P-R interval increment occurs between the first and the second QRS following the blocked P wave. The prolonged A-V conduction occurs during a shorter cardiac cycle which follows a longer one (see page 165).

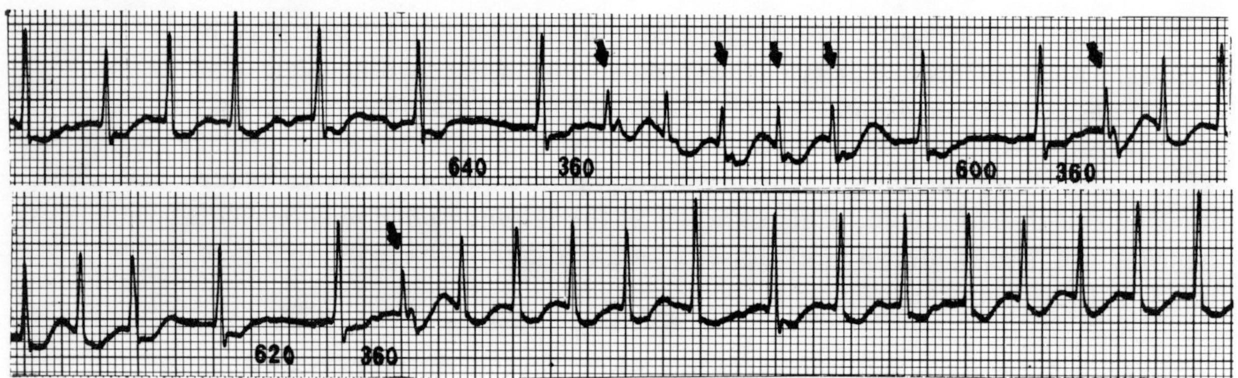

Fig. 94-A - Ashman phenomenon. The phenomenon is indicated by the beats with ventricular aberration which end a "long-short cycle" sequence.

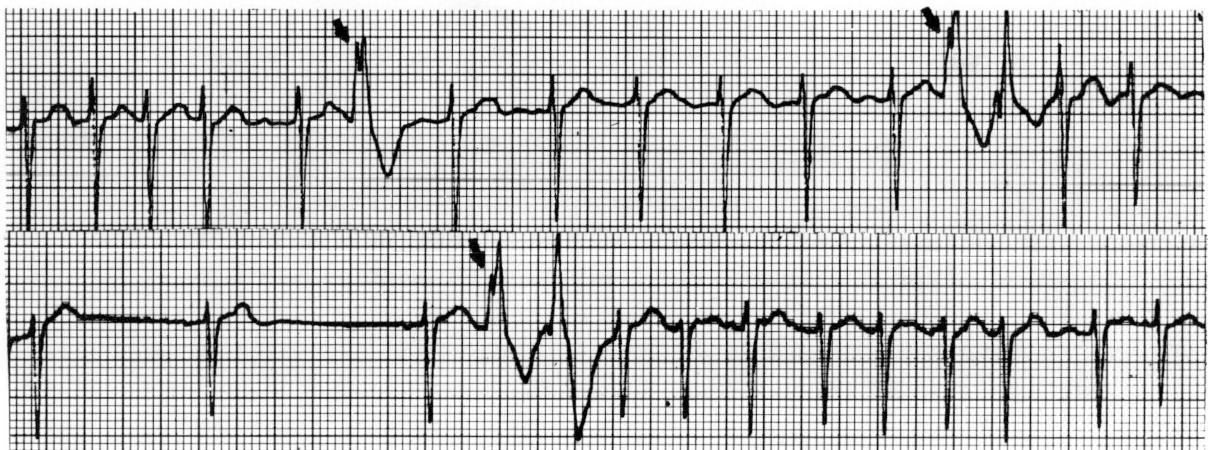

Fig. 94-B - Ashman phenomenon. The bizarre beats of the upper tracing simulate the presence of ventricular extrasystoles. They are, instead, supraventricular beats with aberrant conduction. An Ashman phenomenon is present in the transition between a sinus rhythm and the atrial fibrillation (lower tracing)

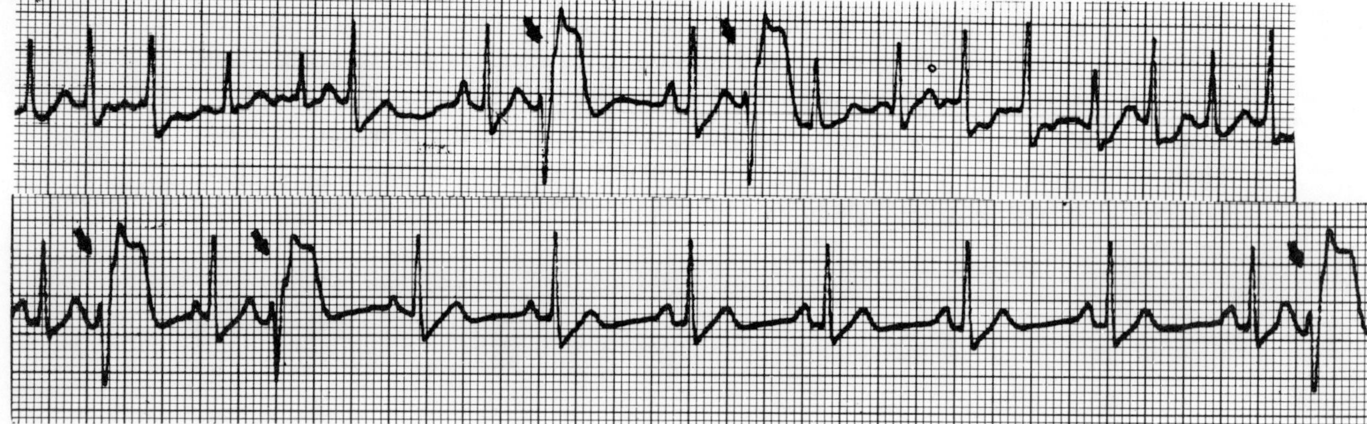

Fig. 94-C - Ashman phenomenon or ventricular extrasystole? The dilemma is solved by the bottom tracing where the patient shows a sinus rhythm.

ASHMAN PHENOMENON

An *aberrantly conducted beat* which closes a shorter cycle following a longer one *(Ashman phenomenon) must be differentiated from a ventricular extrasystole.* The differential diagnosis may have significant therapeutic consequences.

The upper tracing of fig. 94-A shows a brief paroxysm of five rapid and bizarre beats which may suggest a brief paroxysmal ventricular tachycardia. However, several factors indicate the presence of a *ventricular aberration of supraventricular beats:*

a)   the first beat of the paroxysm terminates a shorter cycle which is preceded by a longer one;

b)   other aberrant beats are present in the same tracing and in the bottom tracing (arrows); in every occasion they terminate a shorter cardiac cycle after a longer one.

c)   the initial vector of the aberrant beat is similar to that of other QRS's; this favors the diagnosis of aberration.

The upper tracing of fig. 94-B presents three aberrant beats, with a right bundle branch block configuration, within the irregular rhythm of an atrial fibrillation. Also observe that in the couplets of aberrant beats, both in the upper and lower tracing, the second of the two aberrant beats has a morphology slightly less bizarre and it is immediately followed by a normal QRS. The diagnostic dilemma between ventricular extrasystoles and supraventricular beats with Ashman phenomenon, is solved when recording the transition from a sinus rhythm into an atrial fibrillation (lower tracing). The first and the second beat of the paroxysm clearly shows a ventricular aberration similar to that of the beats recorded in the top tracing. *The long-short principle* is operating, and the ventricular aberration appears after a long-short sequence in all three cases. The conduction is restored to normal in the following beats.

The upper tracing of fig. 94-C shows an atrial fibrillation briefly interrupted by two sinus beats. These are followed by two bizarre and aberrant beats which close a shorter cycle after a longer one. Therefore, the criteria for an Ashman phenomenon are present. However, the lower tracing clears any doubts. The same patient, this time in a stable sinus rhythm, presents obvious ventricular extrasystoles with a fixed coupling interval. The morphology of the PVC's is identical to that of the anomalous beats of the upper tracing. Once again the interpreter is challenged by a simulation. The possibility of comparing the tracing with a previous one is a determining factor in the diagnosis of the arrhythmia. Furthermore, the tracing shows another differential criteria between Ashman beats and ventricular premature beats: *fixed coupling favors PVC's, variable coupling favors ventricular aberration.*

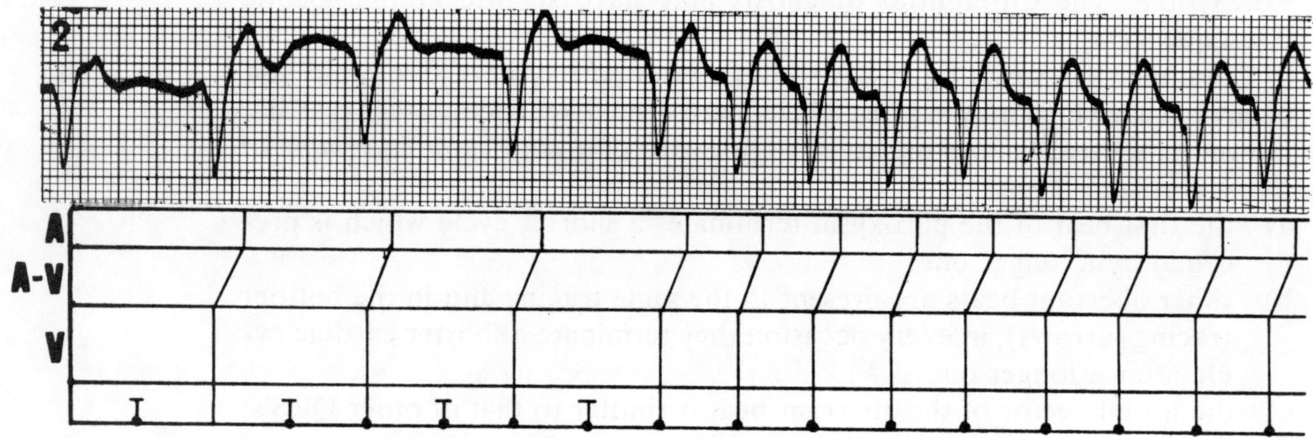

Fig. 95-A - Exit block and ventricular tachycardia. See text.

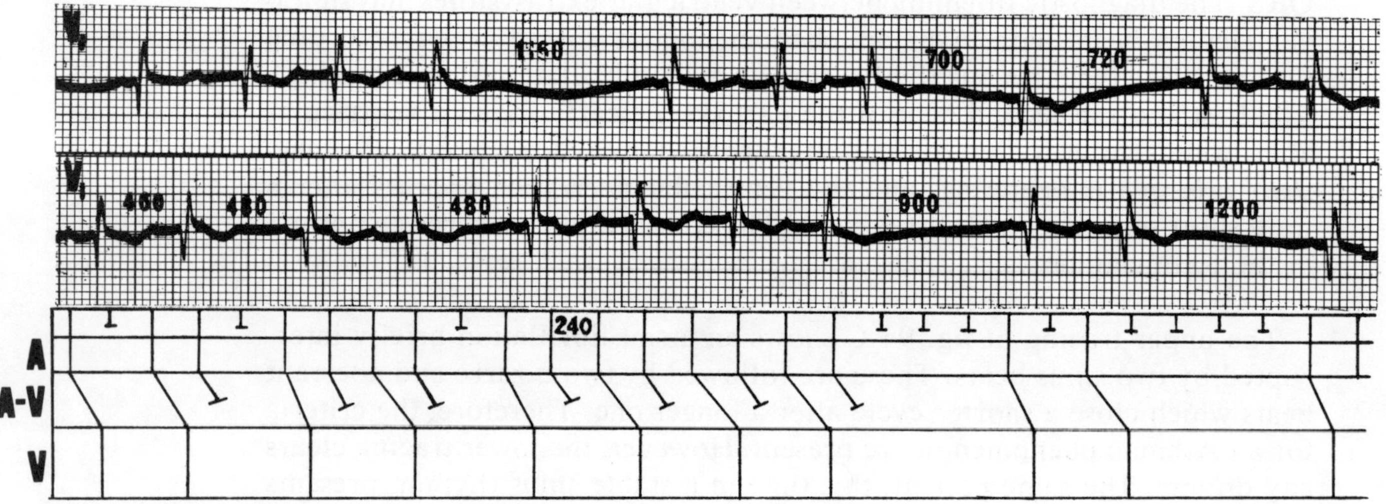

Fig. 95-B - Exit block and supraventricular tachyarrhythmia. See text.

EXIT BLOCK

The *exit block* has been defined as *"a missed propagation of an ectopic impulse into the adjacent myocardial tissue"*. This is, therefore, an unusual conduction disturbance which does not involve the specialized cardiac conduction system, but which occurs into the myocardial tissue surrounding an ectopic ventricular, junctional or atrial focus. The extravagant electrophysiologic phenomenon has been already seen in ventricular parasystoles and in parasystolic ventricular tachycardias (see page 83 and 145), where the exit block explained the protective mechanism surrounding the ectopic focus. To complicate the situation, this parasystolic protective mechanism would also induce an "entrance block"; this would be due to a physiologic refractory state of the myocardium surrounding the parasystolic focus induced by the continuous bombardment of rapid impulses. Of the several ectopic impulses, only one is able to penetrate the adjacent myocardium. This fact would result in a parasystolic rate which is several times slower than the ectopic firing rate (exit block of 4:1, 5:1, etc.). The absence of an *exit block* around a parasystolic focus would reveal the true nature and rate of the ectopic pacemaker. When this happens, the rhythm usually degenerates into a dangerous ventricular tachycardia (see page 83).

An example of *ventricular tachycardia, with periods of 2:1 exit block,* is presented in fig. 95-A. It may be observed that the QRS complexes are bizarre and wide and that atrial activity is not evident. The rate of the first five beats is 75/min. Starting at the fifth beat, the ventricular rate suddenly doubles (150/min.) while the QRS morphology remains unchanged. Therefore, a ventricular tachycardia which, in a few seconds, doubles its rate may have the following explanation (see diagram): the firing rate of the ventricular tachycardic focus would be equal to 150/min. and a 2:1 exit block would be present in the first five beats.

An *atrial tachyarrhythmia, with periods of exit block,* is presented in fig. 95-B. Atrial waves, with a rate of 270/min., are easily recognized in both tracings. Furthermore, a basic 2:1 A-V ratio alternates with periods of 3:1 A-V block. Both tracings show pauses varying from 460 to 1200 msec., where the baseline is isoelectric and no atrial activity is present. The duration of the asystolic pauses is approximately two to five times longer than the interval between two consecutive atrial waves (240 msec.).

Therefore, *a variable and intermittent exit block* (of 2:1 and 4:1) is present in the propagation of the ectopic impulses into the atria. The exit block is due to a markedly prolonged refractory period surrounding the atrial ectopic focus and is equivalent to the exit block commonly seen in parasystolic ventricular foci and in ventricular tachycardias.

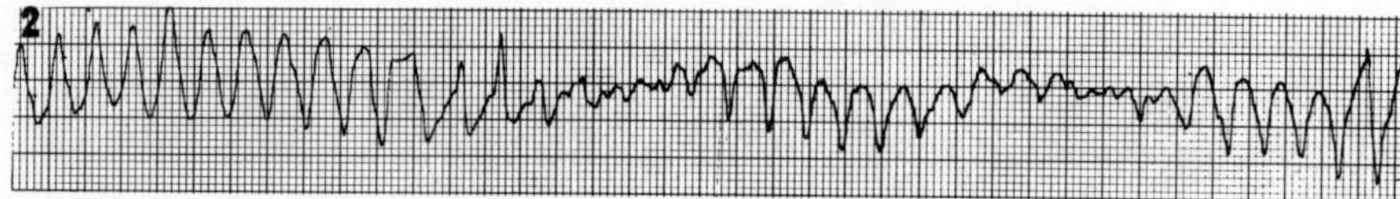

Fig. 96-A - Ventricular fibrillation.

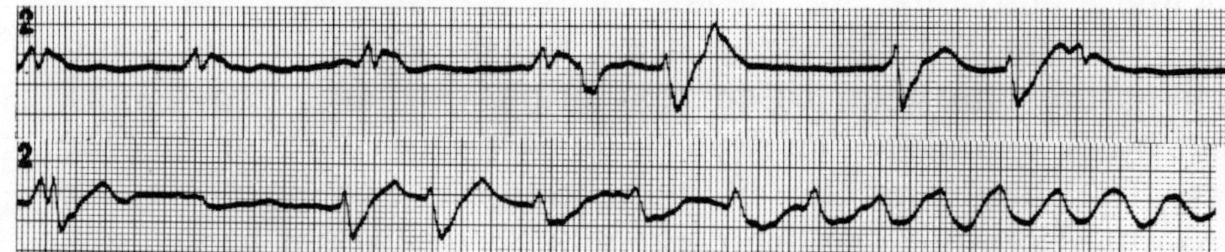

Fig. 96-B - Agonal rhythm.

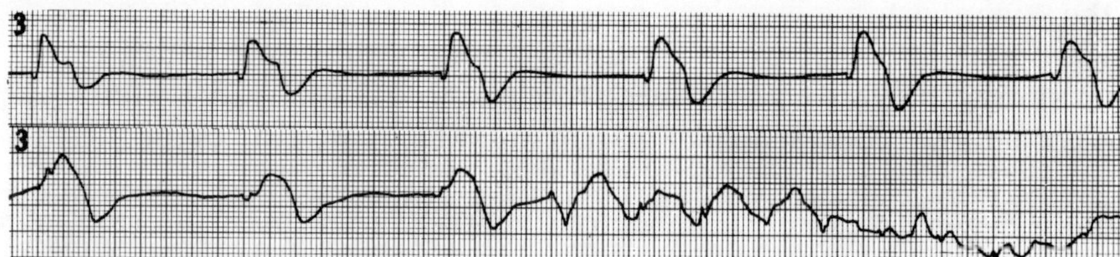

Fig. 96-C - Agonal rhythm.

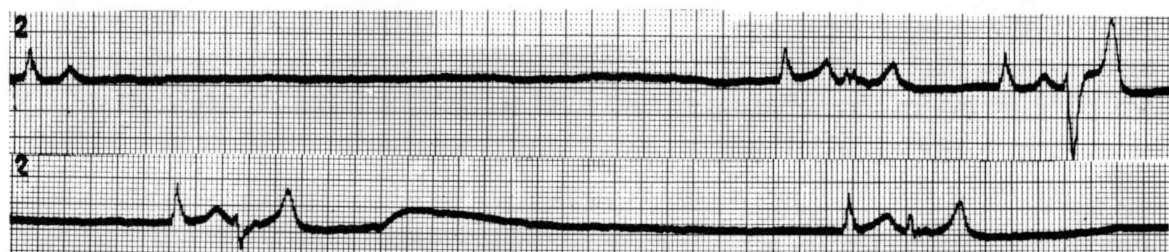

Fig. 96-D - Agonal rhythm and ventricular asystole.

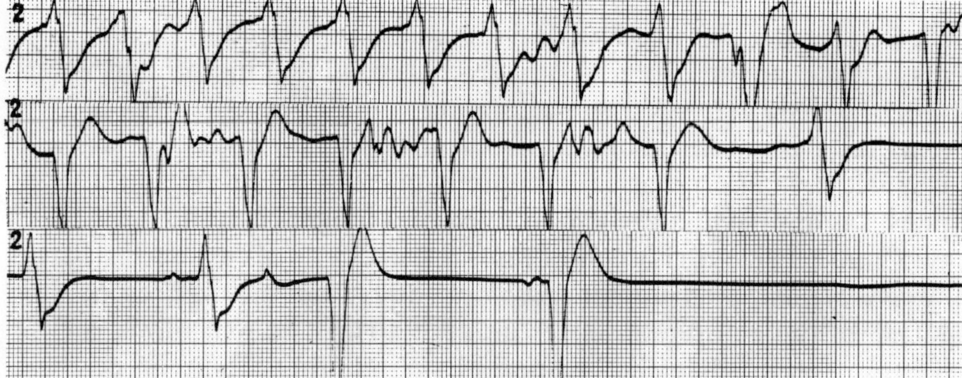

Fig. 96-E - Ventricular tachycardia deteriorating in ventricular asystole.

EXTREME RHYTHMS (THE DYING HEART)

These include rhythms which do not result in hemodynamically effective ventricular contractions.

They are:

1) *Ventricular fibrillation:* the ECG presents abnormal ventricular complexes in the form of irregular "zig- zag" with variable amplitudes (fig. 96-A). The amplitude of the fibrillatory waves has a clinical significance since it is well known that cardioversion is more successful with high fibrillatory waves.

2) *Agonal rhythms:* they usually print their sinister message in the form of widened, bizarre, irregular QRS complexes with extremely low rate. They may end with a ventricular tachycardia or fibrillation as in the case of fig. 96-B and 96-C, or may degenerate in ventricular arrest or asystole (fig. 96-D and 96-E).

3) *Ventricular arrest or asystole:* in this situation there is a total absence of mechanical or electrical ventricular activity. The ECG records an isoelectric line and no ventricular complexes.

In fig. 96-D the idio-ventricular beats have an extremely low rate and are associated with multiform ventricular extrasystoles. The rhythm threatens the appearance of an asystole.

Fig. 96-E presents a ventricular tachycardia, with grossly distorted QRS complexes. The rhythm becomes progressively slower and terminates in a ventricular asystole.

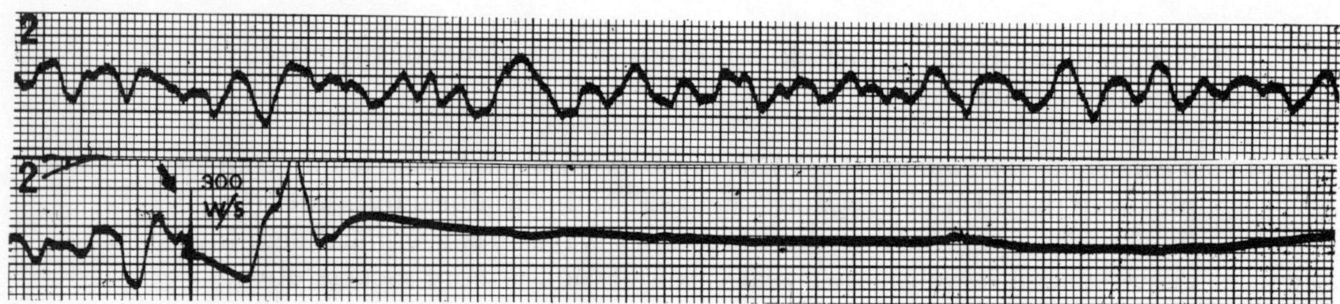

Fig. 97-A - Ventricular fibrillation. The attempt of cardioversion (bottom tracing) transforms the ventricular fibrillation in asystole.

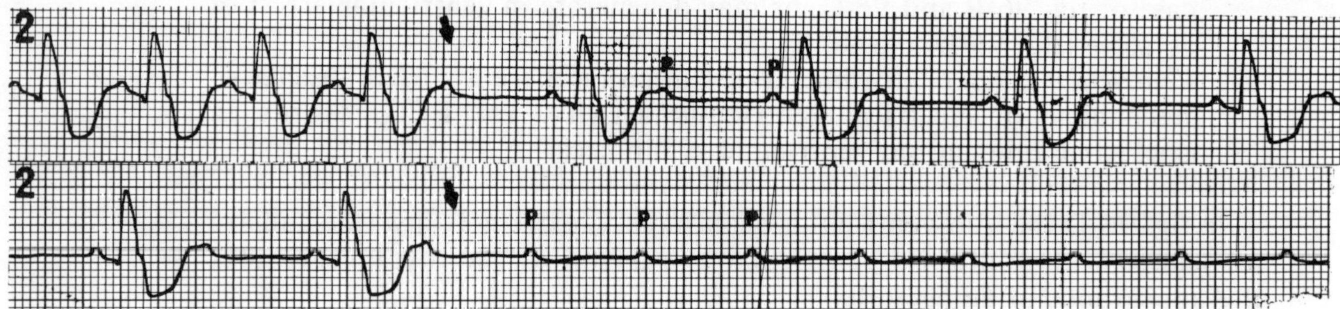

Fig. 97-B - Sinus rhythm, second degree A-V block (upper tracing) and complete A-V block (bottom tracing).

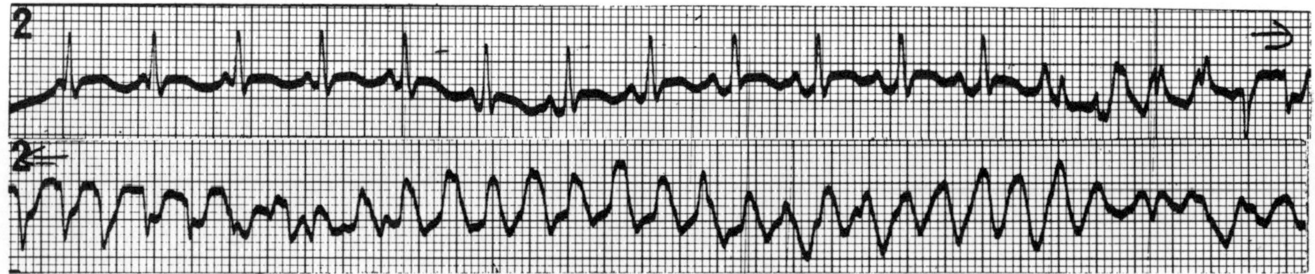

Fig. 97-C - A-V dissociation and ventricular fibrillation.

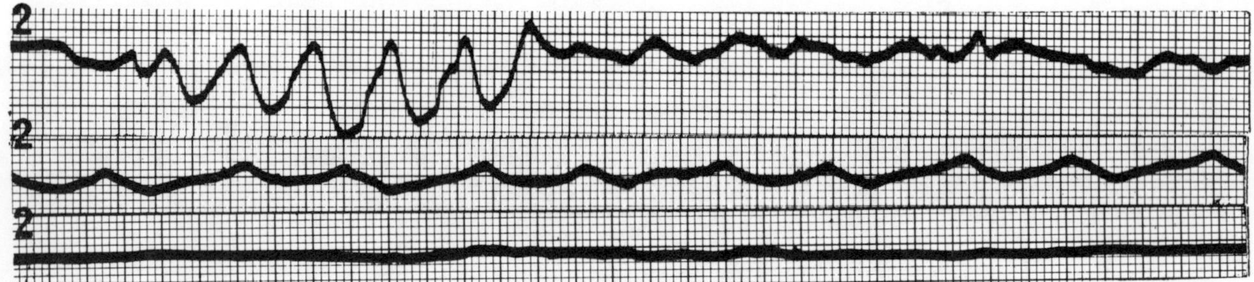

Fig. 97-D - Agonal rhythm.

The tracings on the opposite page show several ways in which the heart terminates its vital function.

An electrical cardioversion is attempted in the lower tracing of fig. 97-A, and transforms a ventricular fibrillation in asystole. From an hemodynamic standpoint there is not much difference between the two situations, since the heart does not generate effective contractions in either condition.

The continuous tracing of fig. 97-B shows a dramatic situation which develops in a few seconds. A normal sinus rhythm suddenly shows a 2:1 A-V block. (The first arrow indicates the moment in which the cardiac rate is suddenly halved.) A few seconds later, a third degree A-V block appears and all the sinus beats are blocked in the A-V junction. Undisturbed sinus P waves are recognized (second arrow), and ventricular activity is absent for the lack of intervention of junctional or idio-ventricular escape beats.

Fig. 97-C shows an A-V dissociation between a sinus and a junctional rhythm. This degenerates first in a ventricular tachycardia and then in a fibrillation.

The agonal type chaotic ventricular activity (upper tracing of fig. 97-D) is gradually transformed into electrical asystole (lower tracing).

ARTIFICIAL PACEMAKERS

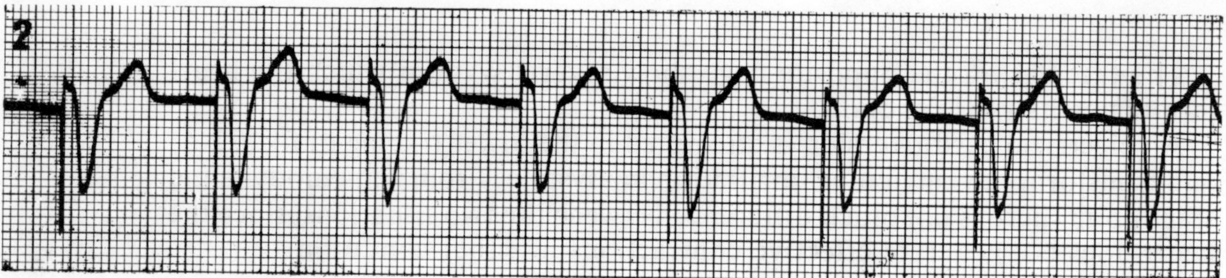

Fig. 98-A - Artificial pacemakers. Fixed rate pacing.

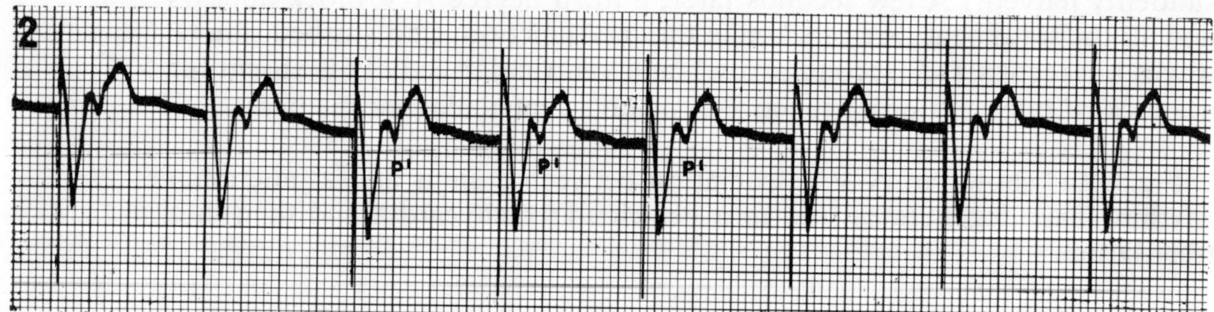

Fig. 98-B - Artificial pacemakers. Fixed rate pacing with retrograde atrial activation (P¹).

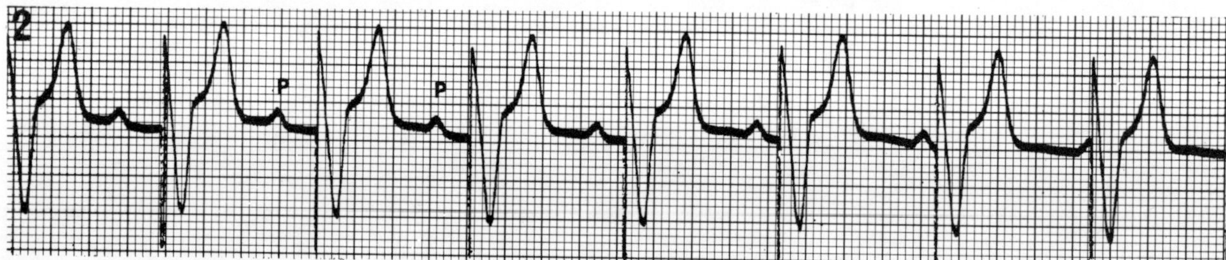

Fig. 98-C - Artificial pacemakers. Fixed rate pacing. The sinus P waves and the ventricular complexes are independent.

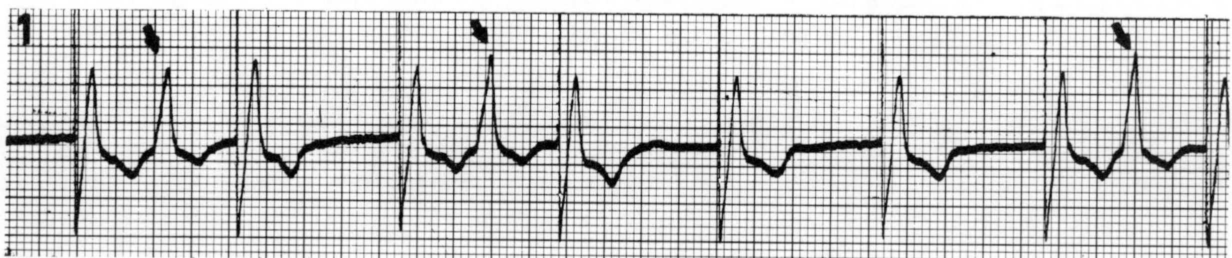

Fig. 98-D - Artificial pacemakers. Ventricular extrasystoles (arrows) interrupt the otherwise regular fixed rate pacing.

ARTIFICIAL PACEMAKERS (AP)

In the age of symbiosis between electronics and medicine, the number of patients treated with the electrical stimulation of temporary and permanent artificial pacemakers is constantly increasing. Therefore, in today's clinical practice one must become familiar with the most commonly used artificial pacemakers and pacing modalities. They are:

A. FIXED RATE VENTRICULAR PACING (ASYNCHRONOUS PACEMAKER)

Fig. 98-A shows a typical *fixed rate ventricular pacing*. The artificial impulse appears on the tracing as a rapid artifact (usually less than 2 msec.) and is followed by an aberrant and wide QRS, similar to that of a bundle branch block. This indicates a slower and aberrant ventricular activation through non-specific pathways. The pacing rate in this patient is 75/min. Sinus activity (P) or retrograde atrial depolarization (P¹) is not present in this tracing.

Fig. 98-B presents a *fixed rate ventricular pacing* of 78/min. (asynchronous pacemaker) with retrograde atrial depolarization. P¹ waves follow each QRS and the ventriculo-atrial conduction time of 0.20 seconds is within normal limits. The presence of retrograde P¹ waves is an interesting and common finding in ventricular pacing. While the anterograde propagation of atrial impulses is blocked in the A-V junction (patient of fig. 98-B was treated for a complete A-V block), the retrograde conduction to the atria may remain perfectly normal.

A patient with a complete A-V block, treated with fixed rate ventricular pacing, may show a sinus activity totally independent from that of the ventricular pacing. Fig. 98-C shows sinus P waves, with the rate of 72/min., dissociated and independent from the ventricular complexes of an asynchronous pacemaker (75/min.).

Spontaneous ventricular activity from extrasystoles or supraventricular impulses does not influence the stimulation rate of a fixed rate pacemaker. Therefore, *competitive rhythms* may be present between spontaneous and paced beats.

Fig. 98-D presents a ventricular pacing with a fixed rate of 72/min. In three different occasions (arrows), ventricular extrasystoles are interpolated between two artificial impulses. The spike which follows the extrasystole does not fall in the absolute ventricular refractory period and, therefore, activates the ventricles. During the "triplets" (pacing-extrasystole-pacing) the heart rate is equal to 150/min. and this may have a negative hemodynamic effect. Furthermore, the pacemaker impulse may fall on the preceding extrasystolic T waves and initiate a repetitive phenomenon ("pacing on T phenomenon").

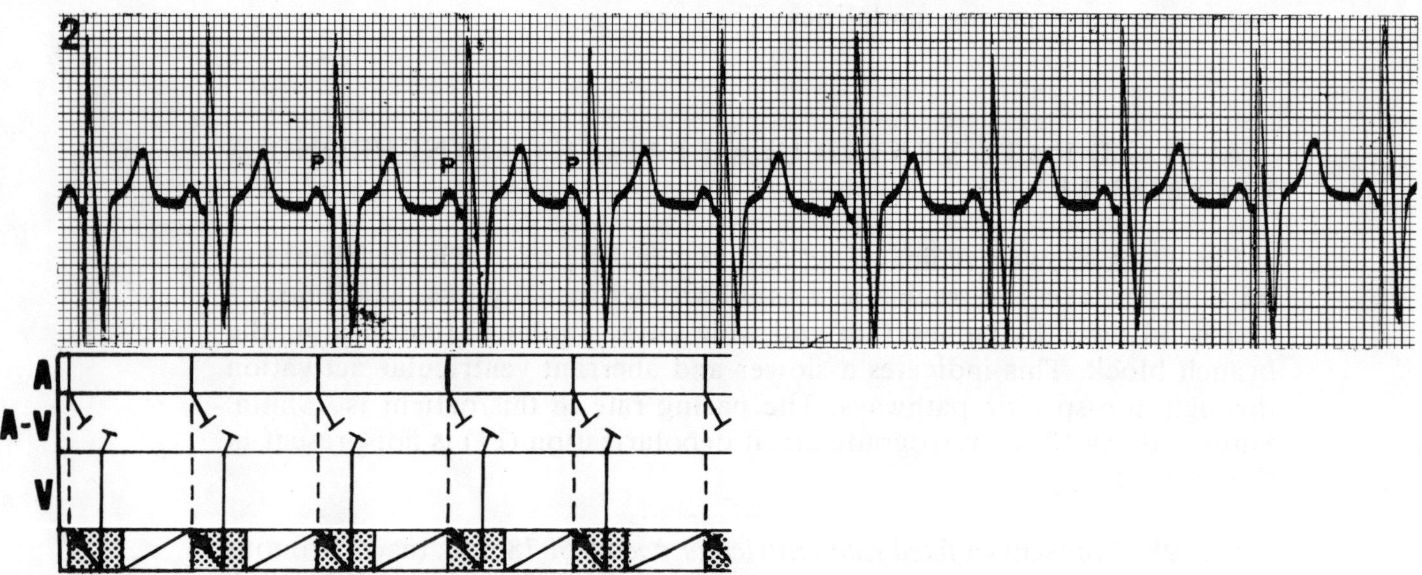

Fig. 99-A - Artificial pacemakers. P-wave synchronous pacing. Sinus P waves precede
each ventricular complex. The P-S intervals (P-spike) are constant (0.16 secs.).

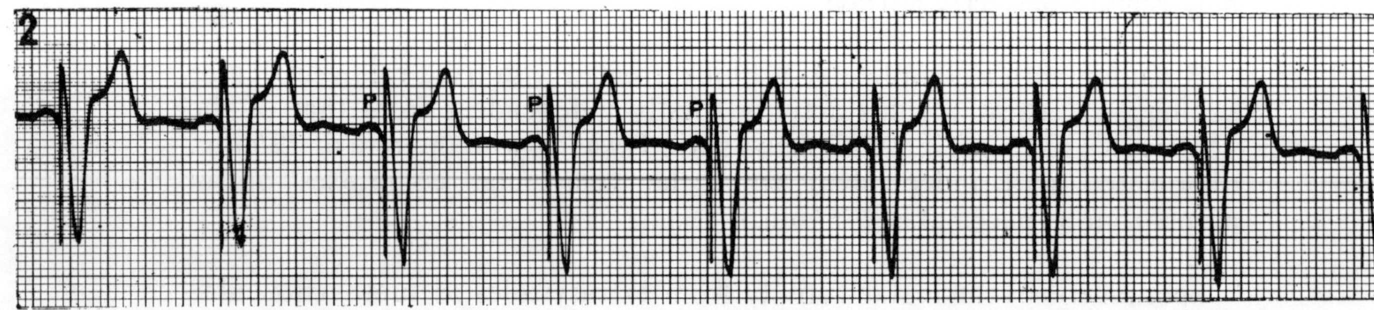

Fig. 99-B - Artificial pacemakers. P wave synchronous pacing.

B. P-WAVE SYNCHRONOUS PACEMAKER

This type of pacemaker is a true A-V prosthesis. Patients with P-wave synchronous pacemakers have a P-wave sensing electrode implanted in the atria and a stimulating electrode in contact with the ventricular myocardium. Ventricular pacing occurs after a predetermined interval of time, similar to the physiologic P-R interval and obtained through a circuit-delay, from the sensing of atrial potentials. In such a way the P-QRS relationship and synchronism are maintained within physiological limits. This type of pacing is the only one which responds to physiological variations of sinus rate.

Fig. 99-A shows a *P-wave synchronous pacemaker*. Sinus P waves are present before each impulse activating the ventricles. The P-stimulus interval (P-S) is equal to 0.16 sec. The diagram illustrates the mechanism of the pacemaker. The P wave, blocked within the A-V junction, is sensed by the atrial electrode. After an interval of time of 0.16 sec. the ventricular electrodes deliver an impulse and activates the ventricles.

A *P-wave synchronous pacemaker* is shown in fig. 99-B. The P-stimulus interval is 0.16 sec. The P-S interval may vary between 0.12 and 0.20 seconds. In the absence of regular atrial activity (atrial fibrillation, sinus arrest, sino-atrial block, etc.), after an interval of time that is predetermined at the moment of implantation, the pacemaker triggers a safety circuit and initiates a fixed rate ventricular pacing.

If the sinus rate is above 125/min., or in the presence of atrial tachyarrhythmias, the pacemaker senses every other P wave and, therefore, halves the ventricular response with a 2:1 block. With an atrial rate faster than 190/min., a 3:1 block is established.

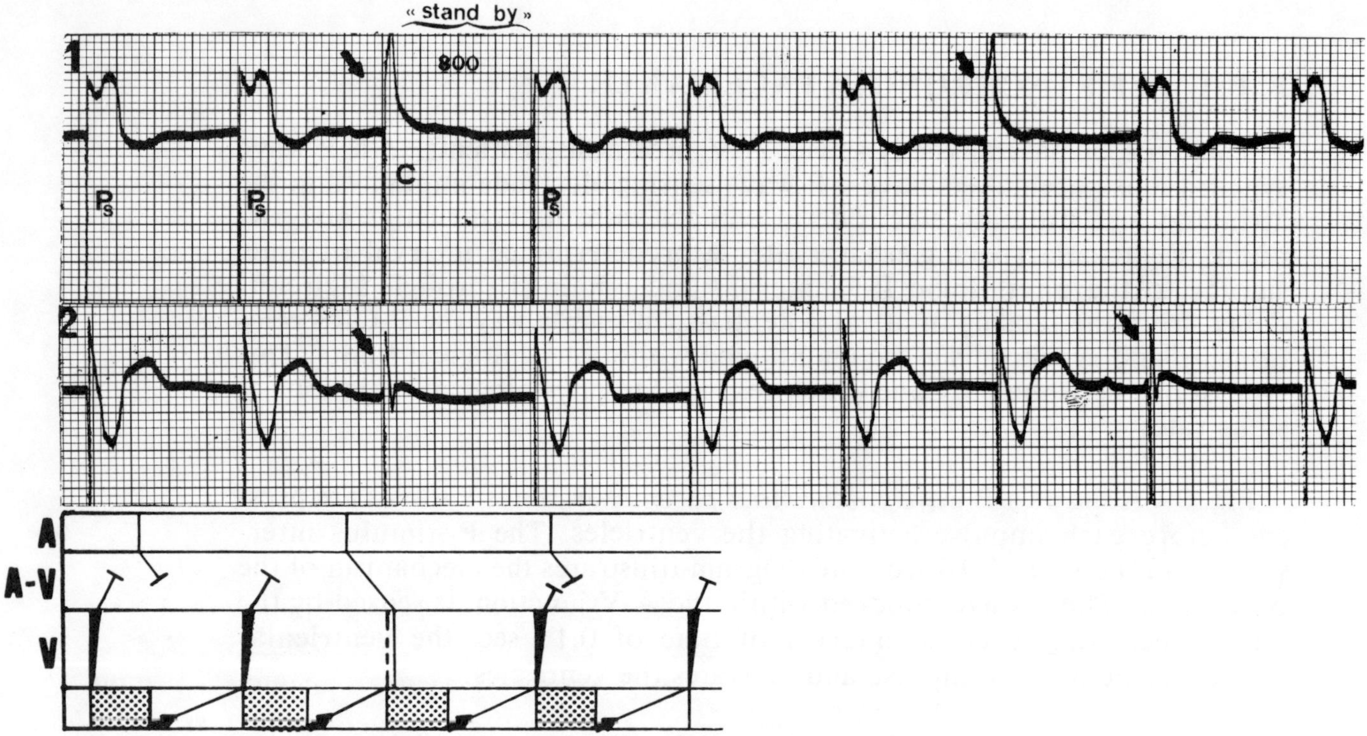

Fig. 100-A - Artificial pacemakers. QRS-synchronous "demand" pacing. An artificial impulse is triggered by the sinus beats conducted to the ventricles (arrows). At the end of a stand-by interval of 800 msec. the pacemaker fires at a fixed rate (Ps).

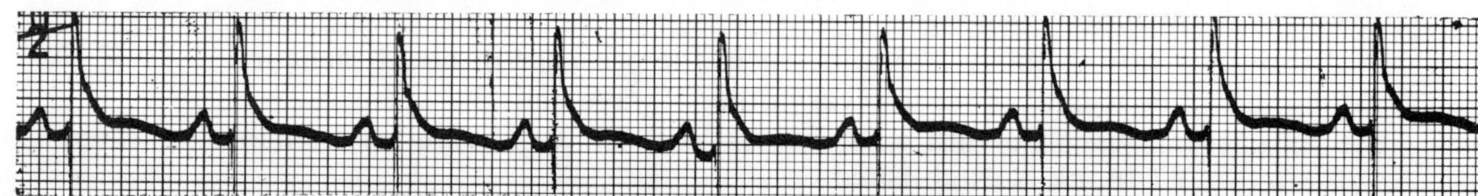

Fig. 100-B - Artificial pacemakers. QRS-synchronous "demand" pacing. The rhythm is a normal sinus rhythm. Spikes fall within the conducted QRS's and, therefore, within the absolute ventricular refractory period. They do not depolarize the ventricles.

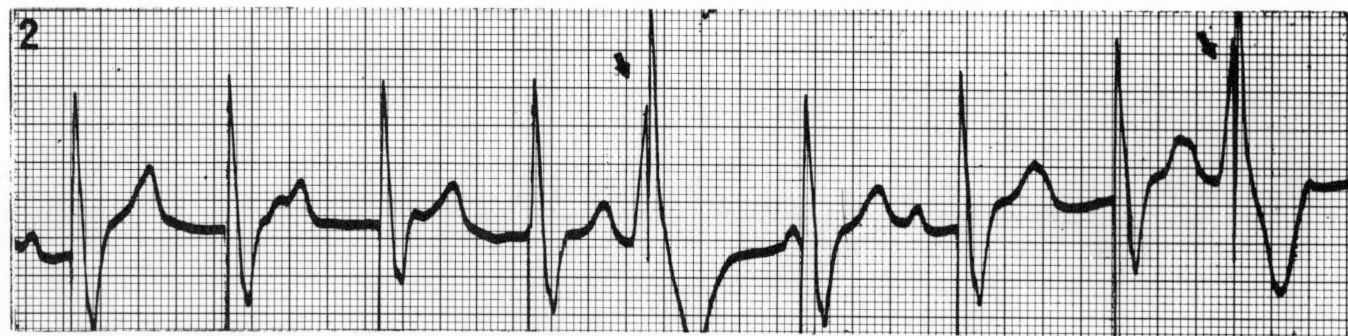

Fig. 100-C - Artificial pacemakers. QRS-synchronous "demand" pacing. The pacemaker senses the ventricular extrasystole (arrow) and delivers an ineffective impulse. The presence of PVC's identify the type of pacing.

ARTIFICIAL PACEMAKERS (AP)

"DEMAND" PACEMAKERS

"Demand" artificial pacemakers perform two types of pacing modalities: QRS-synchronous and QRS-inhibited pacing.

A. QRS - SYNCHRONOUS PACING

The QRS-synchronous pacemaker senses the ventricular potentials of spontaneous beats and immediately delivers an impulse. However, the stimulus falls within the ventricular refractory period and is only able to deform the morphology of the QRS. The impulse delivery during a spontaneous beat discharges the pacemaker and initiates a new recharging cycle; this prevents the appearance of competitive rhythms during the vulnerable period of the ventricular repolarization. If spontaneous ventricular activity is not present, after a predetermined interval of time the pacemaker starts a fixed rate pacing until a new spontaneous rhythm appears.

Tracings of fig. 100-A illustrate the typical behavior of a "demand" *QRS-synchronous pacemaker*. The first two beats of the upper tracing show pacemaker impulses (Ps) with a complete ventricular capture. The third complex is a sinus beat conducted to the ventricle (C). The QRS is preceded by a sinus P wave with a P-R interval of 0.20 seconds. At the beginning of the spontaneous ventricular depolarization, the pacemaker senses the ventricular potentials and delivers an impulse. However, the spike can only deform the recording of the conducted QRS. The conducted beat is followed by a pause with no atrial or ventricular activity. Therefore, after an interval of 800 msec., the pacemaker delivers a new impulse with a complete ventricular capture (Ps). This interval is called *stand-by interval* and is predetermined for each pacemaker at the moment of implantation. If ventricular activity is not present and an artifical stimulation is requested, at the end of the *stand-by interval,* the pacemaker starts a fixed rate pacing (beats indicated with Ps). On the other hand, if ventricular potentials are sensed, the pacemaker delivers the impulse into the absolute ventricular refractory phase following the spontaneous QRS (beats indicated by the arrows). The bottom tracing of fig. 100-A was recorded from the same patient and the diagram illustrates the mechanism of action of the pacemaker. Two conducted QRS's are present and they are deformed by the artificial impulse.

Fig. 100-B presents a sinus rhythm with normal conduction to the ventricles. Since the pacer is continuously triggered by the spontaneous ventricular potentials, all the QRS's are altered by a pacemaker spike. The restoration of a normal A-V conduction in a patient with a permanent pacemaker is not a rare finding and, therefore, the presence of a *"demand" pacemaker* such as the *QRS-synchronous type* eliminates the possibility of competitive rhythms (which would be present when using a fixed rate or synchronous pacemaker).

Fig. 100-C shows a ventricular pacing with a rate of 75/min. P waves are recognizable and are dissociated from the ventricular rhythm. The tracing suggests the presence of an asynchronous pacer. However, two ventricular extrasystoles (arrows) clearly show a superimposed pacemaker spike and, therefore, indicate that a *QRS-synchronous "demand" pacemaker* is operating.

ARTIFICIAL PACEMAKERS

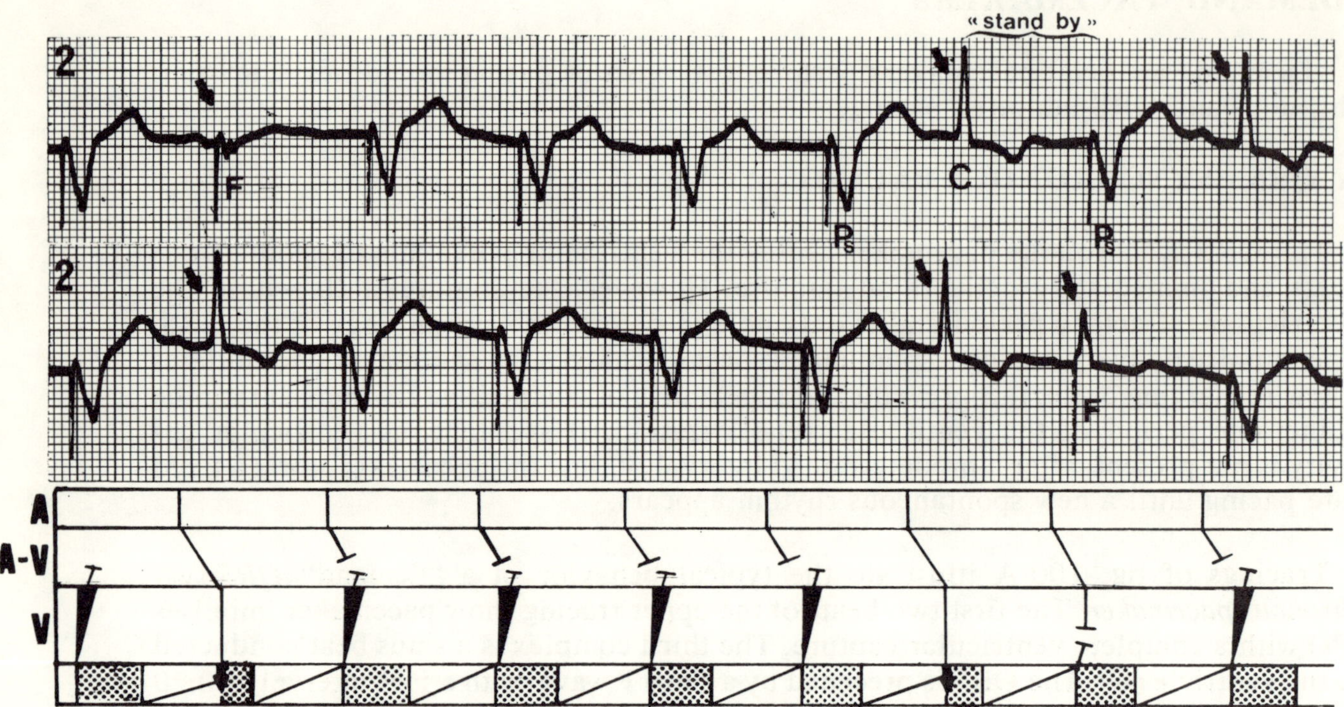

Fig. 101-A - Artificial pacemakers. QRS-inhibited "demand" pacing. The arrows indicate
sinus beats, conducted to the ventricles (C), inhibiting the pacemaker. F
= fusion beats.

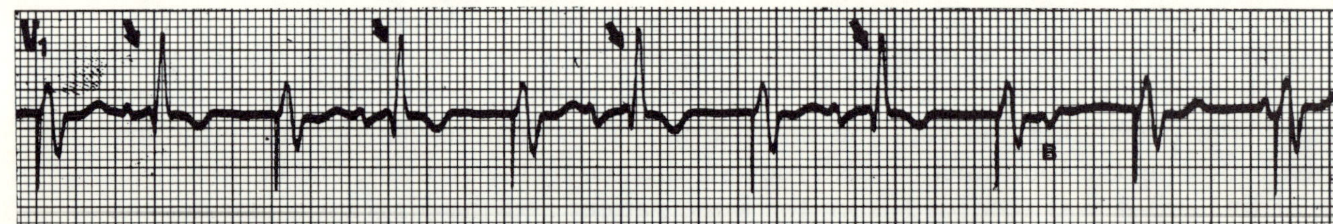

Fig. 101-B - Artificial pacemakers. QRS-inhibited "demand" pacing. Every other QRS
complex is a sinus beat, conducted to the ventricles, and with a P-R interval of
different duration. Sinus beats inhibit the pacemaker and determine a
bigeminal rhythm. B = blocked P wave.

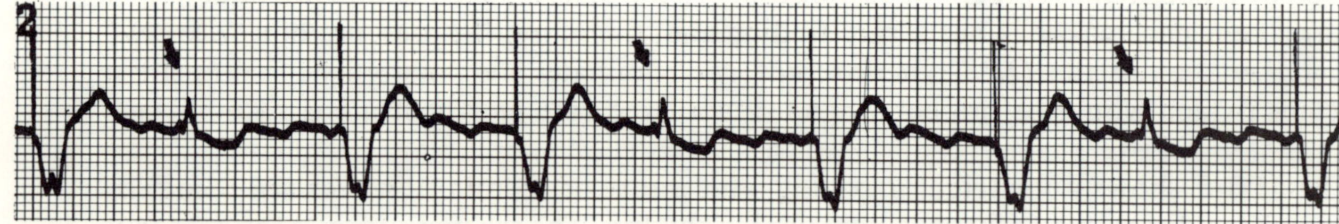

Fig. 101-C - Artificial pacemakers. QRS-inhibited "demand" pacing. The basic rhythm is
an atrial flutter. Occasionally, atrial impulses are conducted to the ventricle
(arrow) and inhibit the pacemaker.

ARTIFICIAL PACEMAKERS (AP)

"DEMAND" PACEMAKERS

B. QRS-INHIBITED PACING

This is also a "demand" or "stand-by" type of pacemaker. However, it works in a totally opposite fashion than the QRS-synchronous pacer. If spontaneous ventricular activity is not present, the pacemaker stimulates the ventricles at a fixed rate. When a spontaneous QRS appears, the pacer senses the ventricular potentials and *it is inhibited*. This means that the *pacemaker is discharged without delivering an impulse*, and initiates a new recharging cycle. If spontaneous ventricular activity continues to be present, the pacemaker is continuously inhibited and the ECG will not show any pacemaker spikes. When spontaneous ventricular activity is absent, after a *stand-by interval,* which is predetermined at the moment of implantation, the pacemaker starts a *fixed rate or automatic pacing*.

Tracings of fig. 101-A are typical of a QRS-inhibited pacing. During the conduction of a sinus beat to the ventricles (C), the pacemaker is inhibited and the spike does not appear on the ECG. The two beats indicated with "F" are fusion beats. The pacemaker *stand-by* interval has expired and, therefore, it delivers an artificial impulse, just when an almost simultaneous sinus impulse reaches the ventricles. The ventricular activation is divided between the sinus and the artificial impulses (fusion beat).

Fig. 101-B shows a bigeminal rhythm. The patient has a QRS-inhibited pacemaker and some of the sinus P waves are conducted to the ventricles (arrows). The sinus beats inhibit the pacemaker and the bigeminal rhythm is formed by a sinus and an artificial beat. The variable length of the P-R intervals of the sinus beats is due to: a) position of sinus P waves in relation to the preceding pacemaker QRS complex; b) concealed retrograde V-A conduction of the pacemaker beats. A P wave is slightly more premature and it is blocked within the A-V junction (B). This happens because the artificial impulse penetrates into the A-V tissue in a retrograde fashion (see page 196). The last three beats reveal the automatic pacing rate (88/min.).

A QRS-inhibited "demand" ventricular pacing is present within the atrial flutter of fig. 101-C. The A-V ratio of the flutter is variable and the beats conducted to the ventricles (arrows) do not show a pacemaker spile. When the A-V block determines an asystolic pause longer than the pacer's stand-by interval, the pacemaker captures the ventricles with an automatic beat.

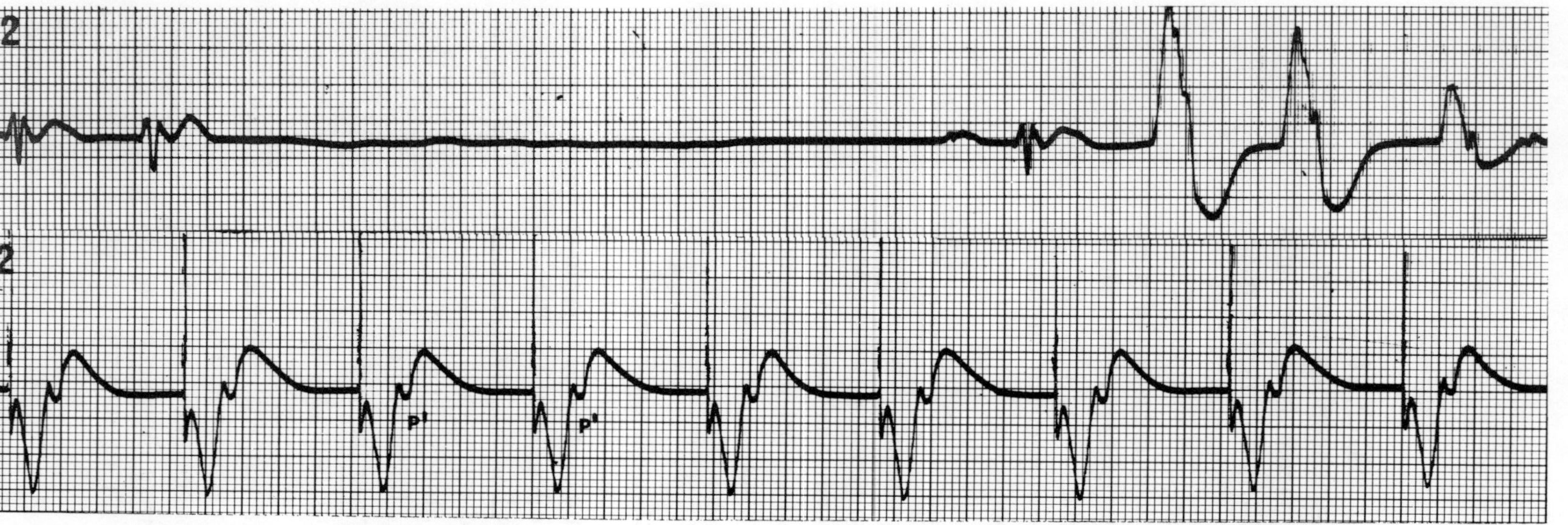

Fig. 102-A - Artificial pacemakers. Transthoracic emergency pacing of a patient with prolonged asystoles (upper tracing). The artificial impulses obtain a good ventricular capture and determine retrograde P¹ waves (bottom tracing).

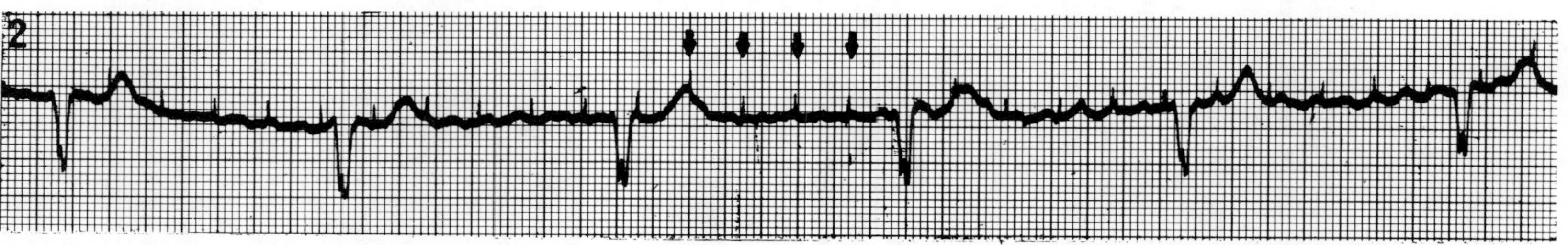

Fig. 102-B - Artificial pacemakers. "Runaway pacemaker". The arrows indicate rapid firing pacemaker spikes (140/min.) which do not capture the ventricles. Idio-ventricular beats maintain the cardiac rhythm.

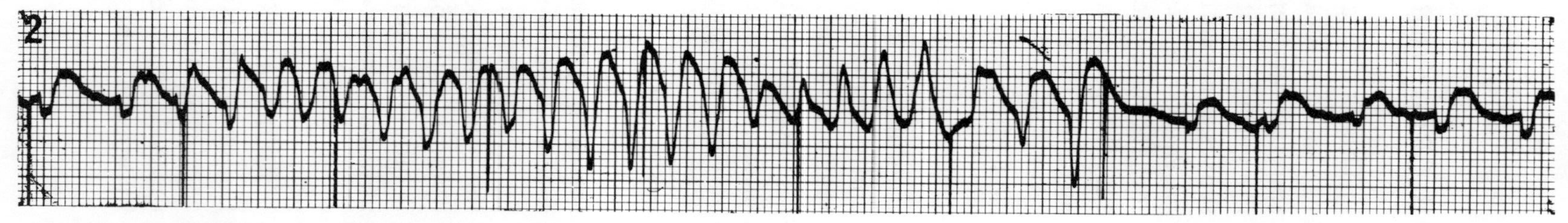

Fig. 102-C - Artificial pacemakers. Fixed rate pacing and ventricular fibrillation.

Tracings of fig. 102-A illustrate an emergency artificial pacing obtained with an intra-myocardial electrode introduced transthoracically. This type of pacing is performed in a situation of extreme emergency, as is indicated by the upper tracing of fig. 102-A. A prolonged asystole (5 secs.) is followed by several ventricular extrasystoles. The rhythm is promptly re-established with the transthoracic insertion of a wire into the myocardial tissue and connected to an external battery. A fixed rate pacing is performed with a complete ventricular capture. P^1 waves are present after each QRS and indicate a good retrograde conduction of the impulse to the atria.

Fig. 102-B presents a rapid artificial pacing (240/min.) without ventricular capture. An idio-ventricular rhythm is simultaneously present with a rate of 40/min. This situation is extremely dangerous and is metaphorically called "runaway pacemaker". The rapid firing of spikes indicate battery exhaustion and may stimulate the endocardium with disastrous consequences (for ex. degenerating into ventricular tachycardia and fibrillation).

Fig. 102-C shows the coexistence of a ventricular fibrillation and ineffective pacing (70/min.). This is a situation of extreme importance because it has been reported that a ventricular fibrillation, in a patient with a pacemaker, may not trigger the alarms of a Coronary Care Unit. This happens because the regular pacemaker spikes are interpreted as heart beats by the monitors and the alarms remain silent.

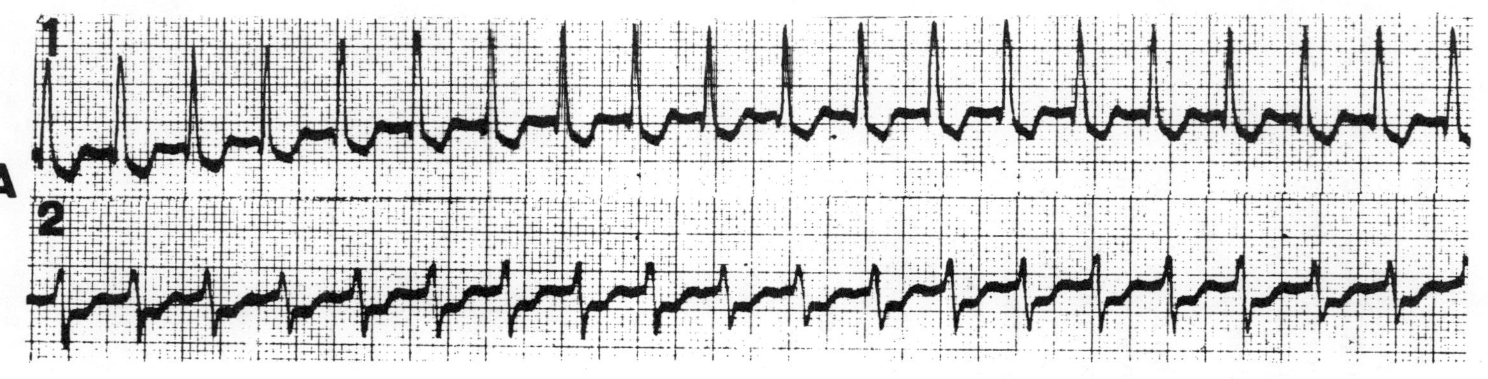

Fig. 103-A - Control standard leads. The rhythm is tachycardic and the underlying mechanism is not clearly evident.

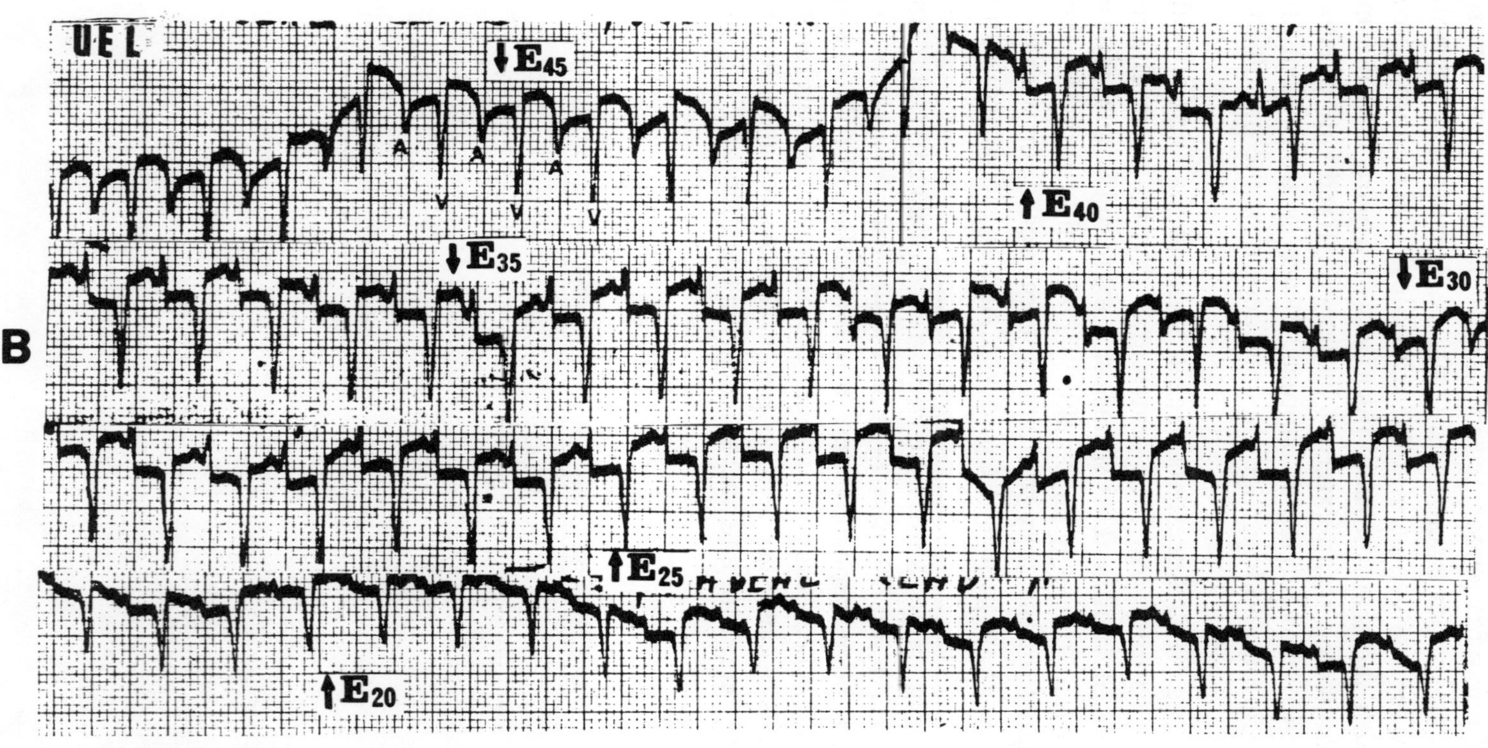

Fig. 103-B - Unipolar esophageal leads (UEL). E45, E40, etc. represent the distance in centimeters between the esophageal electrodes and the patient's nostrils. P waves (A) and the QRS complexes (V) are easily recognized. The rhythm is a sinus tachycardia with a first degree A-V block.

ESOPHAGEAL LEADS

The once commonly used *esophageal leads* have been today replaced by the great simplicity and better quality of the intracavitary leads. Esophageal leads are utilized to decipher those arrhythmias whose mechanism is not clear on the surface ECG.

A classical example of *esophageal leads* recording is presented in tracings A and B of figs. 103-A and 103-B. Tracings A show the recording of L1 and L2 of a not well defined supraventricular tachyarrhythmia. A unipolar esophageal lead (UEL) is recorded by positioning the tip of the catheter into the esophagus at different levels from the patient's nostrils.

Tracings B are recorded while the esophageal catheter is gradually pulled back from a distance of 45 cm. At E45 the atrial activation waves (A) may be clearly distinguished from the ventricular waves (V). The atrial waves appear as negative deflections and are separated from the ventricular complexes, which are of a greater amplitude and show an elevation of the ST segment. With a pull back of 5 cm. (E40) the atrial waves become clearly biphasic. At the E35 level the catheter tip is very close to the posterior atrial wall, and this is the area in which atrial activation potentials become very clear and sharply separated by the ventricular one. At a more proximal level (E30) the atrial waves become more positive and their amplitude gradually decreases. At E20 level the atrial potentials are barely visible while the ventricular ones are still clearly recorded. Thus, the esophageal leads clarify the mechanism of the arrhythmia which is a *sinus tachycardia with a first degree A-V block*.

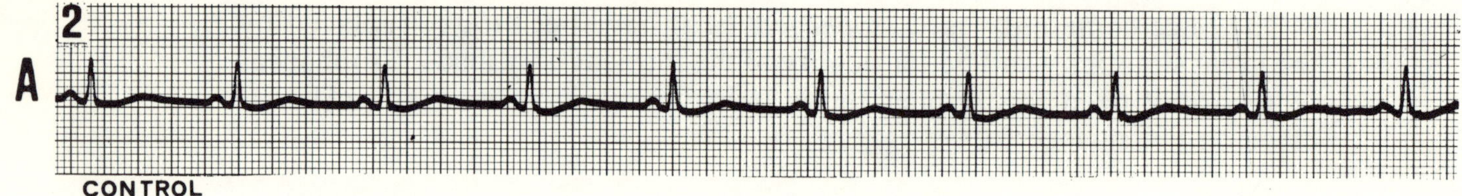

Fig. 104-A - Normal sinus rhythm.

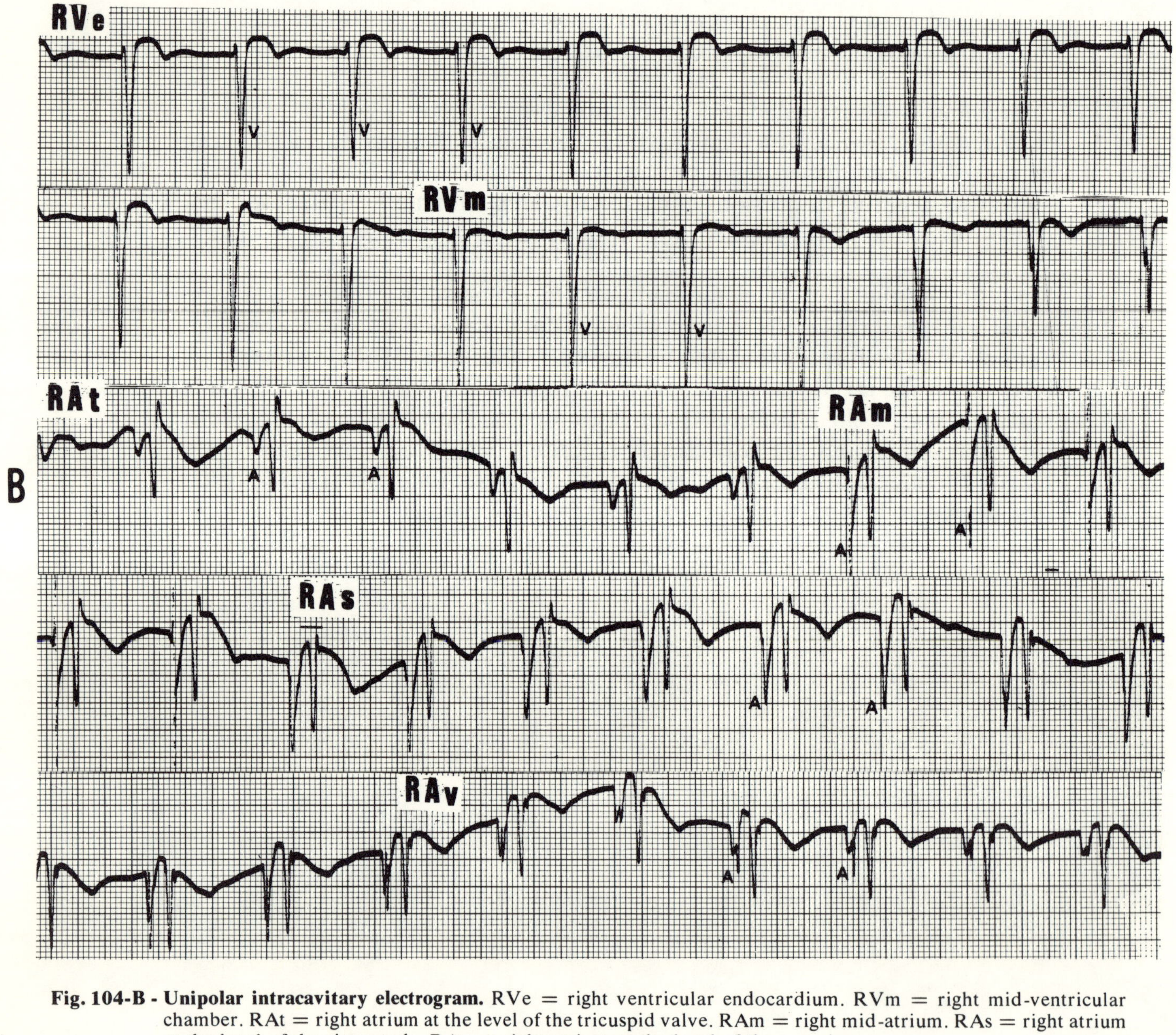

Fig. 104-B - Unipolar intracavitary electrogram. RVe = right ventricular endocardium. RVm = right mid-ventricular chamber. RAt = right atrium at the level of the tricuspid valve. RAm = right mid-atrium. RAs = right atrium at the level of the sinus node. RAv = right atrium at the level of the superior vena cava.

INTRACAVITARY LEADS

They are commonly called *intracavitary cardiac electrograms*. They may be
of two types:
   a) *unipolar electrograms*.
   b) *bipolar electrograms*.

A - UNIPOLAR ELECTROGRAMS

The recent development of cardiac catherization techniques has made
this type of intracavitary recordings very popular in clinical practice. Intracavitary electrograms are often indispensable in clarifying the mechanism of complex arrhythmias.

A typical recording of a *right atrial and right ventricular unipolar
electrogram* is presented in figs. 104-A and 104-B. Tracing "A" shows a normal sinus rhythm in a control tracing recorded in L2.
Tracings "B" shows a recording from a catheter introduced into the right
ventricular apex under fluoroscopic control. The electrograms is recorded
while the operator slowly pulls back the catheter first from the ventricle
into the right atrium, and then into the superior vena cava. When the
catheter tip is in direct contact with the right ventricular endocardium
(RVe), ventricular activation potentials are recorded (V); they appear as
negative and high amplitude S waves, and are preceded by small r waves.
The ST segment elevation is caused by the slight pressure of the tip of the
catheter on the ventricular endocardium. At this level, the atrial potentials
are so small that they are not visible on the tracing.
When the tip of the catheter is slowly pulled back and is left floating into
the middle right ventricular chamber (RVm), RS complexes are recorded
and the ST segment becomes flat on the base line. The different configuration of the ST segment in RVe and RVm position is clear cut, as can be observed in the top two tracings of fig. 102-B. At the level of the tricuspid
valve (RAt), atrial activation potentials start to appear (A) while the
amplitude of the ventricular potentials is noticably reduced. In the mid portion of the right atrium (RAm) the atrial activation waves have the highest
amplitude and are biphasic. The RAm is the preferred site for recording
atrial unipolar electrograms (AUE). Moving toward the superior vena cava,
and in the proximity of the sinus node (RAs), the atrial activation waves appear as negative deflections. At the level of the superior vena cava (RAv)
they show a W shaped configuration and a smaller amplitude. However,
remember that the configuration of the atrial unipolar electrogram may
change, and sometimes markedly, in relation to the position of the
electrode, the respiratory phases and the location of the atrial activation
focus.

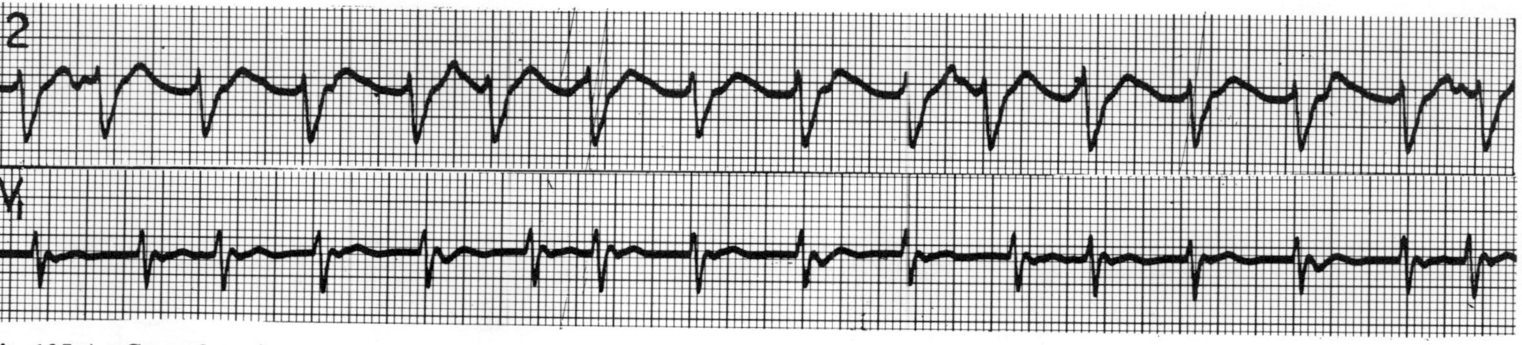

Fig. 105-A - Control tracings.

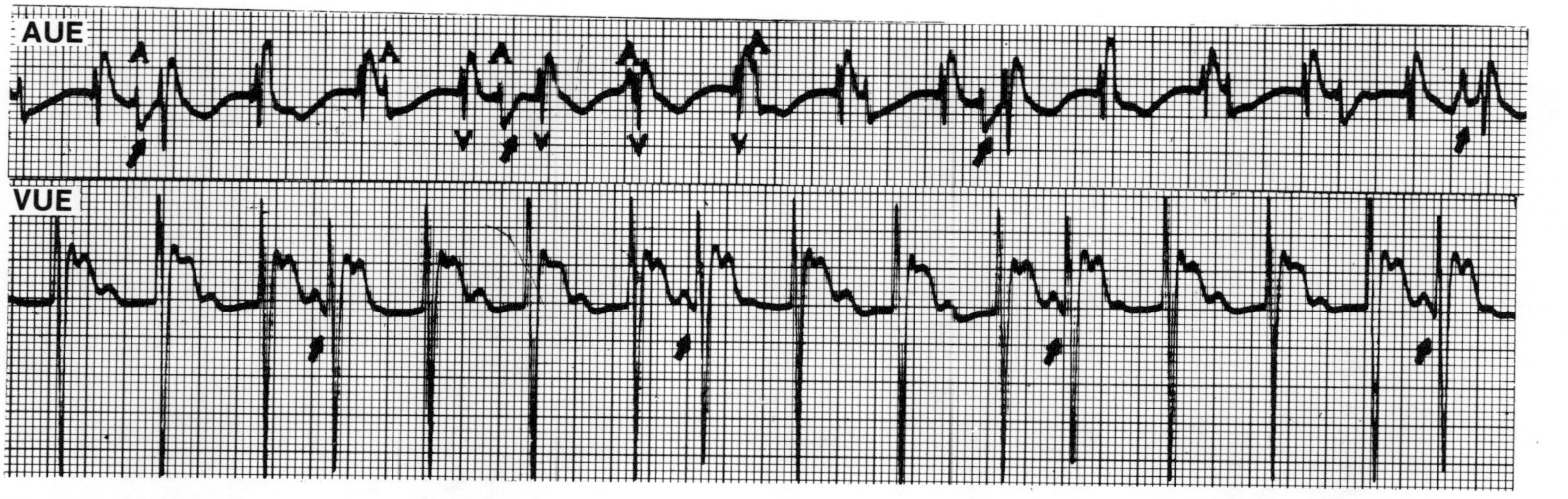

Fig. 105-B - Unipolar intracavitary electrograms. The atrial unipolar electrogram (AUE) reveals a dissociation between atria (A) and ventricles (V). Ventricular capture beats are also present (arrows). The tracings are not simultaneous.

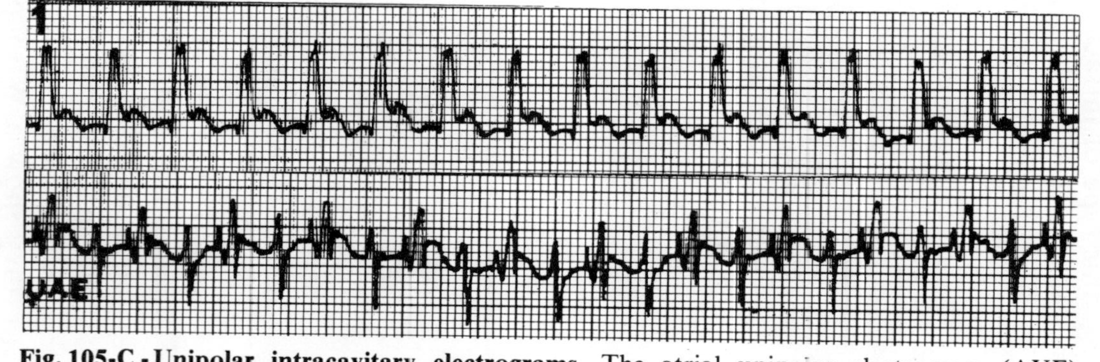

Fig. 105-C - Unipolar intracavitary electrograms. The atrial unipolar electrogram (AUE) indicates a sinus tachycardia with a first degree A-V block.

UNIPOLAR ELECTROGRAMS

Tracings of figs. 105-A and 105-B present a situation in which the recording of intracavitary potentials is of decisive importance for a correct diagnosis of the arrhythmia.

Fig. 105-A shows an irregular rhythm. P or P¹ waves are not clearly evident. A slight undulation of the base line suggests the presence of an atrial fibrillation.

The *atrial unipolar* (AUE) and the *ventricular unipolar* electrograms (VUE) of fig. 105-B reveal the true mechanism of the arrhythmia:

a) Atrial activation waves are clearly visible in the AUE (A). Their rate is 85/min., and it is slower and independent from the ventricular rate measured from the V waves (120/min.). Therefore, an *atrio-ventricular dissociation* is present.

b) Some of the ventricular complexes have definitely shorter V-V intervals (arrows). This is evident also on the surface ECG. When this happens, the QRS is preceded by a P wave with a variable P-R interval. These are *ventricular capture beats,* which confirm the diagnosis of A-V dissociation (see page 122).

The rhythm of the upper tracing of fig. 105-C (L2) is not very clear and suggests the possibility of a paroxysmal atrial tachycardia with a 2:1 A-V block. The *atrial unipolar electrogram* (AUE) reveals the mechanism of the arrhythmia. The rhythm is a sinus tachycardia with a first degree A-V block.

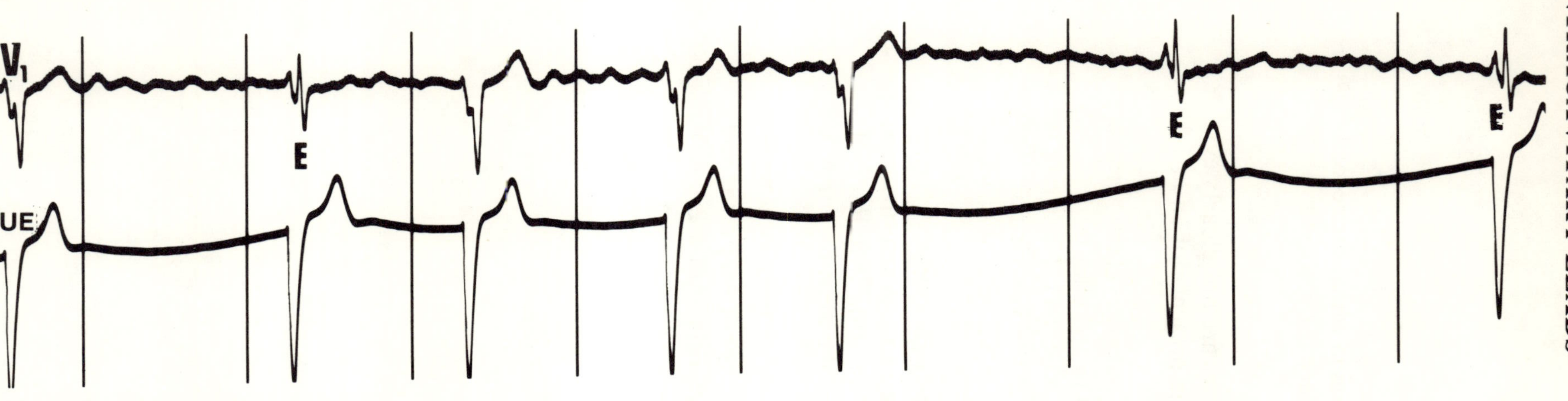

Fig. 106-A - Unipolar intracavitary electrograms. The atrial fibrillation, with a high degree of A-V block, allows for the emergency of ventricular escape beats (E). The latter are not recognizable in the ventricular unipolar electrogram (VUE). Tracings are simultaneous.

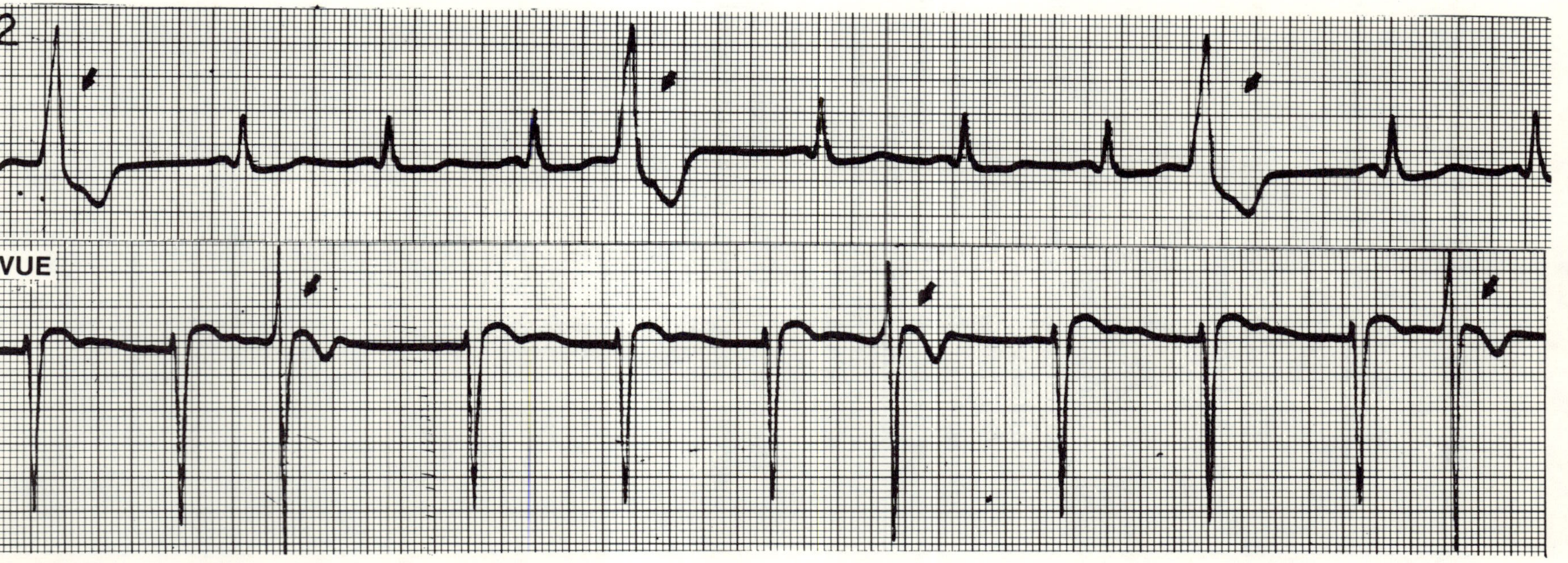

Fig. 106-B - Unipolar intracavitary electrograms. Tracings are not simultaneous. Both the ventricular unipolar electrogram (VUE) and the control L2 show ventricular extrasystoles with a morphology different from that of sinus beats.

UNIPOLAR ELECTROGRAMS

Fig. 106-A presents the L1 recording of the irregular ventricular response of an atrial fibrillation with a high degree of A-V block. The second complex is a ventricular escape beat (E) and it is followed by three conducted beats and by two ventricular escape beats. Note that the ventricular escape beats appear always after a long asystolic pause, which is due to an intermittent third degree or complete A-V block.

The ventricular unipolar electrogram (VUE), recorded simultaneously to the surface ECG, shows ventricular complexes separated by an isoelectric line. This indicates one of the VUE's limitations. The presence of escape beats may not be recognized by the intracardic potentials, since their morphology is not different than that of supraventricular beats conducted to the ventricles. In such a situation, the recording of atrial potentials would be similar to that of a surface ECG and would show fibrillatory waves with an amplitude similar to that recorded on the surface ECG.

Fig. 106-B shows a sinus rhythm and ventricular extrasystoles with fixed coupling. The recording of the *ventricular unipolar electrogram* (VUE) is not simultaneous and shows a good contact of the catheter tip with the endocardial wall (slight elevation of the ST segment). Ventricular extrasystoles are present within the contest of the sinus rhythm, and appear as biphasic complexes with clearly inverted P waves.

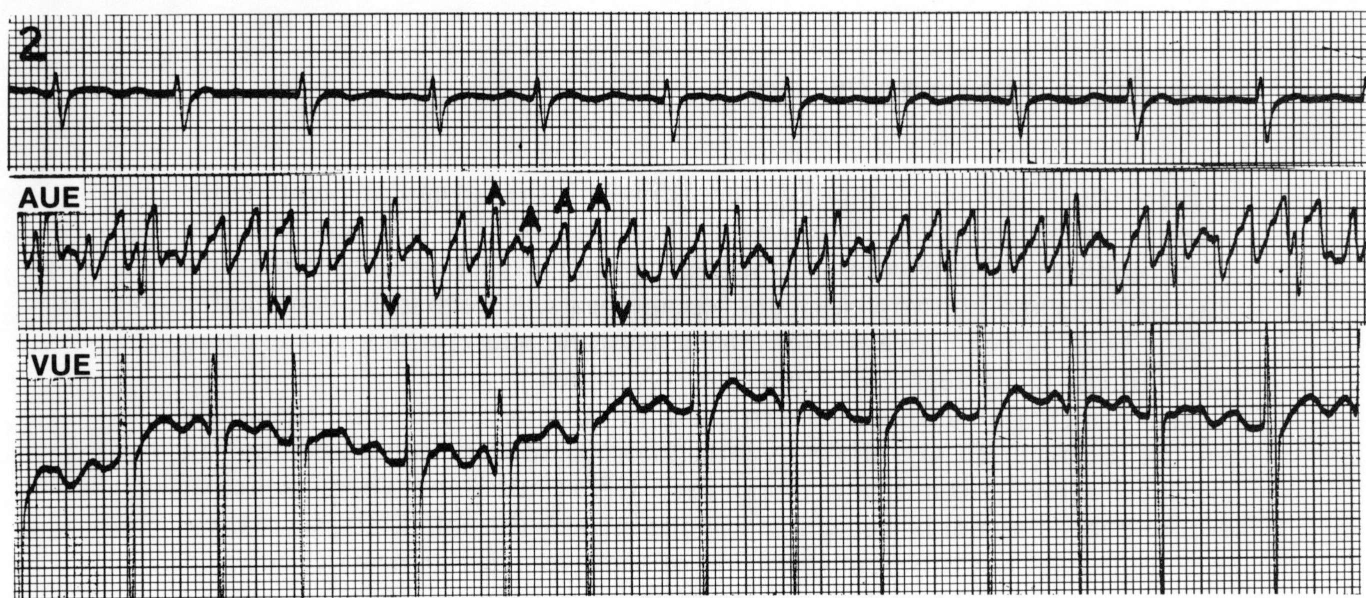

Fig. 107-A - Unipolar intracavitary electrograms. The mechanism of the arrhythmia is not evident in L2. The atrial unipolar electrogram (AUE) reveals the rapid waves of an atrial flutter (A) with a variable A-V ratio. V = ventricular depolarization. Tracings are not simultaneous.

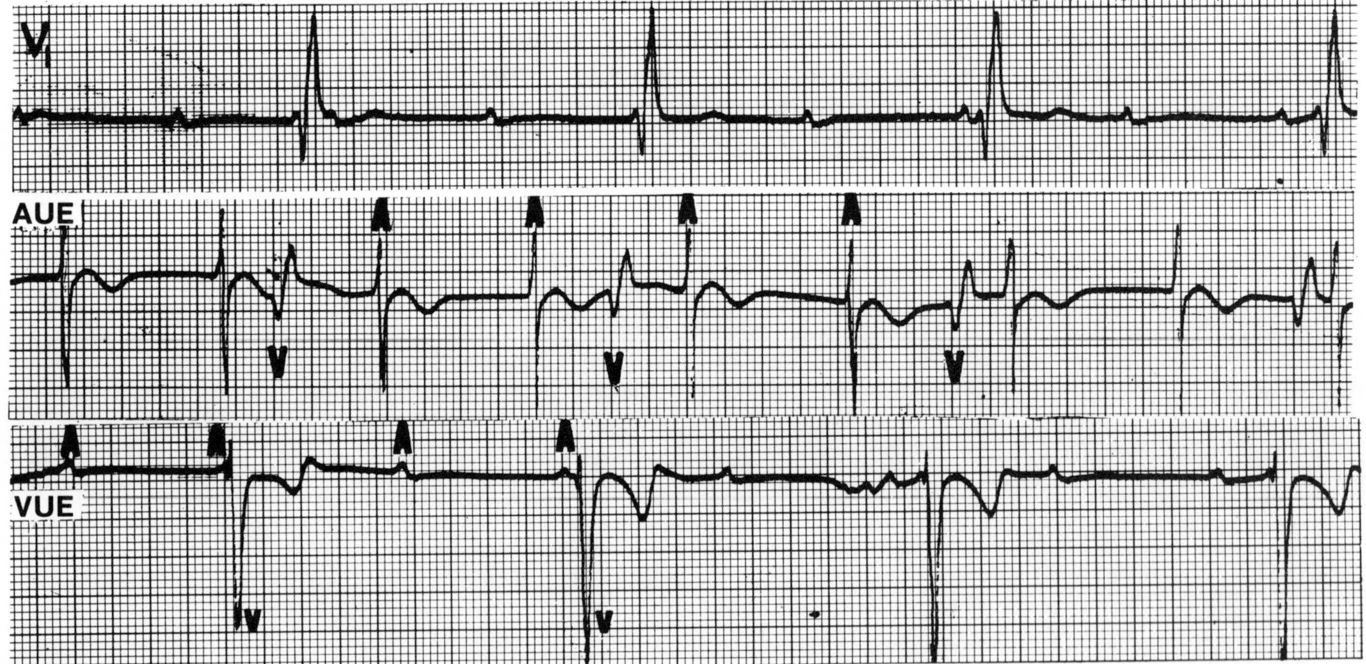

Fig. 107-B - Unipolar intracavitary electrograms.. The atrial (AUE) and ventricular unipolar electrograms (VUE) are recorded during the insertion of a pacing catheter for a complete A-V block. The atrial (A) and ventricular (V) waves are clearly independent. Tracings are not simultaneous.

UNIPOLAR ELECTROGRAMS

Fig. 107-A shows a L2 recording of a rhythm with an irregular ventricular rate and an undulating baseline. The differential diagnosis is between atrial flutter with variable A-V block and atrial fibrillation.

The atrial unipolar electrogram (AUE), which is not simultaneous, clearly shows the regular and rapid atrial activation waves (A) of an atrial flutter with a rate of 300/min. The atrial waves are mixed with ventricular complexes (V) which are irregular for the presence of a variable A-V block.

The ventricular unipolar electrogram (VUE) is of very little help. It only shows the undulation of the baseline between the ventricular complexes.

Fig. 107-B is the recording of an *atrial unipolar electrogram* (AUE) and a *ventricular unipolar electrogram* (VUE) in a patient with a third degree A-V block. The recording of intracavitary potentials is frequently used as a guide for positioning a catheter into the right ventricular chamber in the absence of a fluoroscopic control. Lead V1 shows the complete independence of P waves and QRS complexes. The atria are under sinus control (75/min.) while the ventricles, for the presence of a complete A-V block, are governed by an idio-ventricular pacemaker with a rate of 32/min.

The atrial unipolar electrogram (AUE) is recorded during the insertion of a pacing catheter without fluoroscopy and indicates that the catheter tip is located in the right atrial chamber. The atrial depolarization waves (A) are clearly visible and their rate is faster than the ventricular activation waves (V). Once the catheter crosses the tricuspid valve, the recording drastically changes (VUE). While the atrial waves decrease in amplitude, the ventricular depolarization waves indicate a good contact of the catheter tip with the endocardium. This is the moment when the electrical pacing is usually initiated.

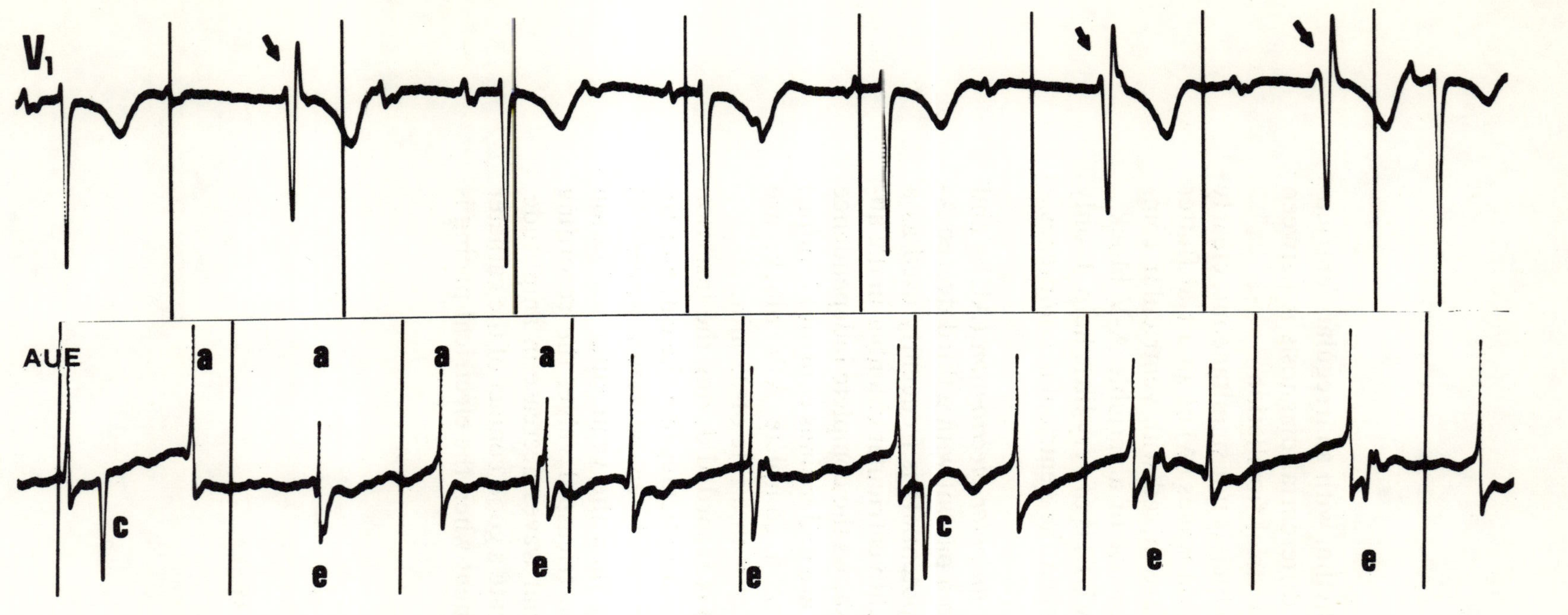
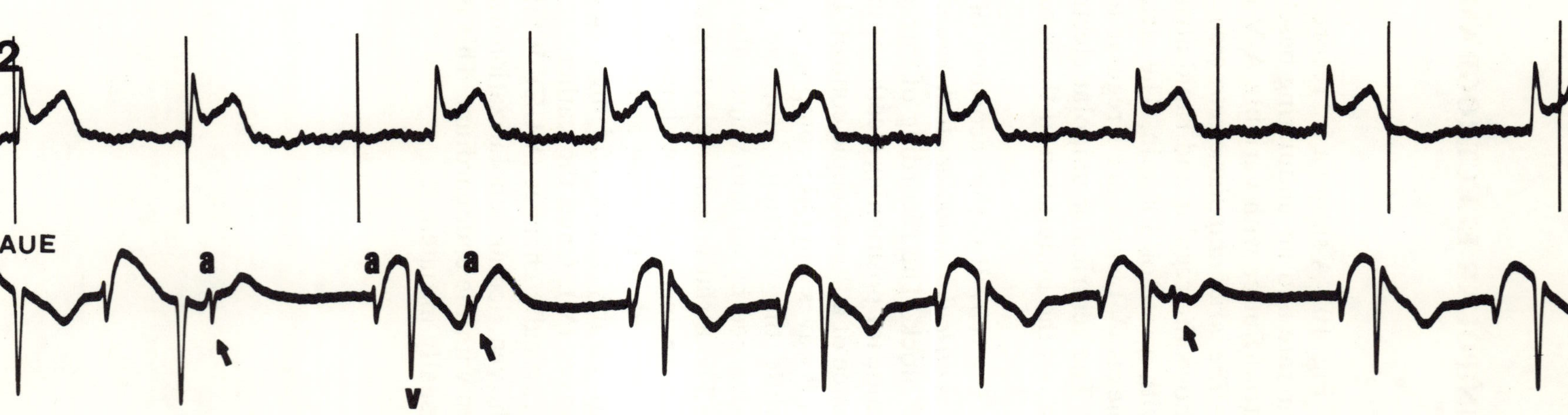

Fig. 108-A - Unipolar intracavitary electrograms. Chaotic atrial tachycardia. Several atrial impulses are blocked and allow for the escape of ventricular beats (arrows). The atrial unipolar electrogram (AUE) shows: a = atrial activation waves; c = atrial impulse conducted to the ventricles; e = escape beat. Tracings are not simultaneous.

UNIPOLAR ELECTROGRAMS

The V1 lead recorded in the upper tracing of fig. 108-A shows QRS complexes with two different morphologies and irregular atrial waves scattered throughout the tracing. Some of the atrial waves seems to conduct to the ventricles with different P-R intervals. The first, third, fourth, fifth, and last QRS are of supraventricular origin while the second, sixth, and seventh QRS (arrow) have a different morphology and are preceded by prolonged asystolic pauses. The latter are ventricular escape beats which follow blocked atrial beats.

The *atrial unipolar electrogram (AUE),* which is not simultaneous, confirms the presence of a *chaotic atrial tachycardia*, with P^1 waves occasionally being conducted to the ventricles (the conducted QRS's are indicated with C). The P^1-R intervals are different in relation to the location of the atrial ectopic foci and the prematurity of the impulses. Several ventricular escape beats (E) follow the blocked atrial waves.

Fig. 108-B shows L2 of a patient with the typical QRS changes of an acute myocardial infarction. The R-R intervals are, at times, regular and the P waves are not clearly visible. The atrial unipolar electrogram (AUE), which is not simultaneous, reveals a sinus rhythm with blocked atrial extrasystoles which are followed by an incomplete compensatory pause. The atrial waves are indicated with "a", while the arrows point to the blocked PAC's. Furthermore, the P-R segment of the atrial waves is clearly elevated. It is commonly believed that this may be due to a disturbance in the atrial repolarization (Ta wave) and, therefore, would indicate an acute injury of the atrial wall.

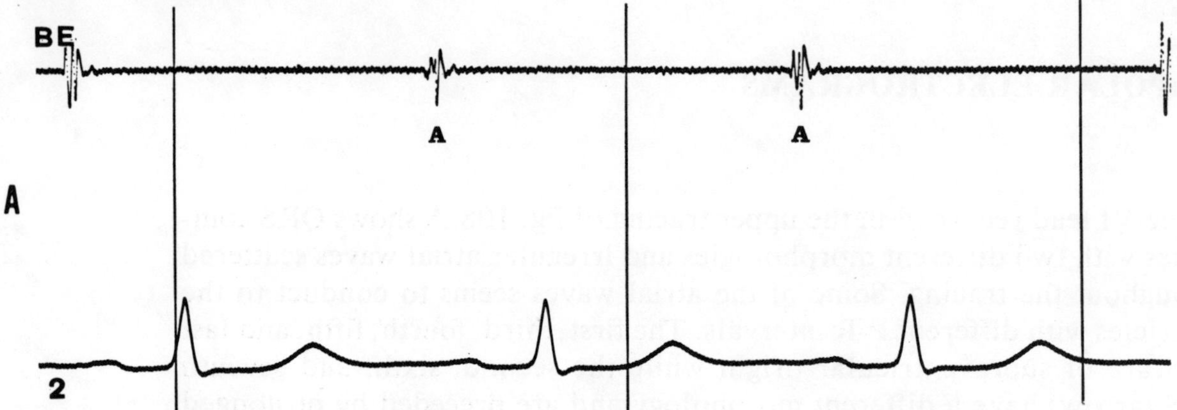

Fig. 109-A - **Bipolar intracavitary electrograms.** The bipolar electrogram (BE) records the atrial activation waves (A) simultaneously to the P waves (L2). The tip of the catheter is in the right atrium.

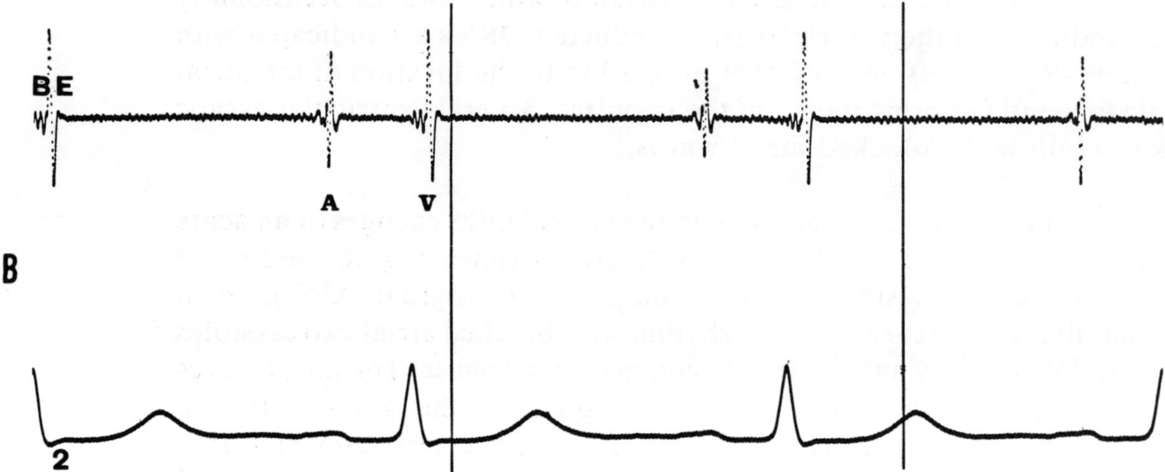

Fig. 109-B - **Bipolar intracavitary electrograms.** The bipolar electrogram is recorded at the level of the tricuspid valve. The atrial (A) and ventricular (V) potentials are simultaneous to the P waves and QRS complexes of the surface ECG.

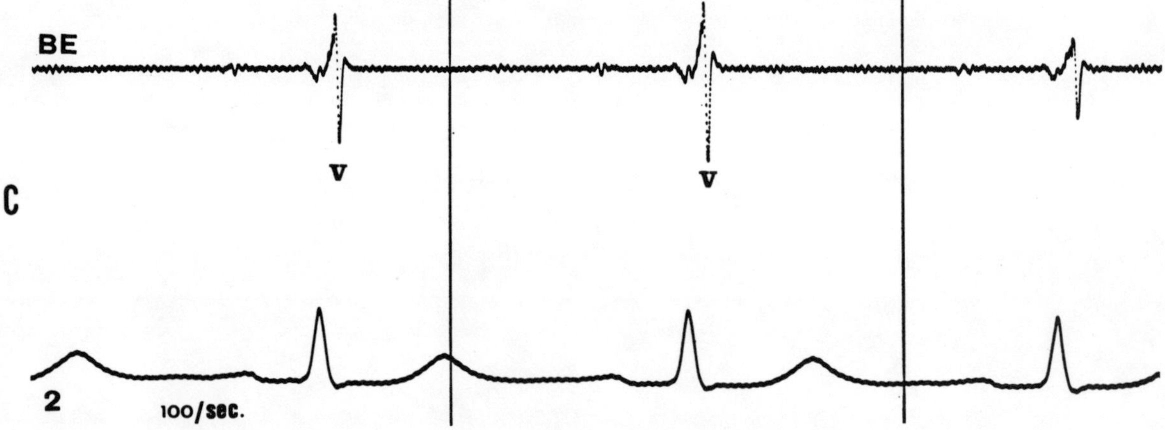

Fig. 109-C - **Bipolar intracavitary electrograms.** The bipolar electrogram (BE) is recorded in the right ventricle. Only ventricular potentials are being recorded.

B - INTRACAVITARY BIPOLAR ELECTROGRAMS

If the tip of the catheter introduced into a cardiac chamber has two electrodes close to each other, the intracavitary potentials which are recorded represent the electrical phenomena occurring between, or in close proximity, of the two electrodes. Therefore, the catheter picks up the depolarization only of those myocardial areas adjacent to the electrodes and does not record what happens in distant areas.

Fig. 109-A shows a classic recording of an *intracavitary bipolar electrogram* (BE) in a patient with a sinus rhythm. L2 is simultaneously recorded. The catheter is positioned under fluoroscopic control in the right atrium and the potentials recorded originate from a myocardial area in close proximity to the two electrodes (A). Other atrial or ventricular areas are not recorded by the narrow field between the two electrodes. The potentials are inscribed simultaneously to the sinus P waves recorded in L2.

In tracing 109-B, the catheter tip is advanced under fluoroscopic control at the level of the tricuspid valve. Atrial potentials (A) of areas close to the A-V junction are recorded simultaneously to ventricular activation potentials (V). The V potentials are of a high septal origin, which is that area of myocardium closer to the exploring poles.

In fig. 109-C the catheter is further advanced into the mid-ventricular chamber. At this level, while the atrial disappear, the ventricular potentials (V) persist and become more evident. The ventricular potentials are simultaneously recorded with the QRS complexes of the surface ECG.

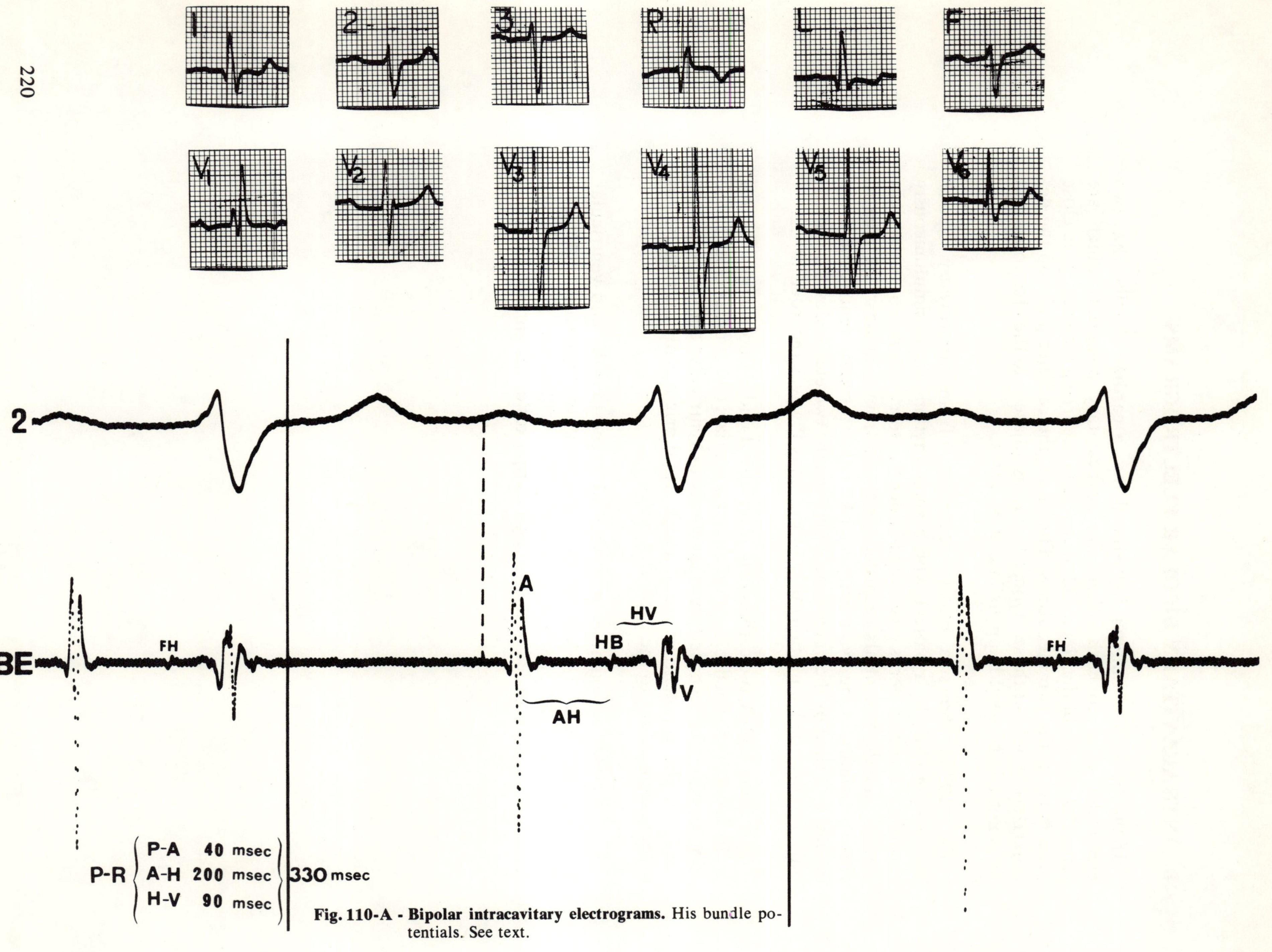

Fig. 110-A - Bipolar intracavitary electrograms. His bundle potentials. See text.

INTRACAVITARY LEADS

BIPOLAR ELECTROGRAMS. HIS BUNDLE POTENTIALS

With the use of multipolar intracavitary catheters, inserted under fluoroscopic control, it is today possible to record electrical potentials of specific conduction tissue (A-V node, His bundle, proximal portions of the right and left bundles). These potentials are not recorded by the surface ECG. In recent years the *technique of His bundle potentials recording* has been perfected and it has opened new ways of diagnosing A-V conduction abnormalities. Without the help of His bundle recording, which enables the exploration of areas electrically "silent" (such as the P-R interval of the surface ECG), an exact localization of abnormal A-V conductions would not be possible.

Fig. 110-A presents the recording of *His bundle potentials* through a *bipolar intracavitary electrogram*. The patient shows a sinus rhythm with a first degree A-V block, left axis deviation and a complete right bundle branch block. The *bipolar electrogram* (BE), recorded at the level of the tricuspid valve, shows several cardiac potentials. They are:
1) potentials of atrial tissue in a close proximity to the exploring electrodes (A).
2) His bundle potentials (H).
3) potentials of ventricular tissue close to the catheter tip (V).

Furthermore, different time intervals can be measured:
a) *P-A interval* (normal = 30-50 msec.); it represents the conduction time of the stimulus from the S-A node to the atrial tissue close to the exploring poles.
b) *A-H interval* (normal = 75-100 msec.); it represents the conduction time of the stimulus from the atria to the His bundle.
c) *H-V interval* (normal = 45-50 msecs.); it represents the conduction time of the stimulus from the His bundle to the ventricular tissue included between the exploring electrodes.

In a patient with an A-V conduction abnormality, the measurement of these intervals, and the comparison with those considered "normal", indicates whether the impulse is delayed or blocked in the proximal A-V junction (atria, junction between the atrium and A-V node and the A-V node itself) or in the distal portions of the His bundle (right or left bundle).

In the case of the patient of fig. 110-A the *P-A interval* (40 msecs.) is normal while both the A-H interval (200 msecs.) and the H-V interval (90 msecs.) are markedly prolonged. This confirms what is recorded on the surface ECG. A first degree A-V block and a right bundle branch block are present, as indicated by the proximal and distal conduction abnormalities on the His bundle recording. In the presence of a complete A-V block, this technique permits one to locate the exact area of the A-V junction where the atrial impulses are being blocked.

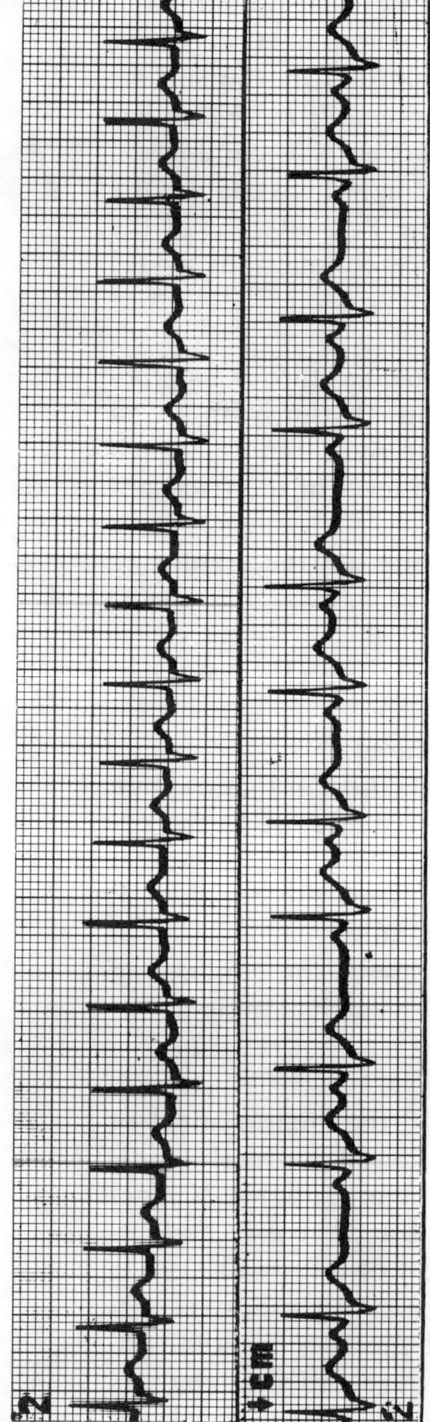

Fig. 111-A - **Carotid sinus massage.** The supraventricular tachycardia is promptly converted into a sinus rhythm. The transition is marked by several premature beats.

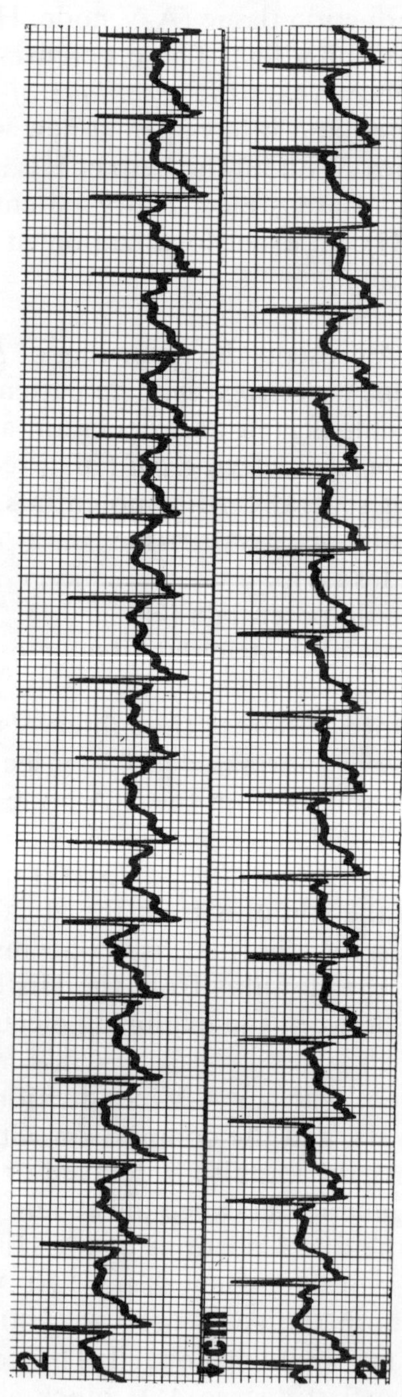

Fig. 111-B - **Carotid sinus massage.** The sinus tachycardia (upper tracing) is transformed into an A-V dissociation for the emergence of a junctional tachycardia.

The *carotid sinus massage* (as the Valsalva maneuver or the ocular compression) is a simple and effective form of vagal stimulation. It is largely used in the emergency treatment of atrial paroxysmal tachycardias or as a diagnostic tool in the diagnosis of atrial flutter and fibrillation.

When applied during an atrial paroxysmal tachycardia the carotid sinus massage may result in the following:

a)   it may be totally ineffective and the tachycardia remains unchanged;

b)   the tachycardia may cease abruptly with a conversion into a sinus rhythm;

c)   may temporarily increase the A-V block and result in a reduction of the ventricular rate.

The upper tracing of fig. 111-A presents an atrial tachycardia, with a 2:1 A-V block, which is promptly converted into a sinus rhythm with a *carotid massage* (cm). Frequent atrial extrasystoles follow the recovery of a sinus rhythm, as is shown in the lower tracing of fig. 111-A, where they are present in the form of atrial bigeminy.

In fig. 111-B the *carotid massage* (cm) is erroneously performed, in the presence of a sinus tachycardia, in a patient under digitalis therapy. The result is surprising. The slight decrease in the sinus rate, caused by the vagal stimulation, gives rise to an A-V dissociation for the emergence of a junctional tachycardia (lower tracing). The sinus P waves are very close to the QRS complexes and, therefore, they cannot conduct to the ventricles because of the simultaneous propagation of junctional impulses.

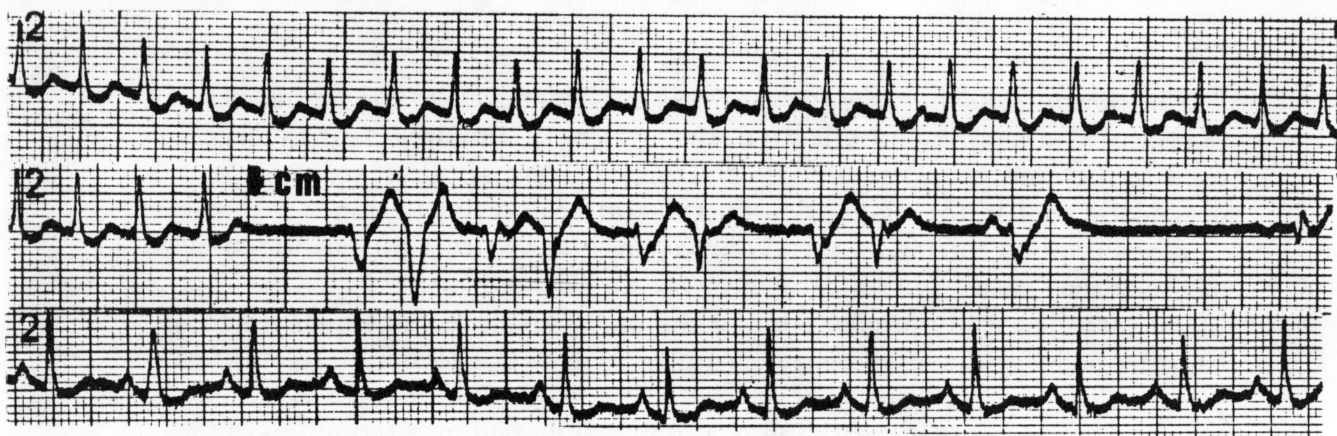

Fig. 112-A - Carotid sinus massage. The transition from a supraventricular tachycardia (first tracing) into a sinus rhythm (bottom tracing) occurs through salvos of multiform ventricular extrasystoles (middle tracing).

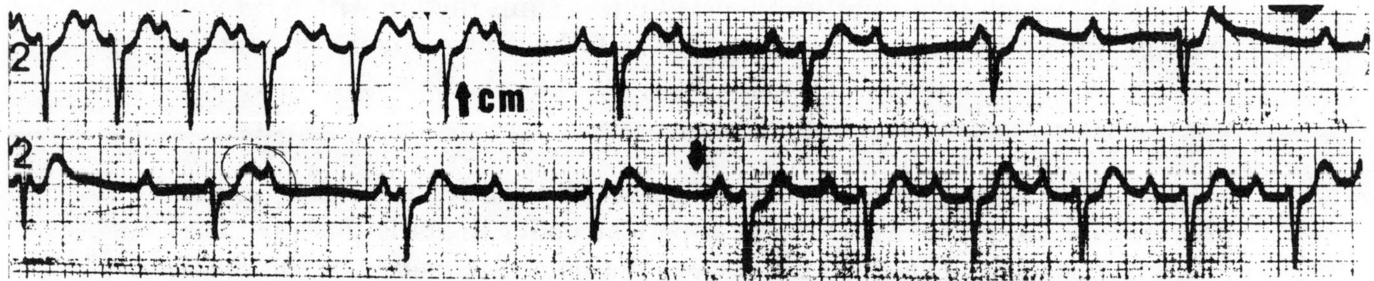

Fig. 112-B - Carotid sinus massage. The vagal stimulation induces a brief period of a third degree A-V block (interval between the two arrows).

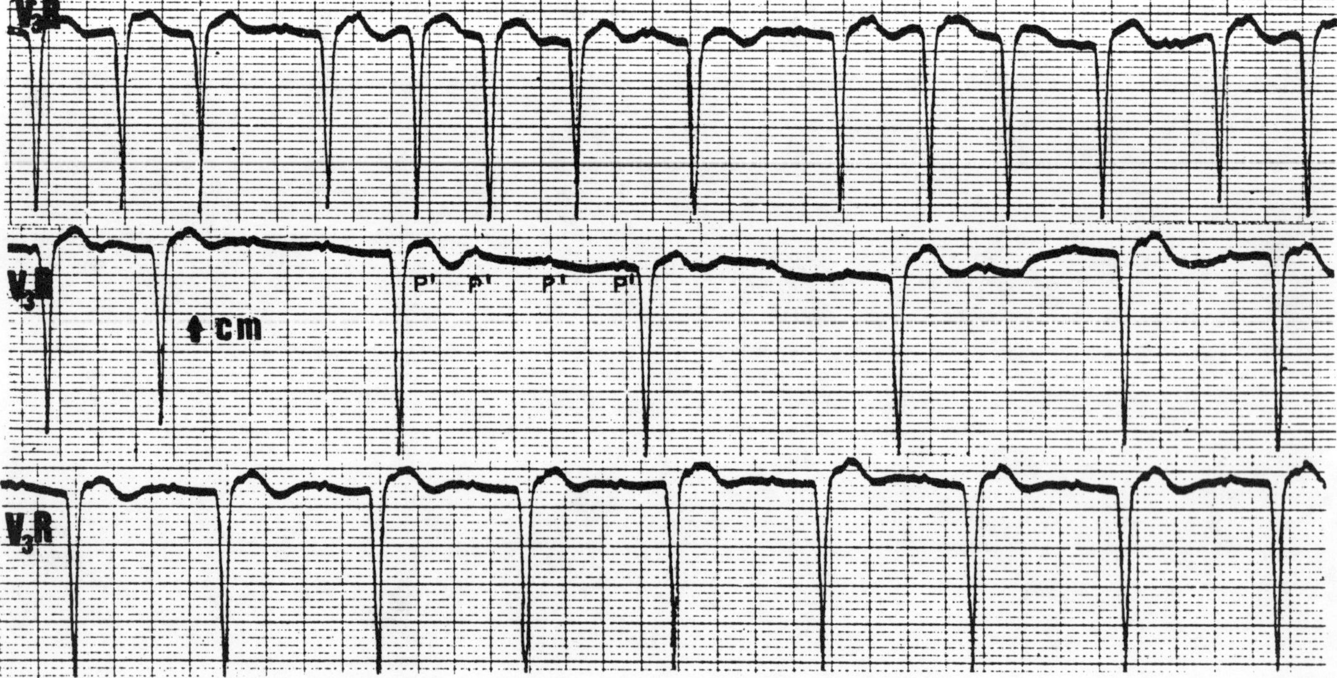

Fig. 112-C - Carotid sinus massage. The atrial tachycardia, with variable A-V block (top tracing), is transformed first into a 4:1 A-V block (middle tracing) and, finally, into a 2:1 A-V block (bottom tracing).

In patients with paroxysmal atrial tachycardias the restoration of sinus rhythm, with a carotid sinus massage, may sometime occur through dangerous transitional rhythms. This may happen because of: a) hypersensitive carotid sinuses; b) digitalis toxicity.

The upper tracing of fig. 112-A shows an atrial tachycardia with a ventricular rate of 200/min. The carotid sinus massage (cm), performed in the second tracing, is followed by a brief asystolic pause and a salvos of multiform ventricular extrasystoles, before the restoration of a sinus rhythm (lower tracing).

In fig. 112-B the application of a carotid massage in the presence of an atrial tachycardia, with a 1:1 A-V conduction and prolonged P^1-R intervals, induces a complete A-V block for almost nine seconds (P^1 waves and QRS complexes are totally independent and the ventricles are controlled by a junctional pacemaker).

The first of the three tracings of fig. 112-C presents an atrial tachycardia with a variable A-V block and an average ventricular rate of 120/min. The carotid sinus massage (cm) immediately increases the A-V block and reveals the rate of the atrial waves (150/min.). After four beats, with a 4:1 A-V block, the rhythm is stabilized in the slower rate presented in the bottom tracing. This shows a 2:1 A-V block and a ventricular rate of 75/min.

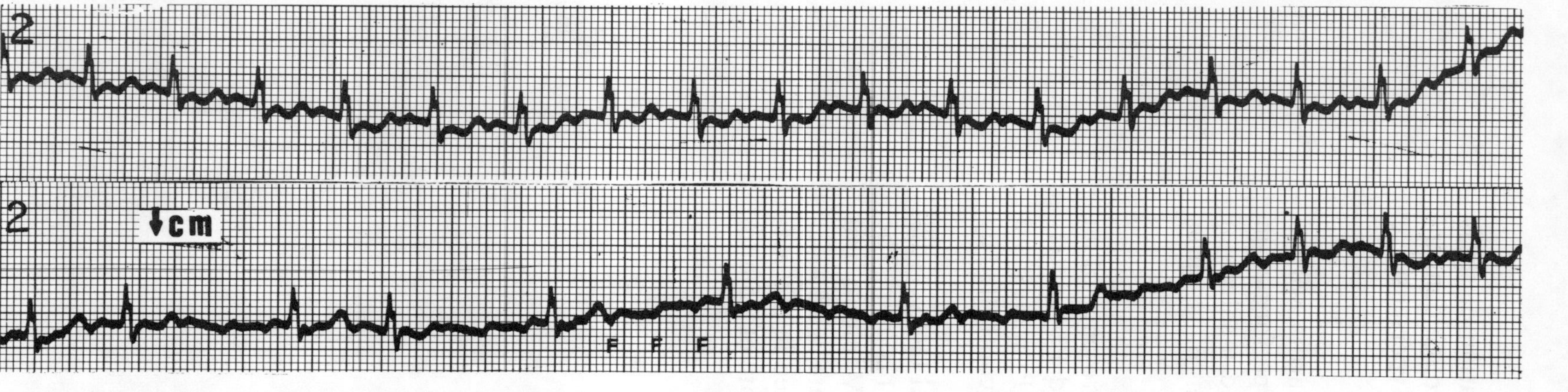

Fig. 113-A - **Carotid sinus massage.** The vagal stimulation increases the A-V block of the atrial flutter; this allows for a better visualization of the F waves.

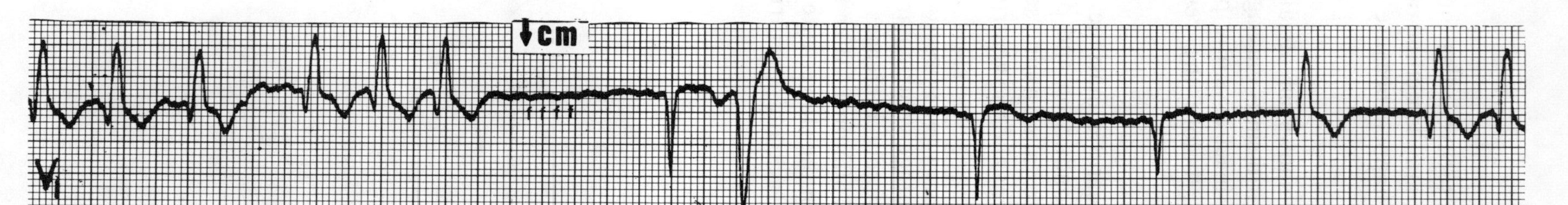

Fig. 113-B - **Carotid sinus massage.** The vagal maneuver performed during an atrial fibrillation results in a complete A-V block and in a brief escape of an idio-ventricular rhythm.

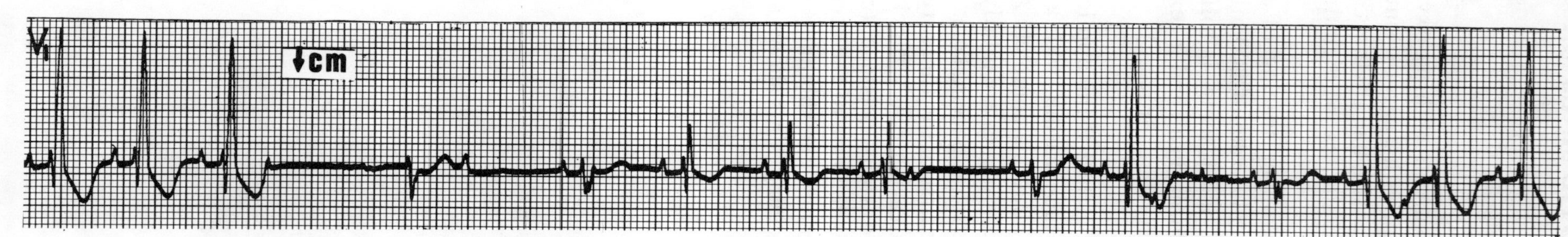

Fig. 113-C - **Carotid sinus massage.** The depressed A-V conduction offers a longer repolarization time to the right bundle. This determines a better conduction of several sinus beats with an incomplete RBBB, before the reappearance of a complete RBBB.

The carotid massage may also be performed in a patient with atrial flutter. The maneuver may confirm an unclear case of flutter, because it permits a better visualization of the atrial waves obtained with a temporary increase of the A-V block.

Fig. 113-A records an atrial flutter with a 2:1 A-V block and a ventricular rate of 130/min. The carotid massage in the bottom tracing increases the A-V block from 2:1 to 4:1 and improves the visualization of the atrial F waves. As soon as the pressure on the carotid sinus is released, both the rhythm and the A-V block return to the level of the control tracing.

A differential diagnosis between an atrial flutter, with a variable A-V block, and an atrial fibrillation is solved with the application of carotid sinus massage (fig. 113-B). The vagal maneuver completely suppresses the transmission of impulses across the A-V junction. The following asystolic pause brings out the fine undulations typical of an atrial fibrillation. The pause is punctuated by several ventricular escape beats, before the conduction of the impulses through the A-V junction is re-established.

The carotid massage performed in the patient of fig. 113-C produces several complexes with different degrees of right bundle branch block. The QRS complexes change from a normal morphology into one of an incomplete right bundle branch block and, finally, into one of a complete right bundle branch block.

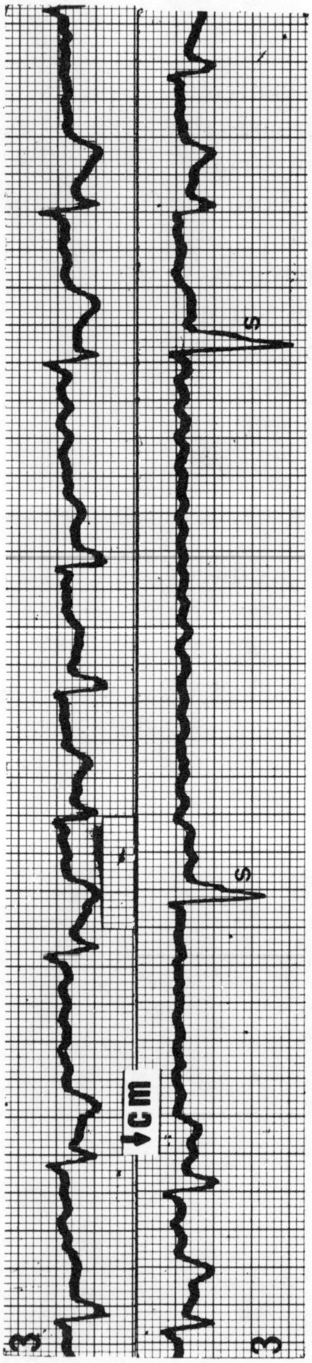

Fig. 114-A - Carotid sinus massage. It determines a complete A-V block and the emergence of two ventricular escape beats (E). Atrial fibrillatory waves are clearly visible.

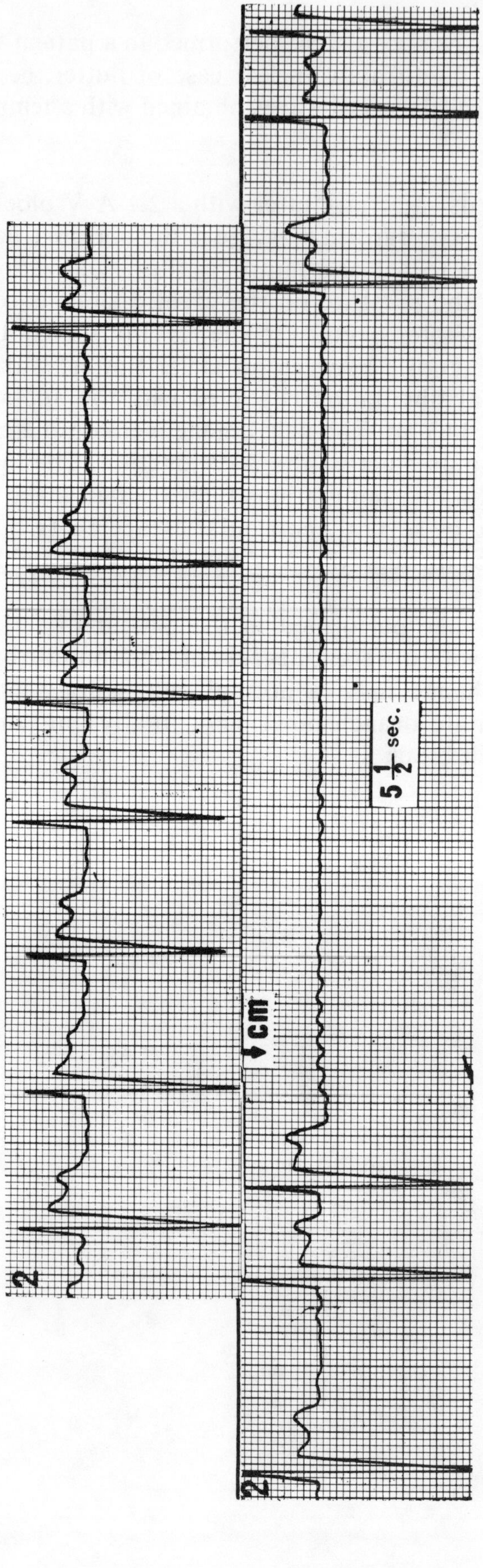

Fig. 114-B - Carotid sinus massage. The prolonged asystolic pause of 5 1/2 seconds is due to the absent A-V conduction of atrial impulses.

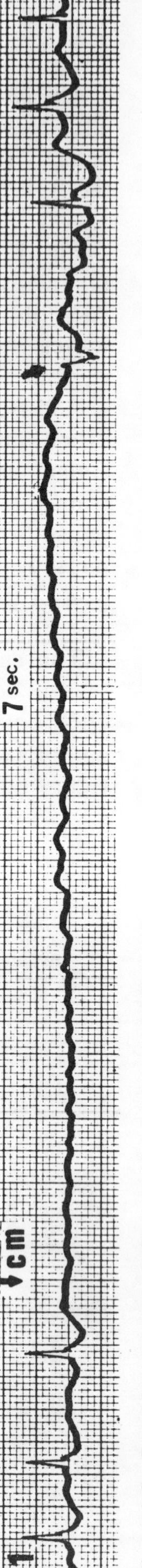

Fig. 114-C - Carotid sinus massage. The asystolic pause is particularly pronounced (7 seconds) and is terminated by a ventricular escape beat (arrow). The atria are fibrillating.

The carotid sinus massage if often used in the presence of an atrial fibrillation. This is done to assay the level of transmission of atrial impulses through the A-V junction after a digitalis therapy. However, this maneuver is not without risks, as is amply illustrated in the tracings of the opposite page.

Fig. 114-A shows the performance of a carotid sinus massage in a patient with atrial fibrillation and a moderate ventricular rate. The vagal stimulation results in a complete block in the conduction of the impulses through the A-V junction, followed by an asystolic pause and two ventricular escape beats (e), before the restoration of a normal A-V conduction.

A similar situation is that of fig. 114-B where the carotid massage determines a long asystolic pause (5 1/2 secs.) before the atrial impulses are again transmitted through the A-V junction.

In fig. 114-C seven seconds elapse before the emergence of ventricular escape beats, after the prolonged asystolic pause induced by a carotid sinus massage.

In the three cases presented the atrial fibrillatory waves are clearly visible during the asystolic pauses. There is no doubt that the digitalis effect on the A-V conduction is dramatically documented. The cases presented illustrate the potential risks of this maneuver and do not advise the application of a carotid massage in patients with atrial fibrillation and a slow ventricular rate.

The information sought through a carotid massage may also be obtained with a physical exercise. The increase in the ventricular rate with exercise is in a closer relation to the functional state of the A-V junction and to the degree of digitalization.

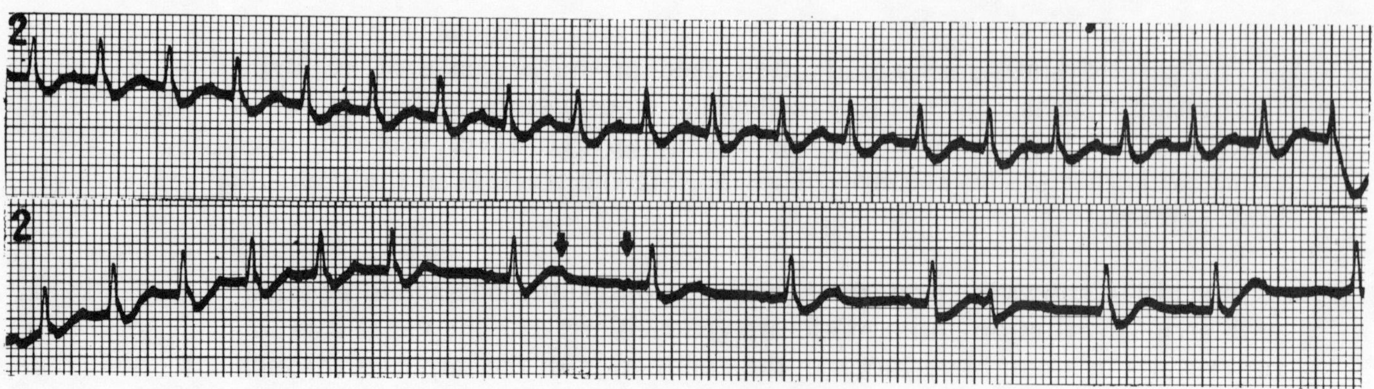

Fig. 115-A - Tensilon. (Edrophonium Chloride). The anticholinesterasic drug increases the A-V block (lower tracing) of the atrial tachycardia.

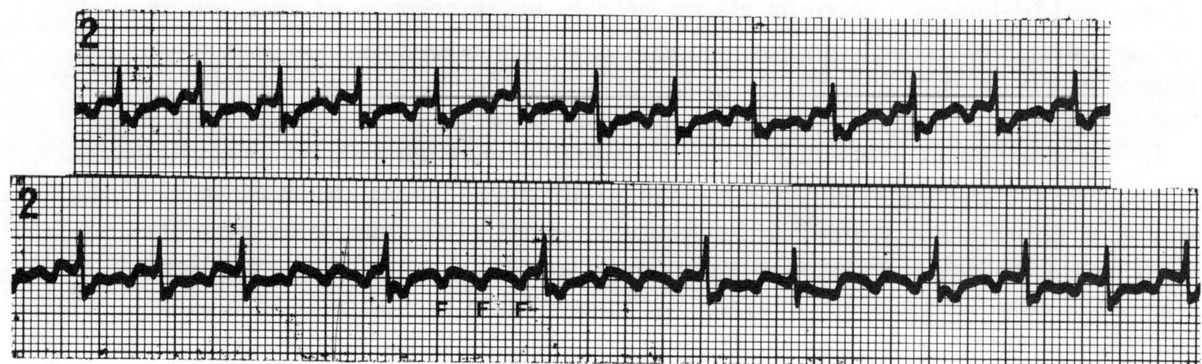

Fig. 115-B - Tensilon (Edrophonium Chloride). The temporary increase of the A-V block brings out the F waves of an atrial flutter.

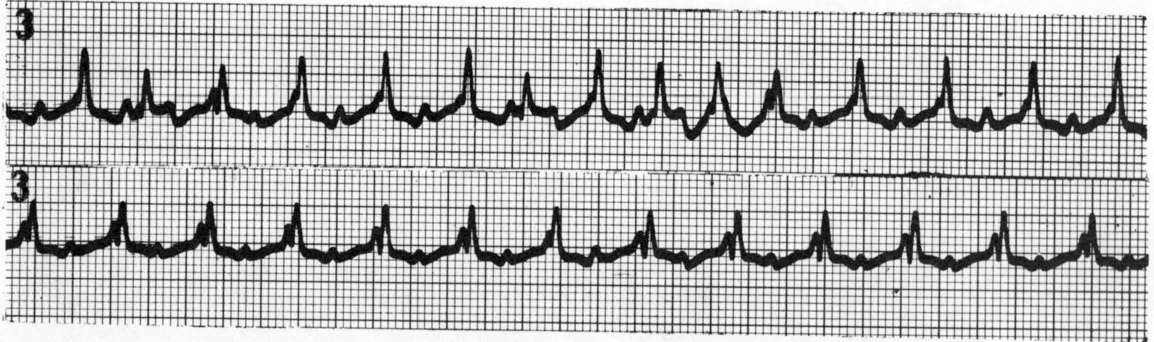

Fig. 115-C - Tensilon (Edrophonium Chloride). The atrial tachycardia, with a variable A-V block, is transformed into one with a stable 2:1 A-V block with IV Tensilon.

Several drugs are used as a diagnostic tool in clinical situations where it is necessary to define the mechanism of tachyarrhythmias and sometimes to abort supraventricular tachycardias. The mechanism of action of the drugs used is very close to that of a carotid sinus massage. They mainly work through a parasympathetic reflex.

A - TENSILON (Edrophonium Chloride).

It is used for the differential diagnosis of myasthenia gravis during an acute myasthenic crisis, and during anesthesia as a curare antagonist. The drug is an *anticholinesterasic* of short duration (5-10 mins.). When administered intravenously, it temporarily increases the A-V block and elucidates the mechanism of a supraventricular tachycardia.

Fig. 115-A shows a case of supraventricular tachycardia with a ventricular rate of 180/min. The administration of IV Tensilon (bottom tracing) induces a temporary increase of the A-V block and a better visualization of the atrial waves (arrows). Therefore, this is an atrial tachycardia with a 1:1 A-V conduction.

In fig. 115-B the diagnosis of atrial flutter is again confirmed through the use of Tensilon. The bottom tracing shows the transition from a 2:1 A-V block to a 4:1 A-V block, as indicated by the "saw-tooth" undulation typical of the atrial flutter.

An atrial tachycardia with an A-V block variable from 2:1 and 1:1, and periods of A-V Wenckebach, is diagnosed by the stabilization of the A-V block on a 2:1 type (lower tracing) with the use of IV Tensilon (fig. 115-C).

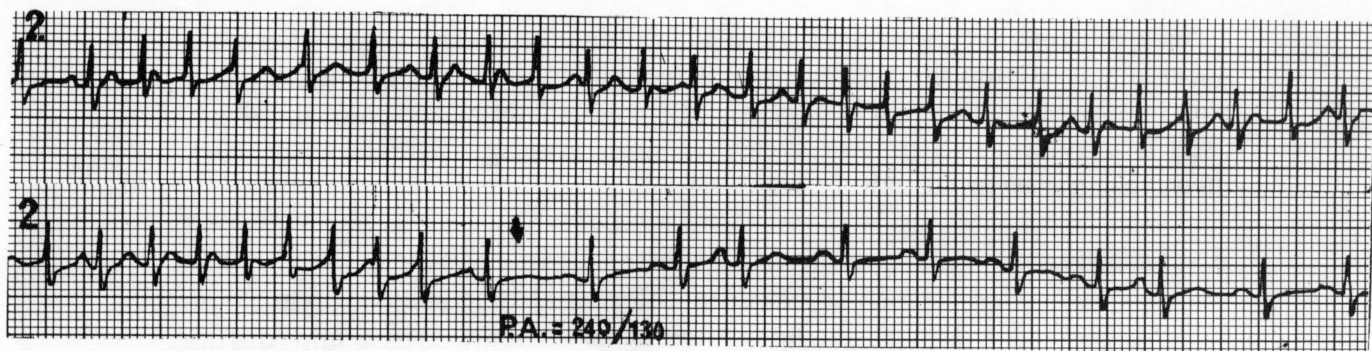

Fig. 116-A - Aramine (Metaraminol). The atrial tachycardia, with variable A-V block, is converted into a sinus rhythm with IV Aramine. The blood pressure values, obtained at the moment of conversion, are reported on the tracing.

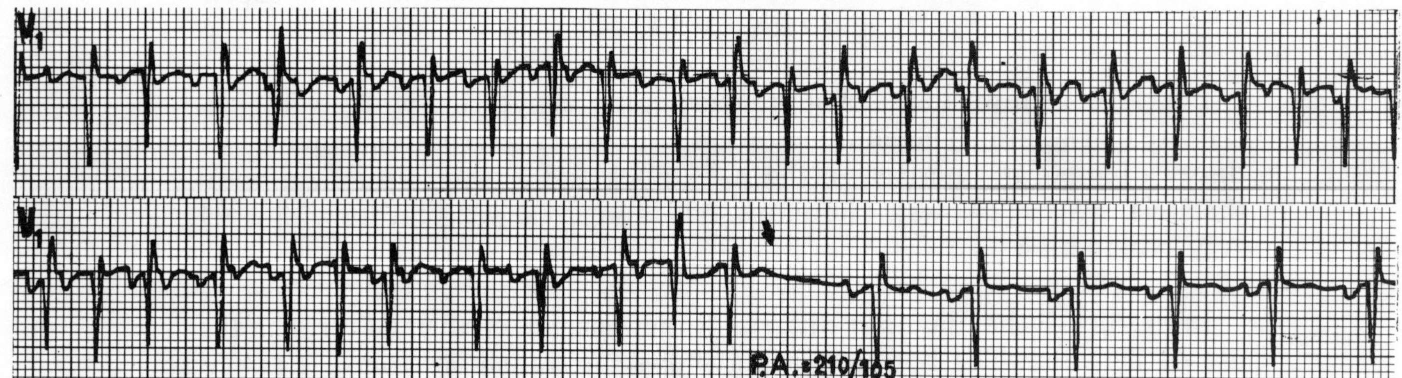

Fig. 116-B - Aramine (Metaraminol). Notice the presence of an A-V Wenckebach phenomenon in the A-V conduction of atrial impulses immediately preceding the cessation of the arrhythmia.

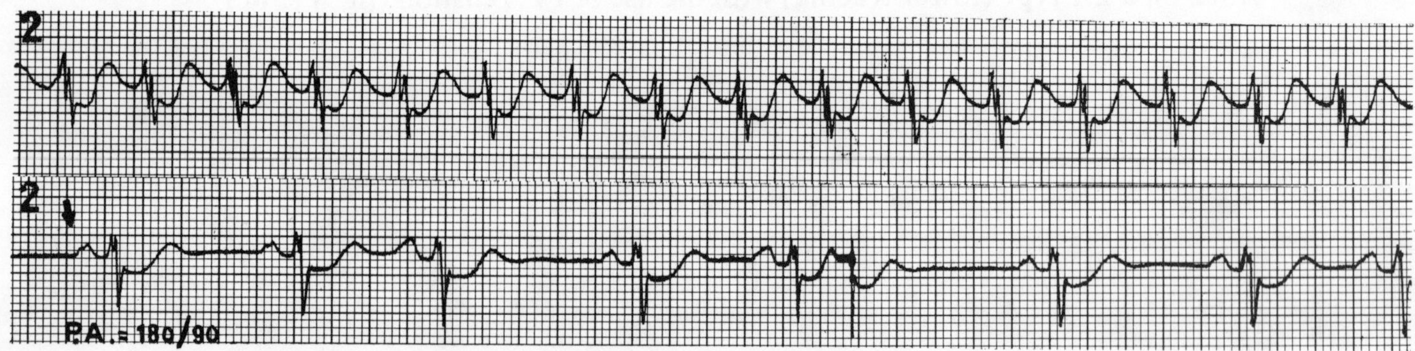

Fig. 116-C - Neosinephrine (Phenylephrine Hydrochloride). The supraventricular tachycardia is converted by IV Neosinephrine into a sinus rhythm with PAC's.

B - ARAMINE (Metaraminol Bitartrate)

C - NEOSYNEPHRINE (Phenylephrine Hydrochloride)

They are both potent pressure amines which produce a rapid and marked increase of both systolic and diastolic blood pressures and of the peripheral vascular resistances.

The antiarrhythmic effect of these drugs is due to a vagal reflex which originates from the aortic and carotid sinus baroceptors and which is triggered by the sudden and marked increase of the arterial pressure. Therefore, these drugs are administered with both EKG and blood pressure monitoring. They are used in emergency situations to stop paroxysmal supraventricular tachycardias only when other vagal maneuvers have failed.

Fig. 116-A shows the cessation of a paroxysmal supraventricular tachycardia with the intravenous administration of Metaraminol (Aramine). The arterial pressure at the moment of conversion into a sinus rhythm is indicated on the tracing.

The patient of fig. 116-B shows a paroxysmal atrial tachycardia, with a variable A-V block, successfully converted into a stable sinus rhythm with IV Metaraminol.

Fig. 116-C shows a supraventricular tachycardia converted into a sinus rhythm with IV Neosynephrine.

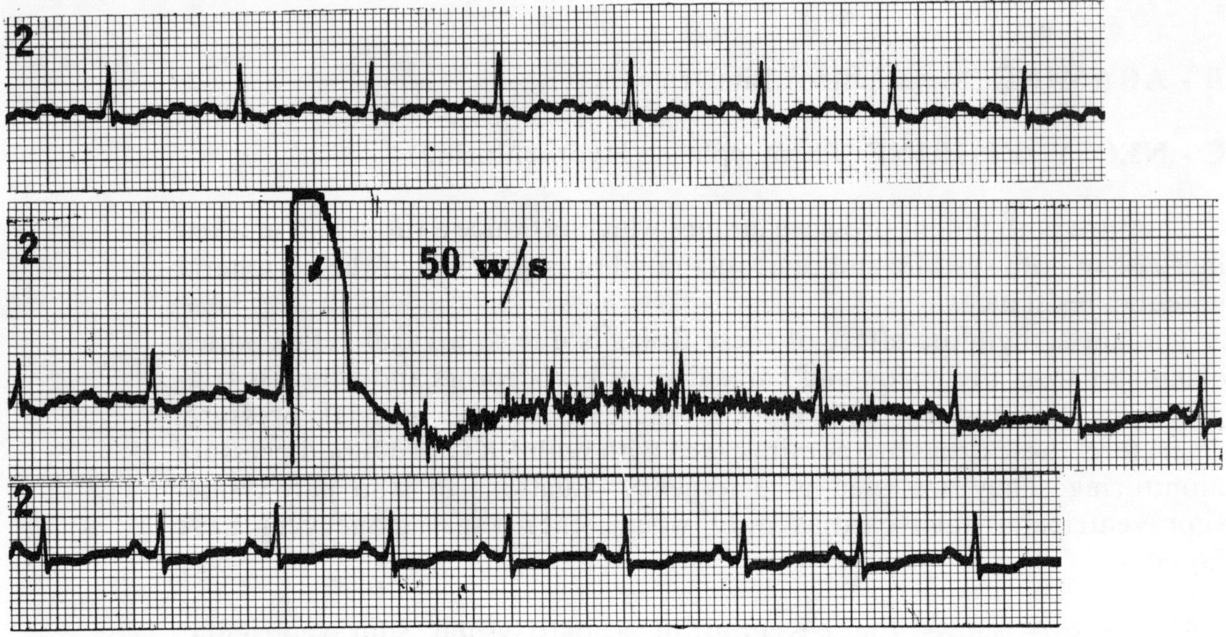

Fig. 117-A - Electrical cardioversion.

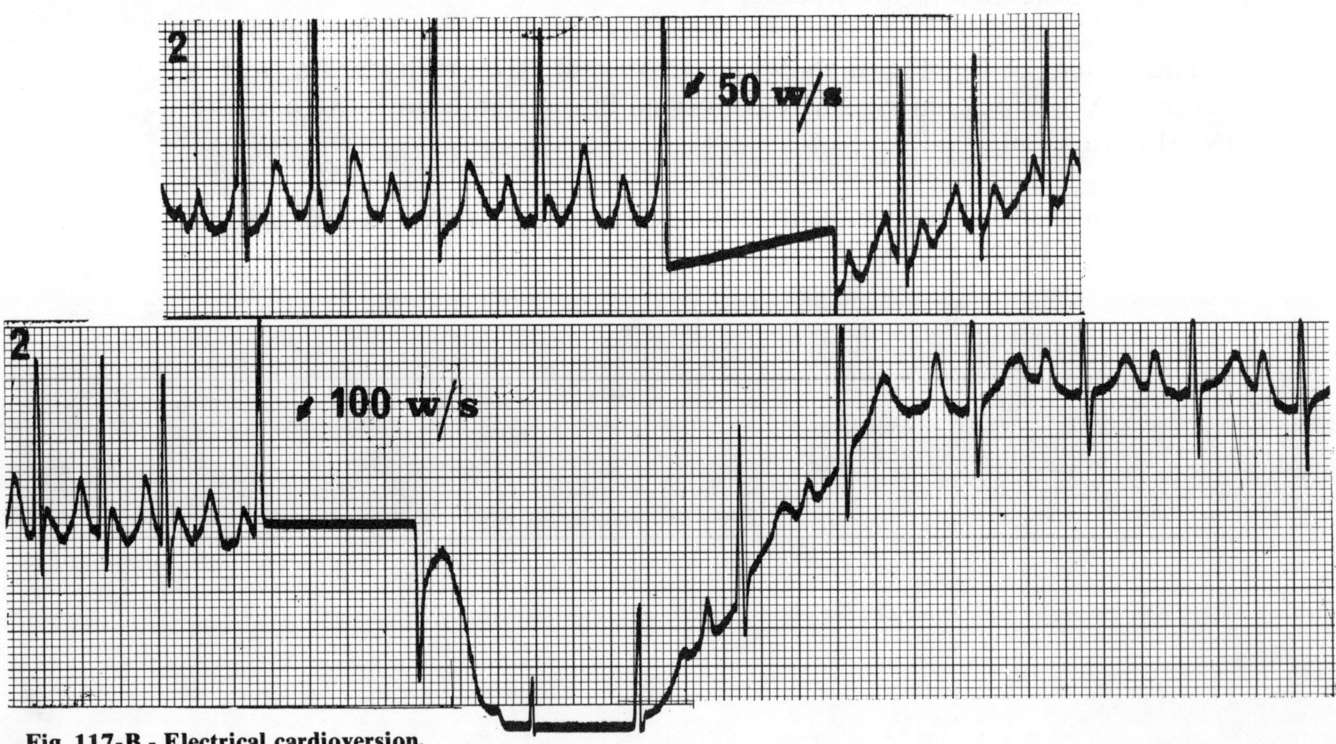

Fig. 117-B - Electrical cardioversion.

CARDIOVERSION AND ARRHYTHMIAS

Cardioversion is the electrical conversion into a sinus rhythm of a number of arrhythmias secondary to abnormal impulse formation. It represents an alternative in the therapy of those arrhythmias which were almost exclusively treated with drugs.

Cardioversion consists in the electrical depolarization of the entire heart through a transthoracic electrical discharge which is synchronized with the R wave of the ECG. The electrical discharge suppresses, for a short interval of time, the formation of impulses in all myocardial cells and, therefore, also in the cells of the ectopic focus which sustains the arrhythmia. This offers the sinus node an opportunity to regain control of the cardiac rhythm. A great amount of clinical experience has been accumulated about cardioversion; today it is a treatment of choice for a certain number of cardiac arrhythmias.

The arrhythmias most commonly treated with *electrical cardioversion* are: atrial flutter, atrial fibrillation and, in some cases, supraventricular tachycardias. The following examples illustrate some of the rhythm disturbances which may be present during and after the restoration of a normal sinus rhythm, in a patient treated with electrical cardioversion.

Fig. 117-A shows a typical case of electrical cardioversion of an atrial flutter with a stable 4:1 A-V block. The atrial rate is 360/min., while the ventricular is 90/min. An electrical discharge of 50 watts/sec., synchronized with the R wave, determines the immediate cessation of the arrhythmia and the prompt restoration of a sinus rhythm. The conversion from an atrial flutter into a normal sinus rhythm is immediate and without transitional arrhythmias. Notice that the electrical impulse falls just during the inscription of the R wave; this guarantees the impossibility of inducing more dangerous arrhythmias, since the stimulus falls into the absolute refractory period of the ventricular excitability. For a few seconds following the discharge, the recording is disturbed by the muscular tremor of the patient. This obscures slightly the P waves and QRS complexes.

Again, fig. 117-B shows a case of atrial flutter which requires two electrical discharges with different energy (50 and 100 watts/secs.) before the conversion into a sinus rhythm.

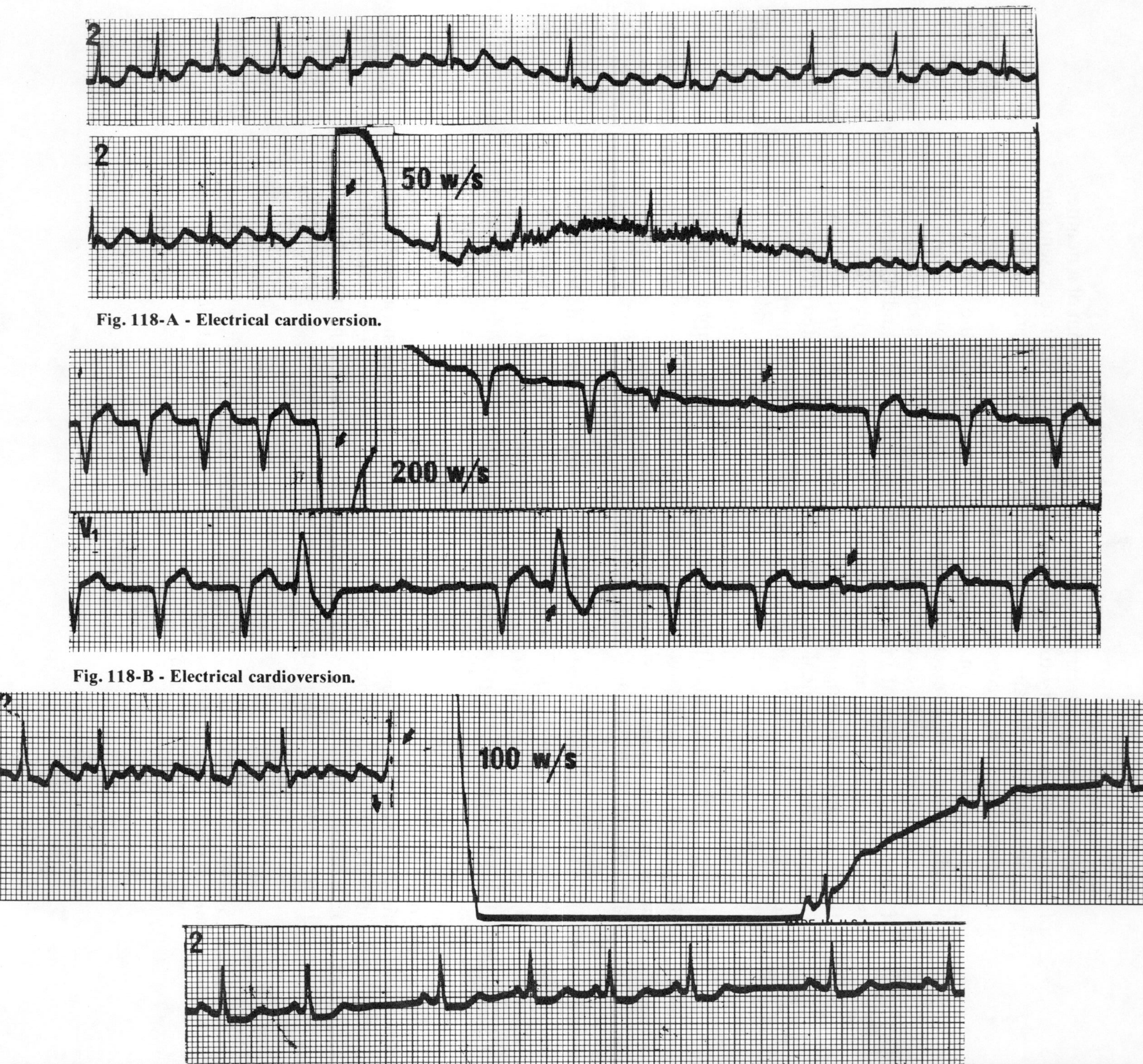

Fig. 118-A - Electrical cardioversion.

Fig. 118-B - Electrical cardioversion.

The atrial flutter of the upper tracing of fig. 118-A records an atrial rate of 280/min. and a variable A-V ratio. An unsuccessful attempt at cardioversion with 50 watts/sec. results in a faster atrial rate (320/min.) and a stable 4:1 A-V ratio.

Fig. 118-B presents an atrial tachycardia, with a 2:1 A-V block, converted into a sinus rhythm with a transthoracic electric shock of 200 watts/sec. The post-conversion tracing shows a sinus rhythm with a first degree A-V block (P-R = 0.30 sec.) and several multifocal ventricular extrasystoles. Some of the PVC's have a fixed coupling interval, while others are of the endiastolic type.

The upper tracing of fig. 118-C shows an atrial flutter, with a variable A-V block, which is transformed into a sinus rhythm with cardioversion (100 watts/sec.). The lower tracing, recorded a few seconds later, shows a brief salvos of premature atrial beats with P[1] waves sharply different from sinus P waves.

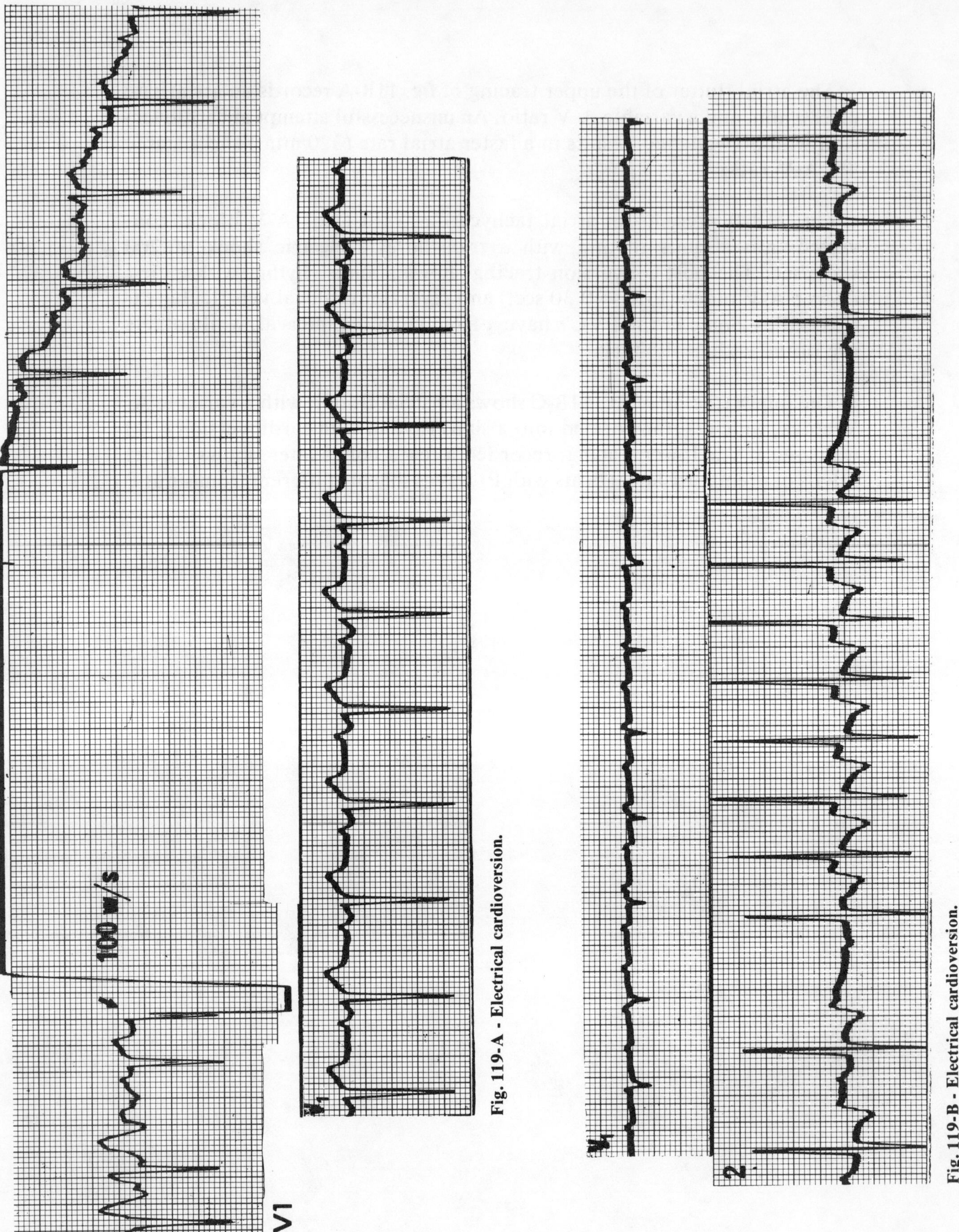

Fig. 119-A - Electrical cardioversion.

Fig. 119-B - Electrical cardioversion.

CARDIOVERSION AND ARRHYTHMIAS

Fig. 119-A presents, again, an atrial flutter with a variable A-V block converted into a sinus rhythm with an electrical discharge of 100 watts/sec. Several seconds elapse between the moment of the electrical discharge and the reappearance of QRS complexes. This is a very common situation which can be observed in standard ECG recording. This is due to the sudden electrical overloading of the ECG machine by the transthoracic electrical discharge, which may deviate the electronic beam, or the stylus, off the screen and simulate an asystolic pause.

Fig. 119-B presents an atrial tachycardia with a variable A-V block due to the presence of an A-V Wenckebach phenomenon. As can be observed in the lower tracing, the arrhythmia is converted into a sinus rhythm with an electrical shock. The sinus rhythm is interrupted by a brief salvo of a supraventricular tachycardia which ceases spontaneously. On other occasions, bursts of PAC's may re-establish the supraventricular tachyarrhythmia in a matter of minutes after cardioversion.

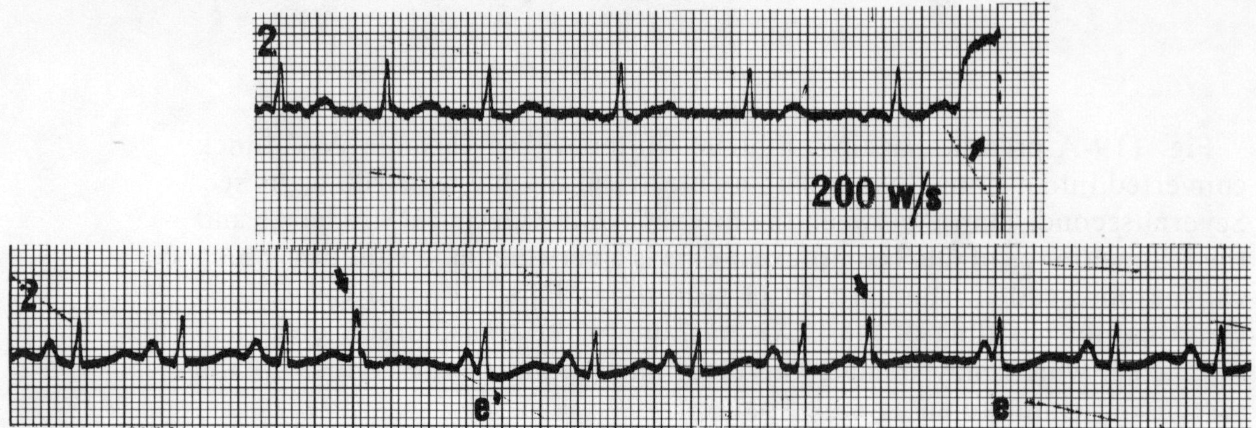

Fig. 120-A - Electrical cardioversion.

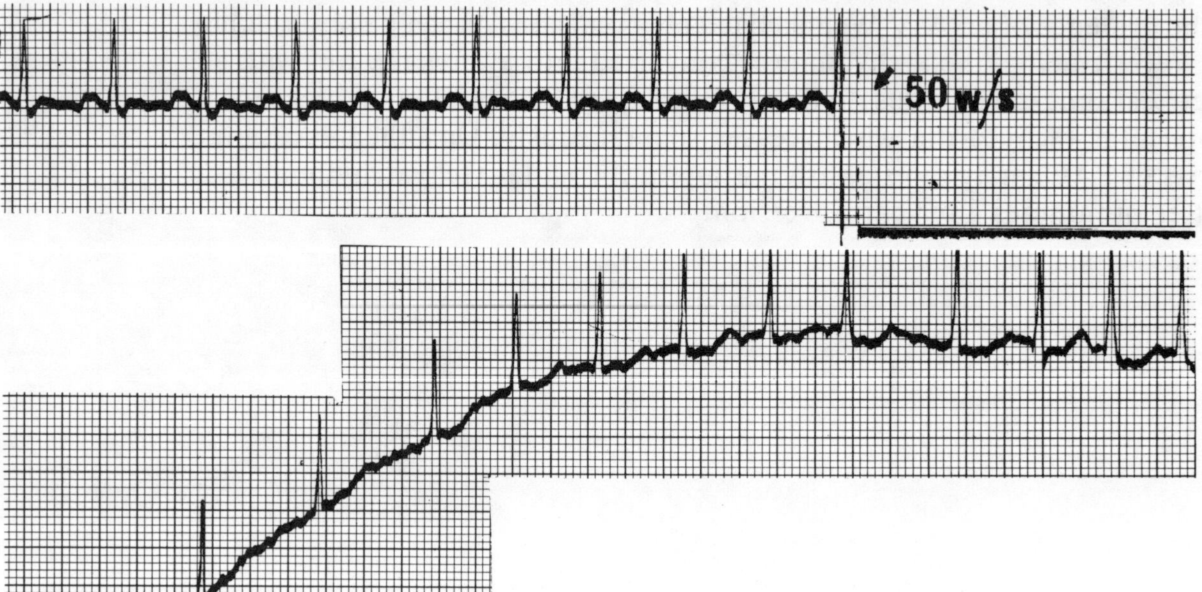

Fig. 120-B - Electrical cardioversion.

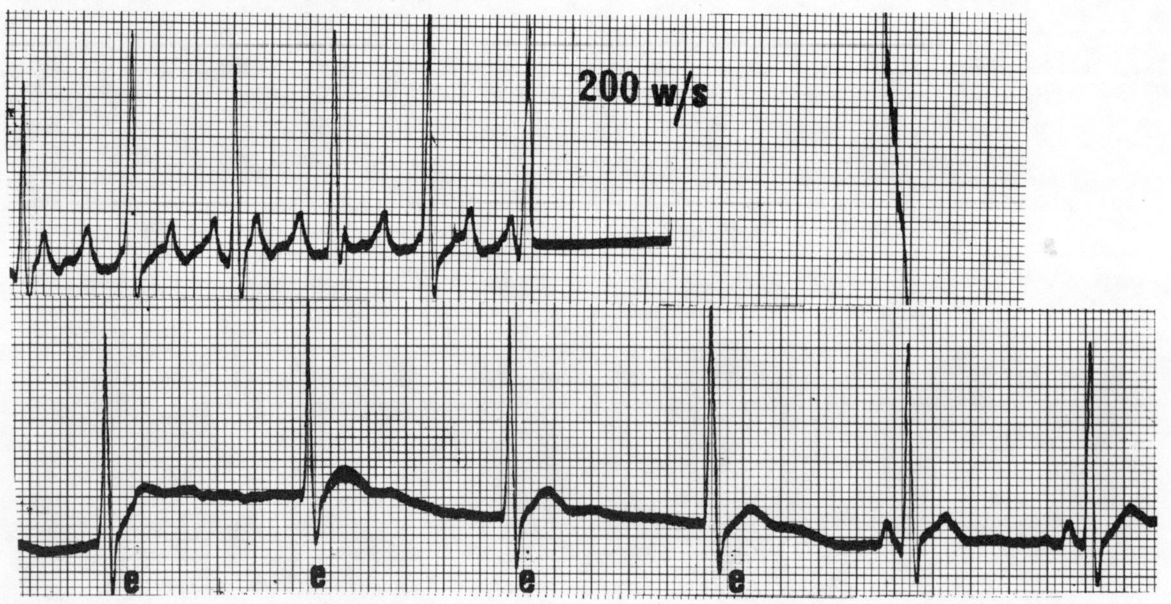

Fig. 120-C - Electrical cardioversion.

A single electrical discharge of 200 watts/sec. transforms the atrial fibrillation of the upper tracing of fig. 120-A into a sinus rhythm, interrupted by an occasional junctional extrasystole (arrows of the bottom tracing). The extrasystoles are followed by junctional escape beats (E) which show an A-V dissociation with sinus P waves. In fig. 120-B, an attempt of cardioversion, with a 50 watts/sec. discharge, transforms the atrial flutter with a 2:1 A-V ratio (upper tracing) into an atrial fibrillation (bottom tracing).

Fig. 120-C shows an atrial flutter being converted into a sinus rhythm with 200 watts/sec. Before the complete re-establishment of a sinus rhythm, several junctional escape beats (e) appear on the tracing and they temporarily suppress the sinus rate.

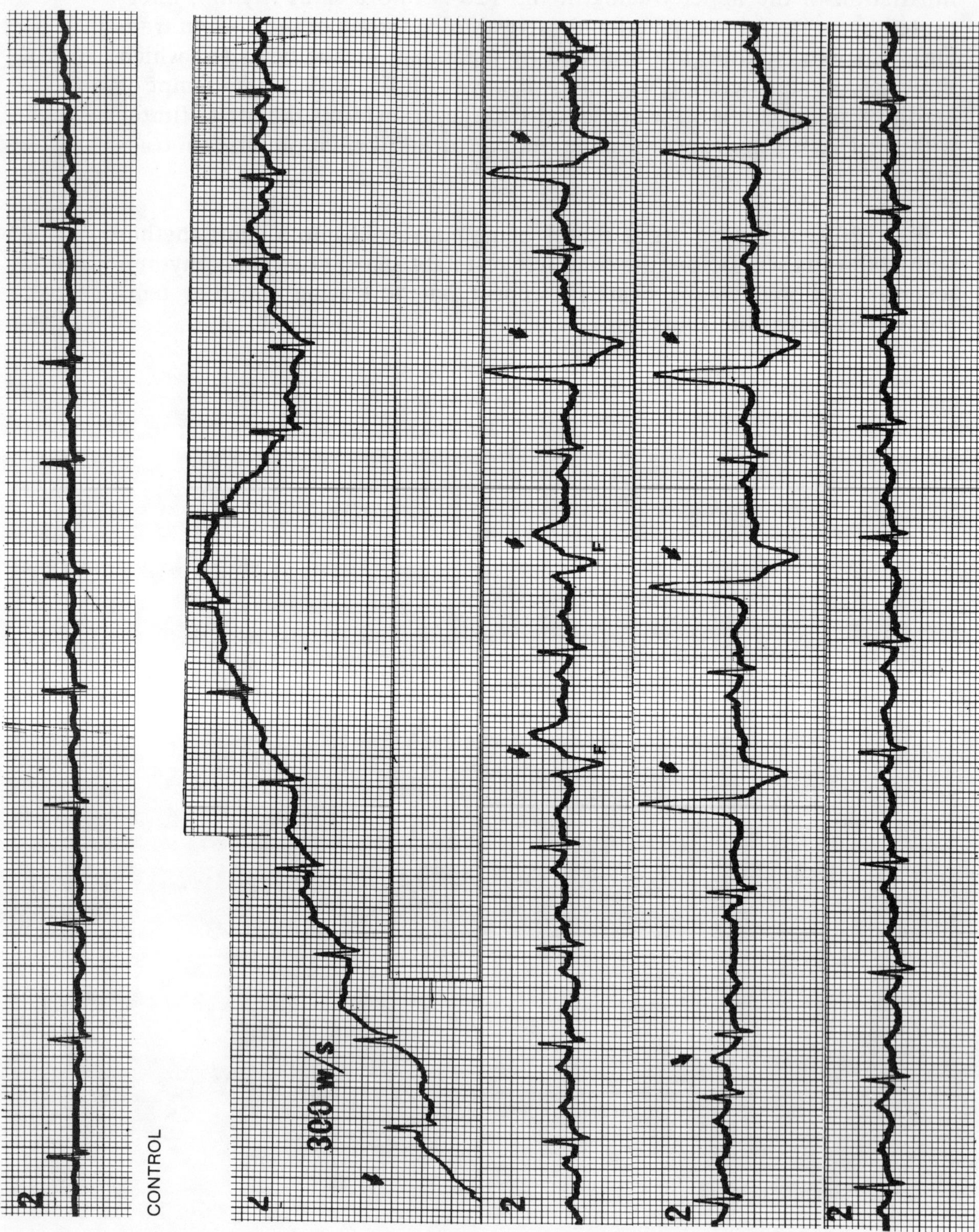

Fig. 121-A - Electrical cardioversion.

Fig. 121-A presents an atrial fibrillation which is converted into a sinus rhythm with a transthoracic electrical discharge of 300 watts/sec. The cardioversion is followed by an immediate restoration of a sinus rhythm which, however, shows several ventricular extrasystoles with variable coupling intervals and fusion beats. Furthermore, the presence of a common interectopic interval suggests a ventricular parasystolic focus.

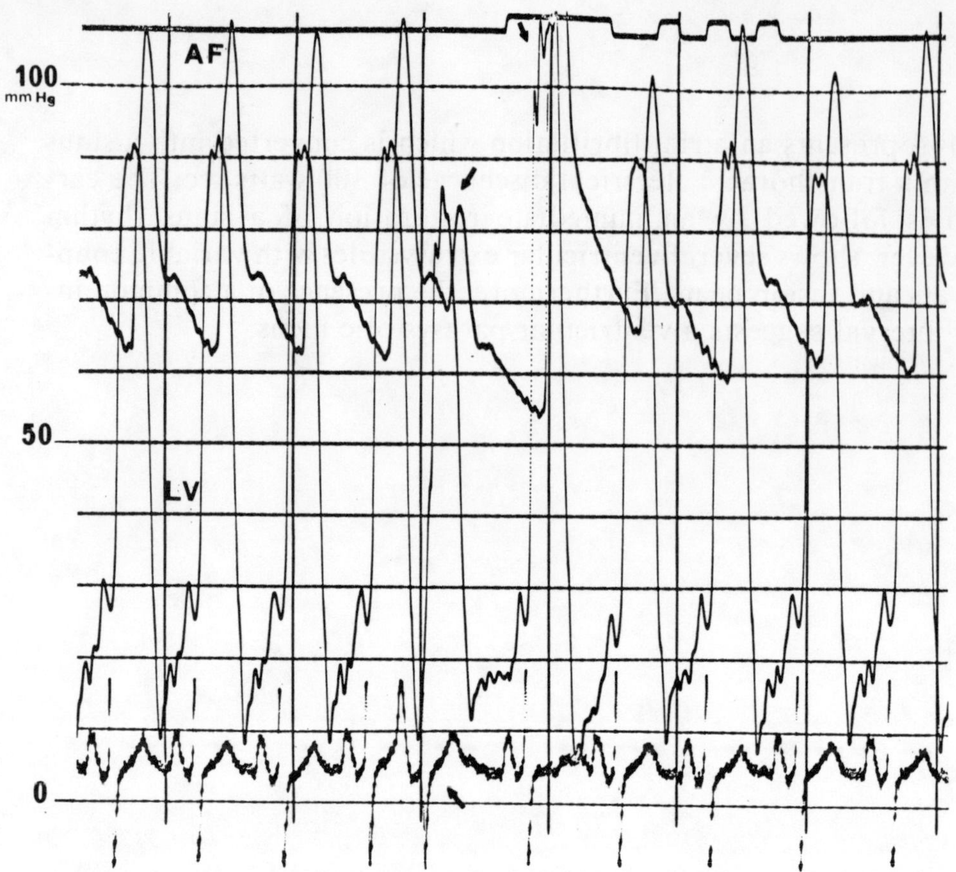

Fig. 122-A - Atrial extrasystole. LV = left ventricular pressure. AF = femoral artery pressure. The pressures are markedly reduced with the atrial extrasystoles (arrow). They increase in the post-extrasystolic beat.

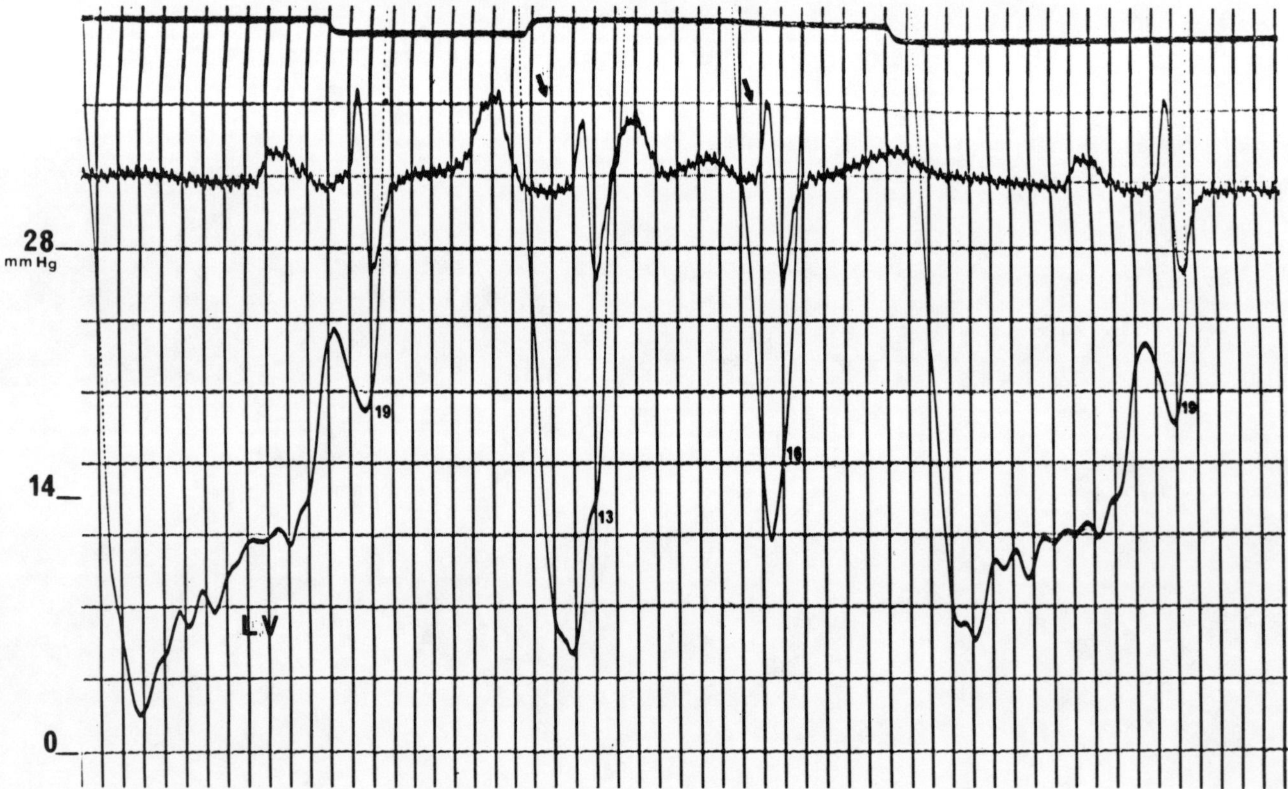

Fig. 122-B - Atrial extrasystole. The endiastolic left ventricular pressure is lower (13 and 16 mm of Hg.) during the atrial extrasystole when compared to that of a sinus beat (19 mm of Hg.).

HEMODYNAMICS OF ARRHYTHMIAS

As a general rule, any type of cardiac rhythm which departs from a regular sinus rhythm has some influence on cardiac hemodynamics and, therefore, on the overall cardiac function.

The hemodynamic mechanisms with which an arrhythmia alters the cardiac function are:

a) variations of the ventricular volume and endiastolic pressure which are reflected in an altered Frank-Starling mechanism.
b) alteration of the state of contractility of the myocardial fibers.
c) alteration of the resistance to the systolic output.

ATRIAL EXTRASYSTOLES

Fig. 122-A presents the simultaneous recording of the surface ECG, the left ventricular pressure (LV) and the femoral artery pressure (FA). The pressure scale is 0-100 mm. of Hg. Note on the ECG recording that the fifth beat is premature and that the P wave is buried in the preceding T wave. The morphology of the QRS is similar to that of a sinus beat; the presence of an incomplete compensatory pause indicates that the premature beat is an atrial extrasystole is capable of generating a very low ventricular pressure when compared to that of a sinus beat. However, the pressure is still able to open the aortic valve and determine a small peripheral pulse. The sinus beat which follows the extrasystole *(post-extrasystolic beat)* has the benefit of a longer diastole and determines a ventricular and a femoral pressures higher than those of sinus beats.

Fig. 122-B shows the recording of the diastolic left ventricular pressures during the interruption of a sinus rhythm by two consecutive PAC's (arrows). The pressure scale is such that each horizontal line is equal to 4mm. of Hg. The pressure value at the end of the extrasystolic diastole *(PAC's end-diastolic pressure)* is lower than during a sinus beat. The ventricles are prematurely interrupted by the extrasystoles during the diastolic filling phase. They raise a lower diastolic pressure and contract on a smaller diastolic blood volume when compared with that of sinus beats.

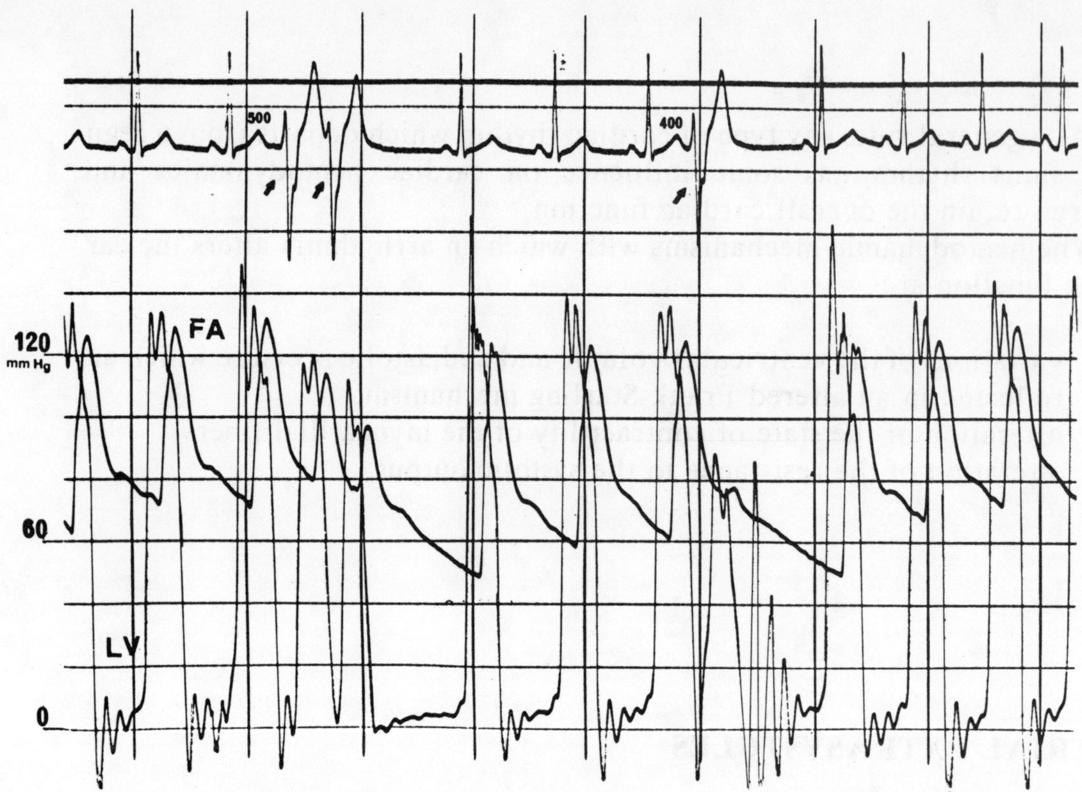

Fig. 123-A - Ventricular extrasystole. The ventricular extrasystole, with a 500 msec. coupling interval, determines a left ventricular (LV) and femoral artery (FA) pressure higher than that of the PVC with a 400 msec. coupling interval.

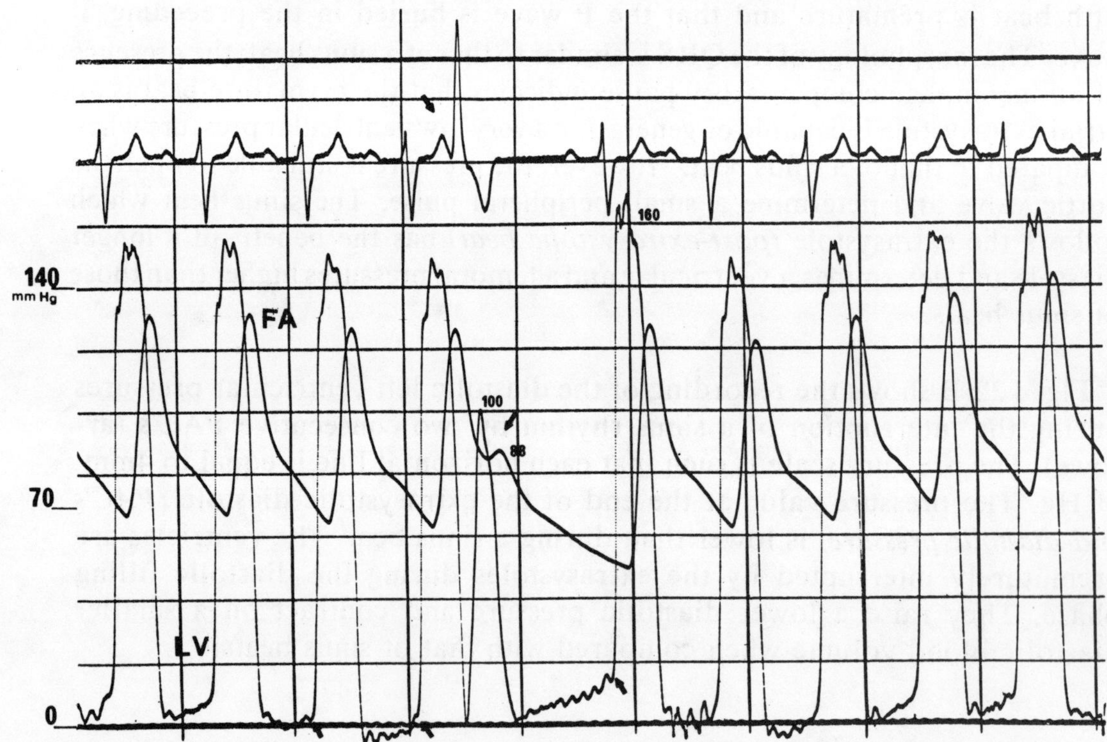

Fig. 123-B - Ventricular extrasystole. In a patient with valvular aortic stenosis, the moderate pressure gradient between left ventricle (LV) and femoral artery (FA) becomes more accentuated during the post- extrasystolic beat. Notice the significant pressure reduction of the extrasystole with an early coupling interval.

VENTRICULAR EXTRASYSTOLES

Ventricular extrasystoles influence cardiac hemodynamics because:
a) the extrasystolic impulse travels through nonspecific intraventricular conduction pathways and it modifies the synchronized sequence of muscular contractions.
b) a PVC induces a contractility potentiation of the post-extrasystolic beat (positive inotropic effect).
c) a PVC may have different coupling intervals with the preceding regular beat. This may determine an interruption of the ventricular diastolic filling at different levels.

Fig. 123-A presents a sinus rhythm interrupted first by a couplet, and then by a single ventricular extrasystole (arrows). The left ventricular (LV) and femoral artery pressures (FA) are recorded simultaneously with the surface ECG (the pressure scale is 0-200 mm. of Hg.). The first extrasystole has a coupling interval of 500 msec. with the preceding beat and it generates enough ventricular pressure to open the aortic valve and induce an adequate peripheral pulse. However, both the LV and FA pressures are reduced when compared to sinus beats. The second PVC of the couplet generates an even lower LV and FA pressure. The following single extrasystole (third arrow) has a coupling interval of 400 msecs. and barely generates a small femoral pulse.

In normal conditions, the ventricular and peripheral systolic pressures of a post-extrasystolic beat will be higher than those of a control beat. In the case of fig. 123-A, the post-extrasystolic pressures do not show a significant difference when compared to the control sinus beat.

Fig. 123-B shows the effect of a ventricular extrasystole, with an early coupling interval, on the pressure gradient between the left ventricle (LV) and the femoral artery (FA). The patient has a mild valvular aortic stenosis. In this situation, the positive inotropic effect of the post-extrasystolic beat is particularly evident since the resistance to the ejection of the systolic volume is of a fixed type (valvular aortic stenosis). The pressure generated by the post-extrasystolic beat is higher than that of a normal beat. This is because of the longer diastolic filling phase which follows the extrasystole which, in turn, determines a higher left ventricular endiastolic pressure (LVEDP) and, consequently, an increase in the ventricular tension and contractility.

This example illustrates the intimate relationship between peripheral resistance, myocardial contractility and ventricular diastolic volumes.

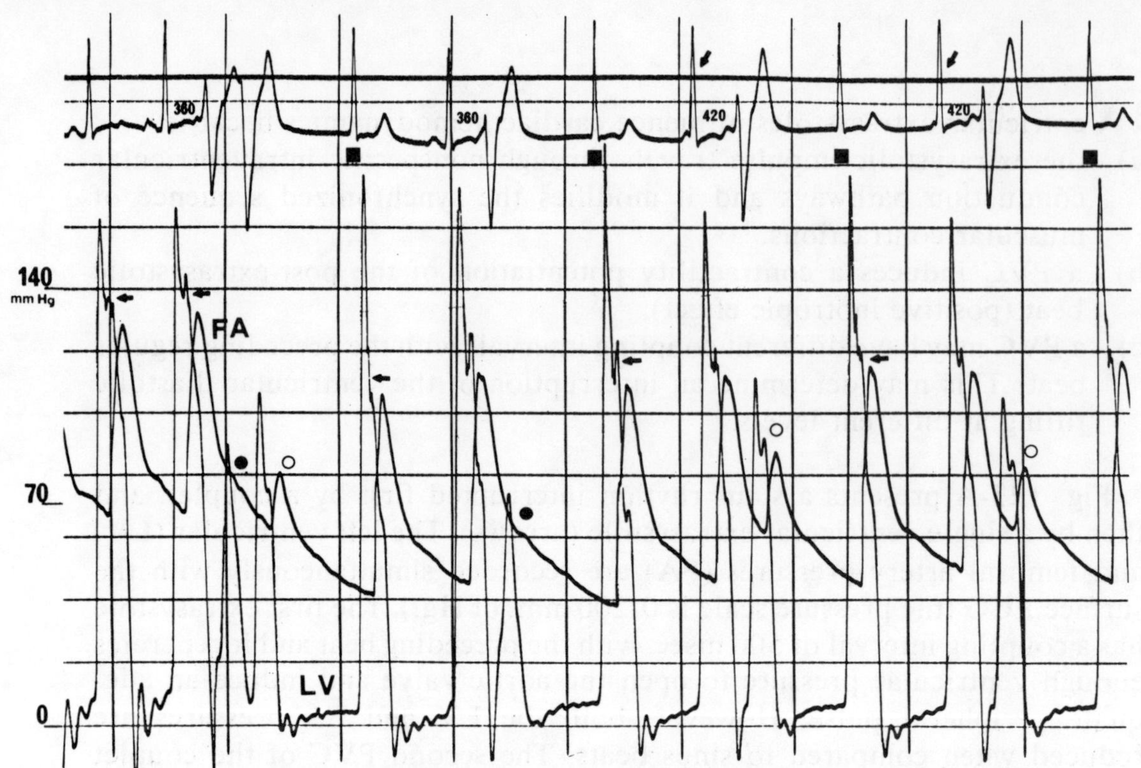

Fig. 124-A - Ventricular extrasystoles, junctional escape rhythm and A-V dissociation.
The first two beats are of sinus origin. LV = left ventricle; FA = femoral artery; ■ = junctional escape beats; 0 = PVC's able to generate a peripheral pulse; ● = early PVC's which do not open the aortic valve. (see text).
tic valve. (see text).

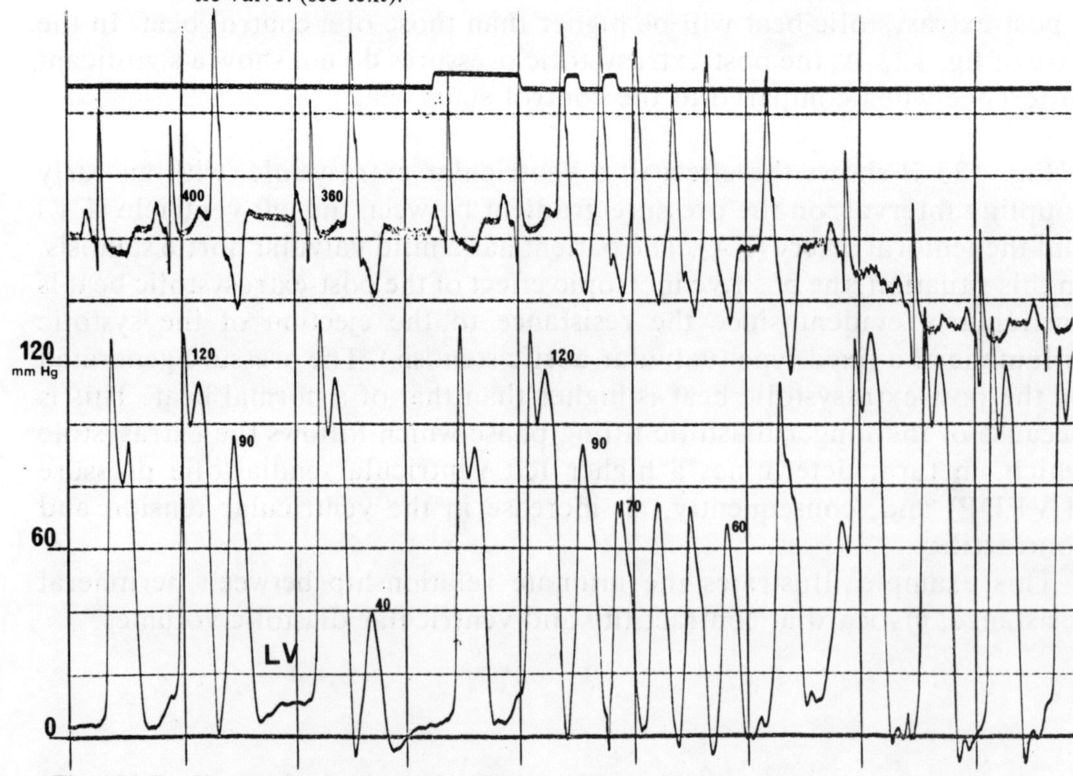

Fig. 124-B - Ventricular tachycardia. LV = left ventricular pressure. Notice the variable pressure levels of the first two ventricular extrasystoles, with 400 and 360 msec. coupling intervals, and the progressive left ventricular pressure decline during the ventricular tachycardia.

VENTRICULAR EXTRASYSTOLES

Fig. 124-A shows the hemodynamic effect of an interesting arrhythmia. The first two beats recorded on the surface ECG are sinus beats. The simultaneous left ventricular (LV) and femoral pressures (FA) have systolic values respectively of 140 and 130 mm. of Hg. They are followed by a pair of ventricular extrasystoles. While the first is too premature (coupling interval = 360 msec.) and does not open the aortic valve, the second PVC raises enough ventricular pressure to generate a femoral pulse. The following pause terminates with a junctional escape beat (dark square). This, in turn, is followed by a sinus beat and again by a ventricular extrasystole with a coupling interval of 360 msecs. The tracing continues with a junctional rhythm with A-V dissociation (arrows), punctuated by PVC's with longer coupling intervals (420 msecs.) Note that the longer the coupling interval the higher the femoral pulse. The ventricular and femoral pressures of the junctional beats are lower than that of a normal sinus beat.

VENTRICULAR TACHYCARDIA

Fig. 124-B shows the behavior of the left ventricular pressure during a brief salvos of ventricular tachycardia. The burst of VT is preceded by two premonitory PVC's, with a variable coupling interval and interrupting a normal sinus rhythm. The ventricular pressures generated by the extrasystoles are lower than those of sinus beats. This is in direct relation with the coupling interval of the PVC with the preceding sinus beat. The shorter the interval the lower the ventricular systolic pressure and vice-a-versa. During the salvo of ventricular tachycardia there is a gradual pressure drop from 120 to 90 and then 70 mm. of Hg. This is followed by a plateau of three beats with 60-70 mm. of Hg. and, finally, by a rapid return to control values with the reappearance of a sinus rhythm.

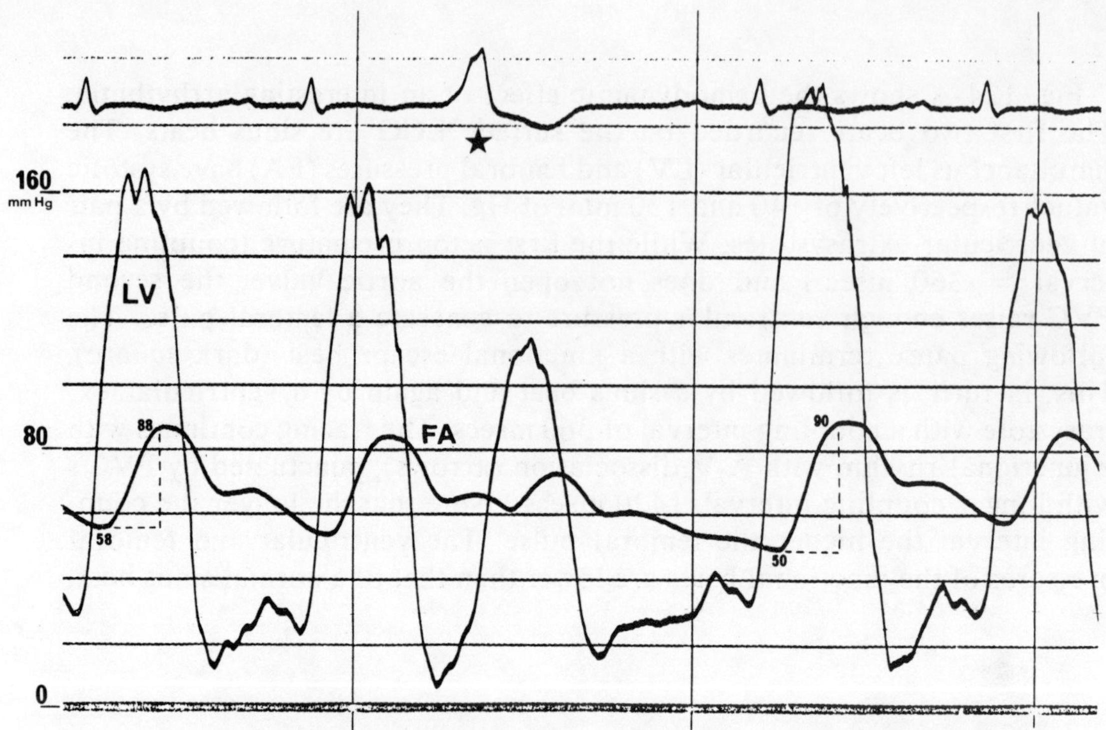

Fig. 125-A - Extrasystoles and valvular aortic stenosis. Notice the lower extrasystolic pressure gradient between the left ventricle (LV) and the brachial artery (BA). The gradient increases markedly in the post-extrasystolic beat. So does the differential pulse of the post-extrasystolic beat when compared with the control beat.

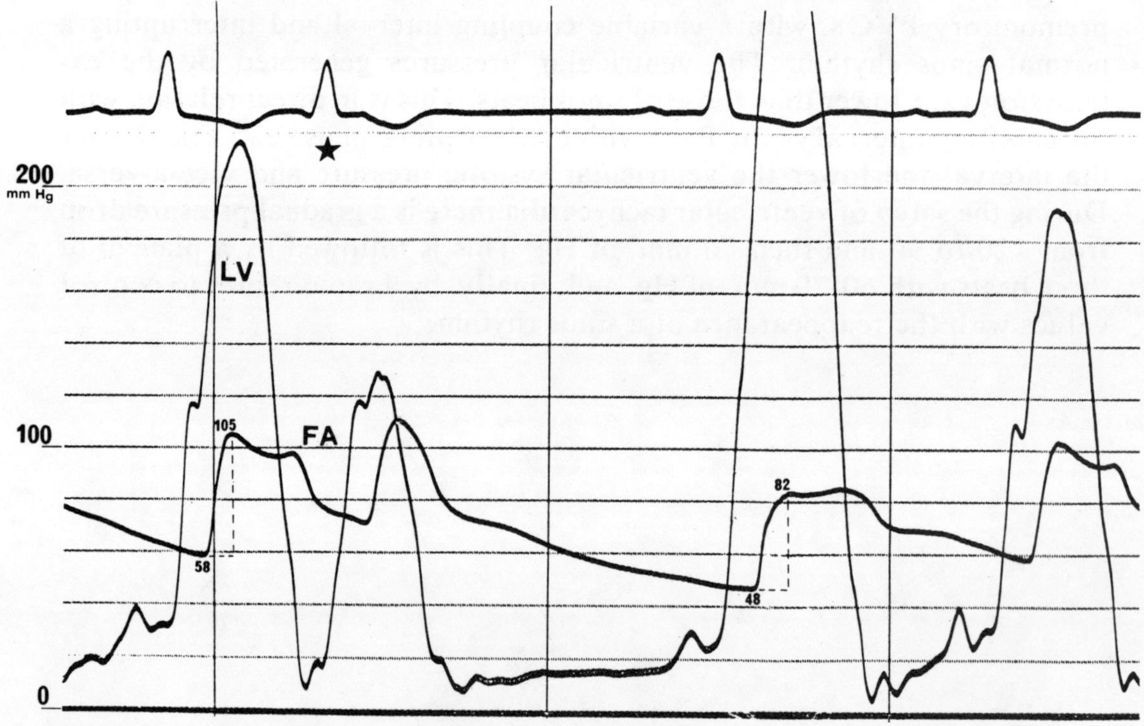

Fig. 125-B - Extrasystoles and idiopathic hypertrophic subaortic stenosis (IHSS). LV = left ventricle; BA = brachial artery. Notice the marked increase in the pressure gradient of the post-extrasystolic beat; this is accompanied by a decreased differential pulse.

VENTRICULAR EXTRASYSTOLES

Idiopathic hypertrophic subaortic stenosis (IHSS) is a pathological condition of the aortic outflow tract. In the presence of IHSS the hemodynamic effects of ventricular extrasystoles are somewhat modified. This example illustrates the positive inotropic effect of the post-extrasystolic diastole on the post-extrasystolic beat. In IHSS the major component of the aortic stenosis is represented by a markedly hypertrophic muscular mass of the septum which reduces the aortic outflow tract and determines an *intra-ventricular pressure gradient* (between the left ventricular chamber and the aortic outflow tract.) It follows that, since the stenosis is not of a fixed but of a dynamic type, any factor which determines an increase in ventricular contractility will induce a greater "strangulation" of the aortic outflow tract.

For a better understanding of the paradoxycal hemodynamic effect of a single or a salvos of PVC's in hypertrophic subaortic stenosis (IHSS), it is useful to compare this situation with the more common fixed valvular aortic stenosis.

Fig. 125-A shows a simultaneous left ventricular (LV) and brachial artery pressure (BA) in a patient with *congenital valvular aortic stenosis* (bicuspid aortic valve). A gradient of about 75 mm. of Hg. is present across the aortic valve. The third complex recorded on the ECG is a ventricular extrasystole (*). The prematurity of this beat induces a fall of the peripheral and ventricular pressures with a consequent reduction of the gradient across the stenotic valve. During the post-extrasystolic pause, the ventricle has a longer diastole and, therefore, develops a higher endiastolic pressure and tension. The ventricular muscle, then, contracts with more energy on a larger volume of blood. Therefore, the post-extrasystolic beat when compared to a control beat will show: a) an increased systolic pressure; b) an increased pressure gradient between LV and BA and, c) an increase in the differential peripheral pressure.

In the case of hypertrophic subaortic stenosis (fig. 125-D), the hemodynamic behavior determined by the extrasystole is pathognomonic for this condition and quite different from that of a valvular aortic stenosis. In fact, when IHSS is suspected clinically one of the rules is to induce some extrasystoles during cardiac catheterization and observe the hemodynamic response. The *post-extrasystolic beat* will show a definite increase in the *ventricular systolic pressure and in the pressure gradient* while at the same time, it will present a drop in the *differential peripheral pressure of the post-extrasystolic beat*. The hemodynamic behavior of IHSS is determined by an augmented contractility of the post-extrasystolic beat and by an increase in the muscular stenosis of the aortic outflow tract.

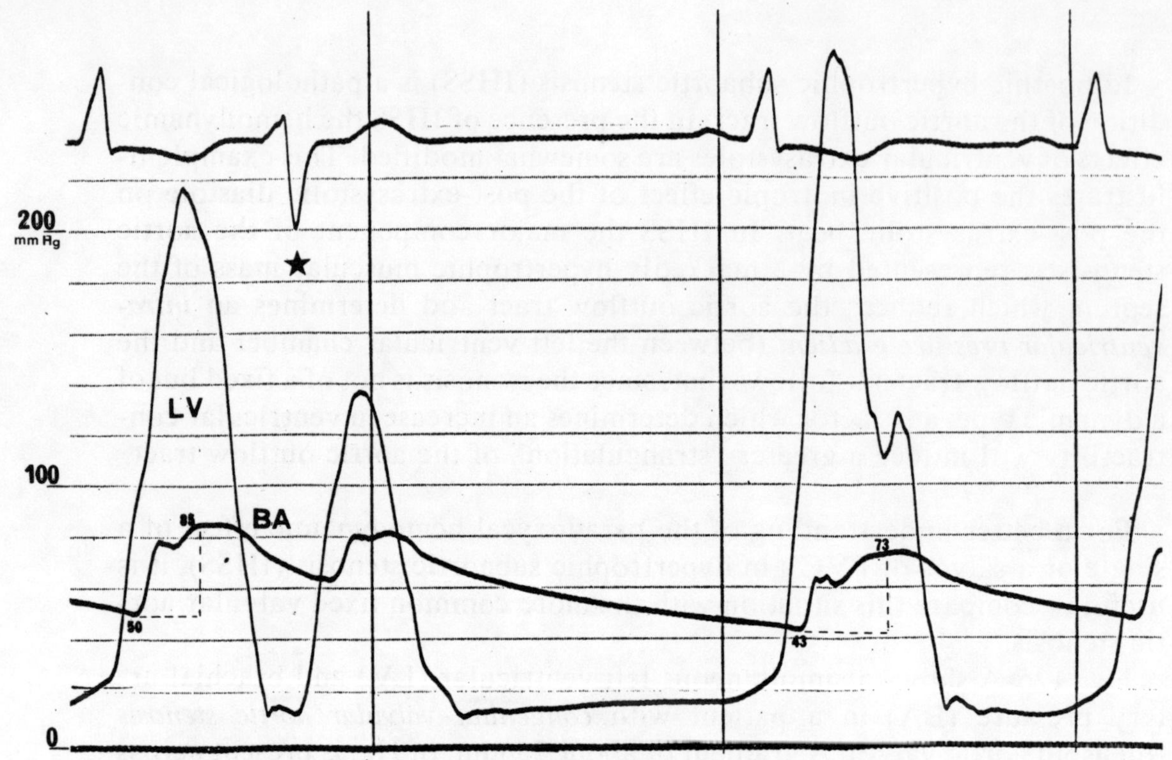

Fig. 126-A - Extrasystole and hypertrophic subaortic stenosis. See text.

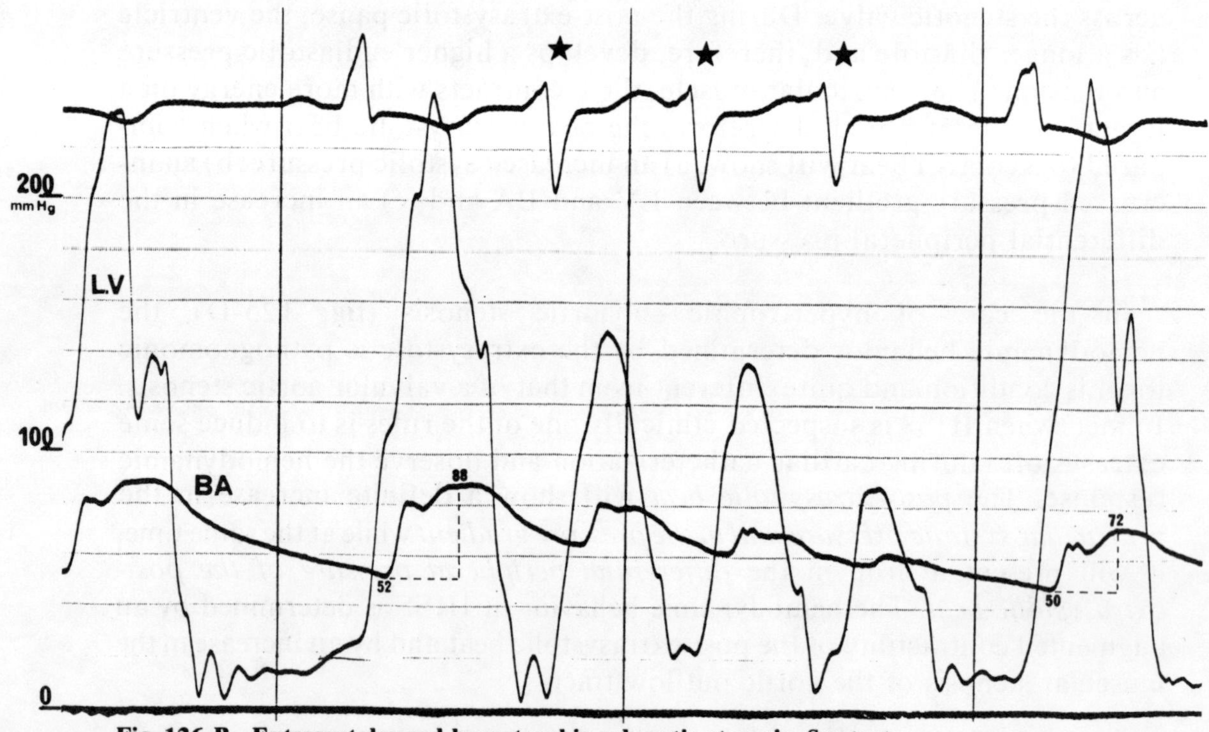

Fig. 126-B - Extrasystoles and hypertrophic subaortic stenosis. See text.

Another patient with hypertrophic subaortic stenosis (IHSS) is presented in fig. 126-A and 126-B.

In fig. 126-A the ventricular extrasystole is indicated by the asterisk and is followed by a long diastolic pause. The post-extrasystolic beat presents a marked increase in the pressure gradient (from 120 to 180 mm. of Hg.) which is determined both by an increased ventricular systolic pressure and by a decreased peripheral pulse systolic pressure.

Fig. 126-B presents the same patient during a salvo of ventricular extrasystoles. It appears evident that a gradual and continuous decrease in the ventricular systolic (LV) and brachial artery pressures (BA) and of the pressure gradient across the stenotic outflow tract occurs with the premature beats. The post-extrasystolic beat again presents the classical finding of hypertrophic subaortic stenosis which is represented by a decrease in the peripheral differential pressure.

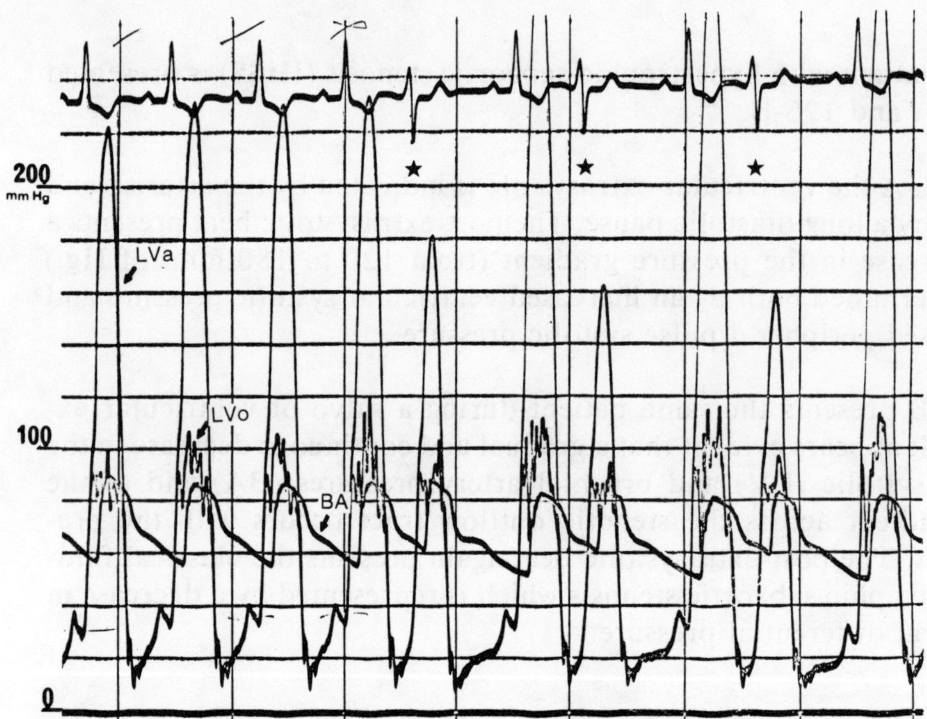

Fig. 127-A - Extrasystoles and hypertrophic subaortic stenosis. LVa = left ventricular apical pressure; LVo = left ventricular outflow tract pressure. See text. text.

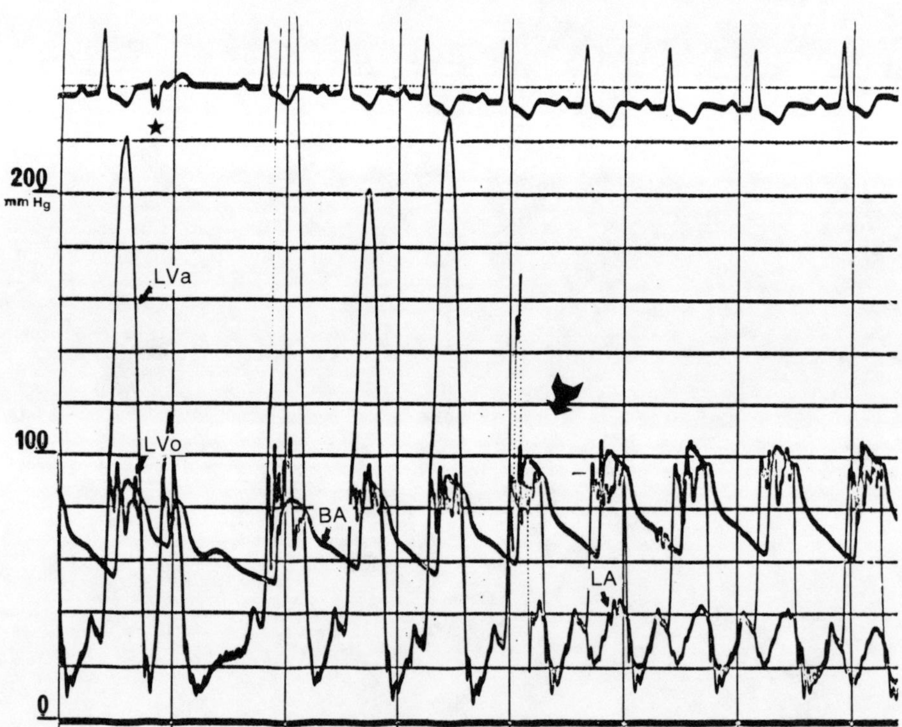

Fig. 127-B - Extrasystoles and hypertrophic subaortic stenosis. The arrow indicates the catheter passing from the left ventricular chamber (LVc) into the left atrium (LA). LVo = pressure in the left ventricular outflow tract; BA = brachial artery.

Fig. 127-A is the simultaneous recording of the pressures of the brachial artery (BA), the left ventricular apical area (LVa) and the aortic outflow tract (LVo) just below the aortic valve. The marked pressure gradient *within the left ventricular chambers* is caused by the hypertrophic subaortic stenosis (gradient between LVa and LVo) and it appears quite obvious. Naturally, a gradient is present also between the LVa and BA pressures. On the surface ECG three extrasystoles are present (*) and they clearly show the hemodynamic effects on the post-extrasystolic beat.

Fig. 127-B belongs to the same patient. The arrow is indicating the moment in which the catheter, which was introduced into the left ventricle through a transeptal approach, is pulled back in the left atrium. The left atrial pressure (LA) is overimposed on the ventricular diastolic pressure.

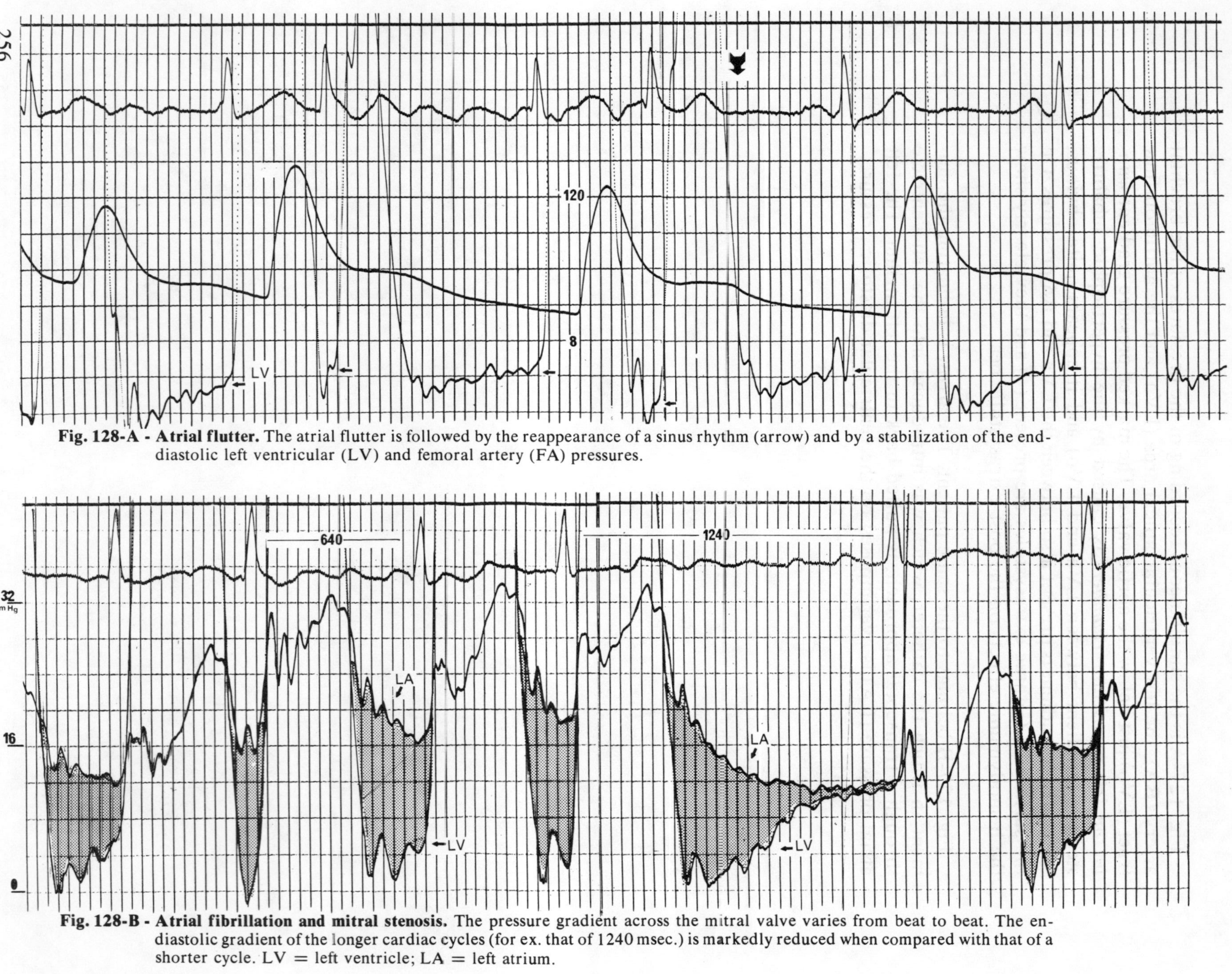

Fig. 128-A - Atrial flutter. The atrial flutter is followed by the reappearance of a sinus rhythm (arrow) and by a stabilization of the end-diastolic left ventricular (LV) and femoral artery (FA) pressures.

Fig. 128-B - Atrial fibrillation and mitral stenosis. The pressure gradient across the mitral valve varies from beat to beat. The end-diastolic gradient of the longer cardiac cycles (for ex. that of 1240 msec.) is markedly reduced when compared with that of a shorter cycle. LV = left ventricle; LA = left atrium.

ATRIAL FLUTTER AND FIBRILLATION

These arrhythmias modify the cardiac hemodynamics through three main factors:

a) the rapid ventricular rate which usually accompanies the atrial tachyar-rhythmia.

b) the irregular ventricular diastolic filling periods.

c) the lack of atrial contribution to ventricular diastolic filling (atrial fibrillation) and abnormal atrio-ventricular synchronism (atrial flutter).

Fig. 128-A shows the spontaneous cessation of an atrial flutter, with a variable A-V block, and the restoration of a regular sinus rhythm (arrow). The surface ECG is recorded simultaneously to the left ventricular (LV) diastolic pressure (pressure scale = 0-40 mm. of Hg.) and the femoral artery pressure (FA), with a pressure scale equal to 0-200 mm. of Hg. In other words, each horizontal line is equal to 4 mm. of Hg. for the left ventricular pressure and to 20 mm. of Hg. for the peripheral pressure. It may be easily noticed that, during the atrial flutter, the ventricular endiastolic and femoral pressures change beat by beat; this is in relation to the different lengths of the ventricular diastolic filling periods determined by the variable A-V block. A shorter cardiac cycle will determine a lower endiastolic and femoral artery pressure; this is compensated by the beat with a longer diastolic interval. With the restoration of a regular sinus rhythm (last two beats) the ventricular and peripheral pressures are stabilized into constant and normal levels.

Fig. 128-B shows the effect of the irregular ventricular rate of an atrial fibrillation on the pressure gradient across the mitral valve, in a patient with moderate mitral stenosis. The left atrial pressure (LA), obtained through a transeptal route, and the left ventricular endiastolic pressure (LV) are recorded simultaneously with the surface ECG. The pressure gradient between the two chambers is indicated by the shaded area. It is interesting to observe the effect of the different lengths of cardiac cycles on the gradient across the mitral valve. For example, the cycle of 640 msec. (between the second and third QRS) determines a gradient which is the highest at the beginning of diastole and remains elevated in mid and endiastole. The cardiac cycle of 1240 msec. (between the fourth and fifth QRS) presents a gradient which is elevated at the beginning of diastole but which gradually drops and disappear at endiastole. This is because of the longer ventricular diastolic filling period which allows for better atrial emptying. Furthermore, the hemodynamic disturbances of atrial fibrillation are not only secondary to an irregular ventricular rate, but also to a decreased atrial contribution to ventricular filling for the absence of valid atrial contractions. It has been clearly shown that valid atrial contractions contribute for at least 20% of the cardiac output.

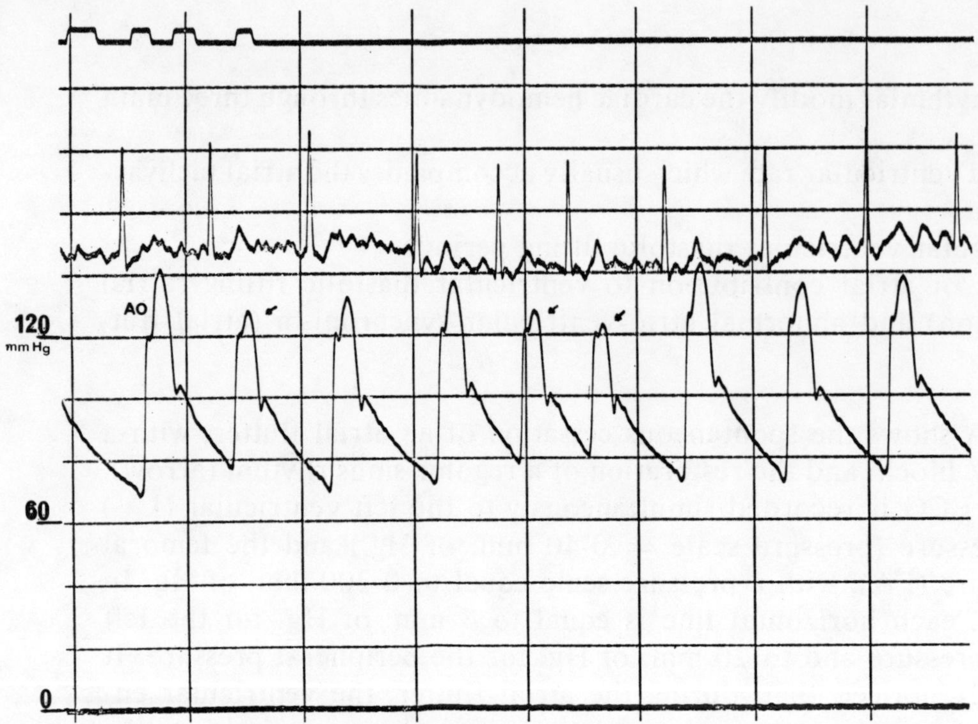

Fig. 129-A - Atrial fibrillation. See text.

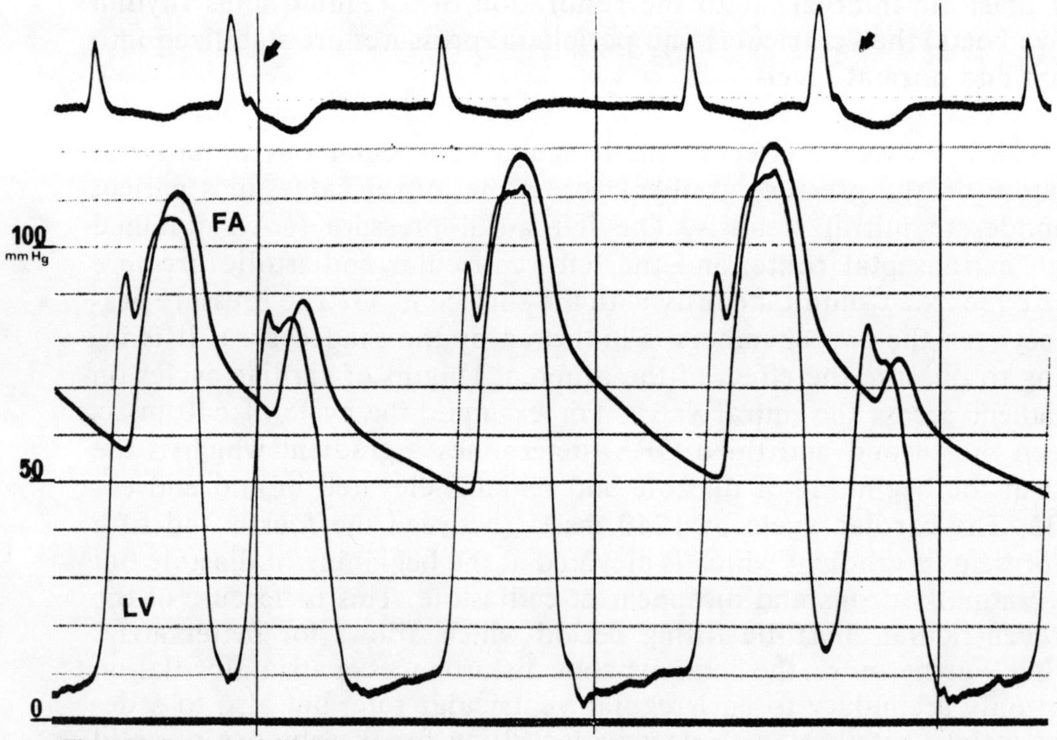

Fig. 129-B - Atrial fibrillation. See text. LV = left ventricle; FA = femoral artery.

ATRIAL FIBRILLATION

Fig. 129-A illustrates the different systolic aortic pressures during the irregular ventricular contractions of an atrial fibrillation. In this tracing it is possible to notice a pressure difference of at least 15-20 mm. of Hg. between the beats with a longer diastolic filling period and those terminating shorter cardiac cycles (arrows).

Some of the impulses coming from the fibrillating atria are transmitted to the ventricles very prematurely in diastole. Therefore, they force the ventricle to contract on a smaller volume of blood. Although these contractions are hemodynamically effective, sometimes they behave like ventricular extrasystoles interrupting a sinus rhythm (see page 246).

In fig. 129-B two supraventricular beats, prematurely conducted to the ventricles during an atrial fibrillation (arrows), generate a peripheral pulse whose amplitude varies in relation to the prematurity of the beat. The peripheral pulse may not be present on palpation and determines the so-called "pulse deficit" (difference between the apical and peripheral rates).

RHYTHMO-QUIZ

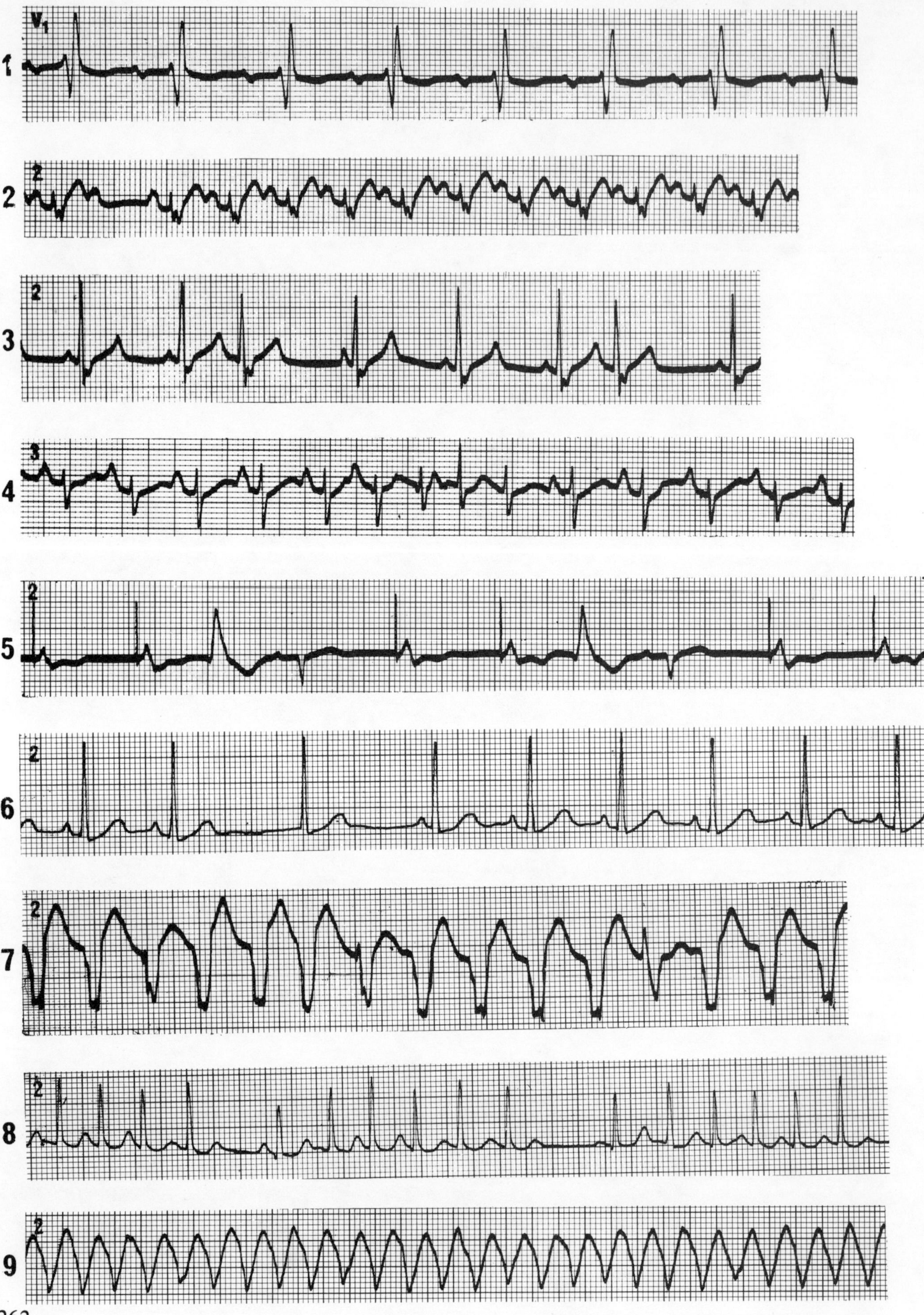

262

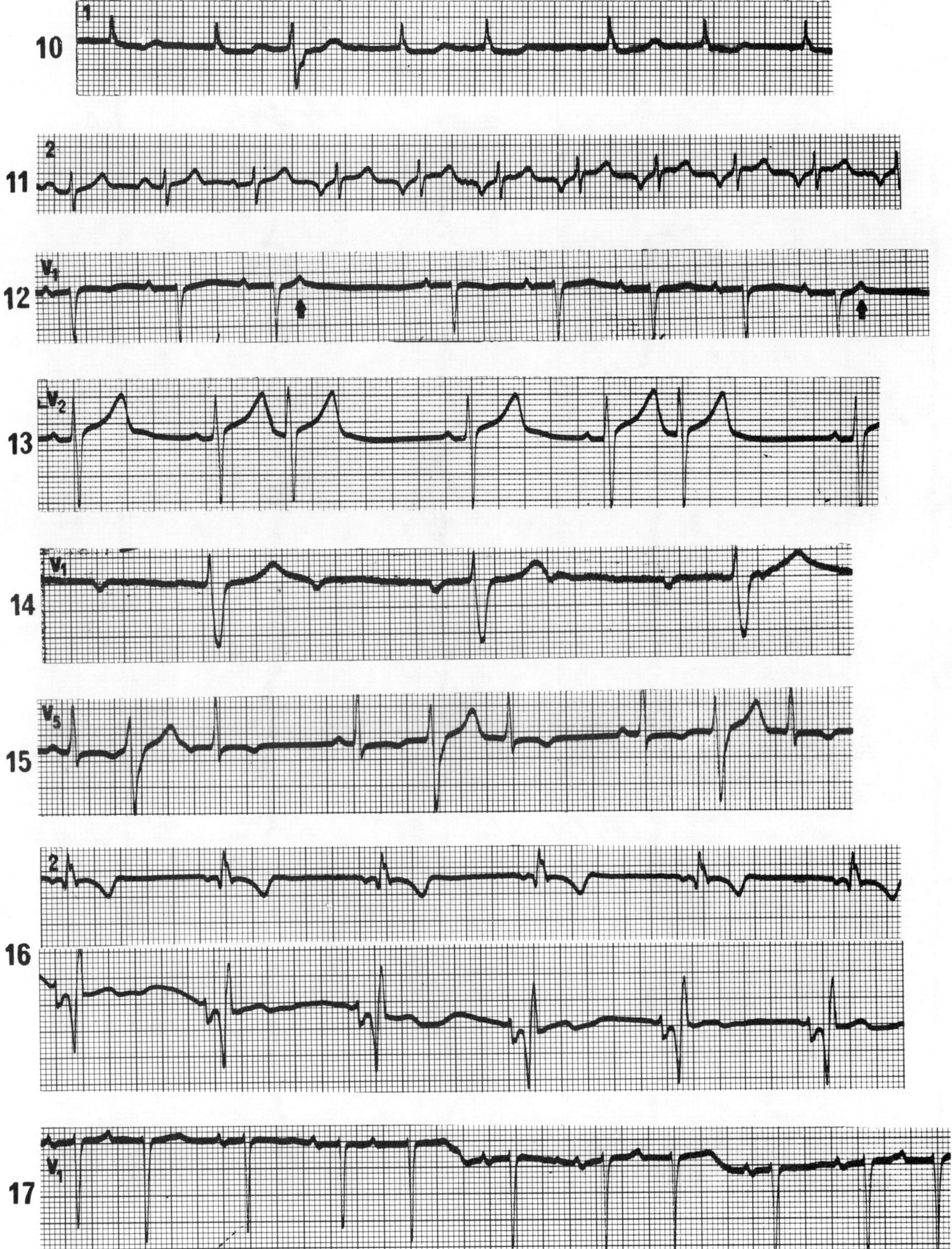

10
1
11
2
12
V₁
13
V₂
14
V₁
15
V₅
16
2
17
V₁

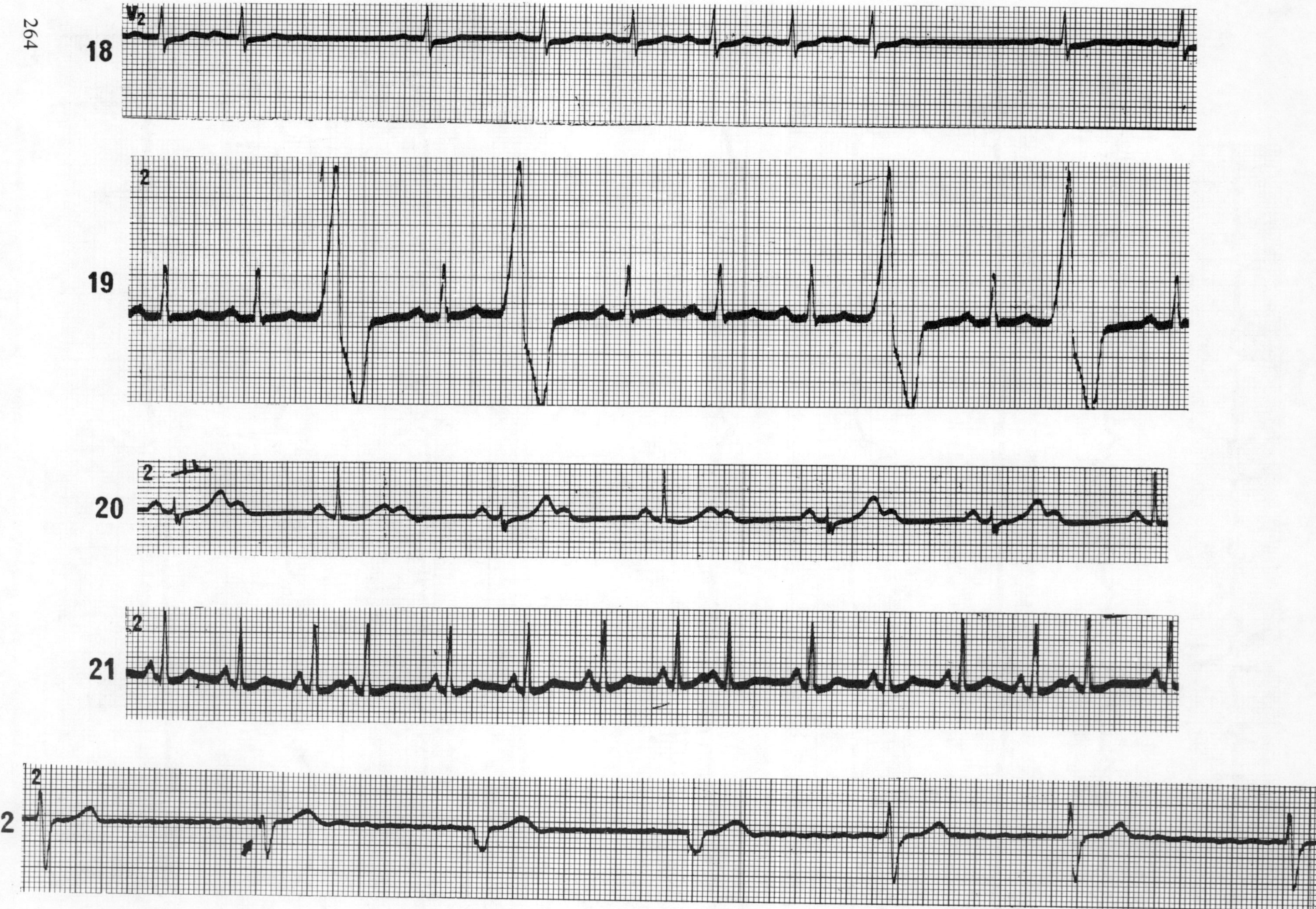
264
V2
18
2
19
2
20
2
21
2
22

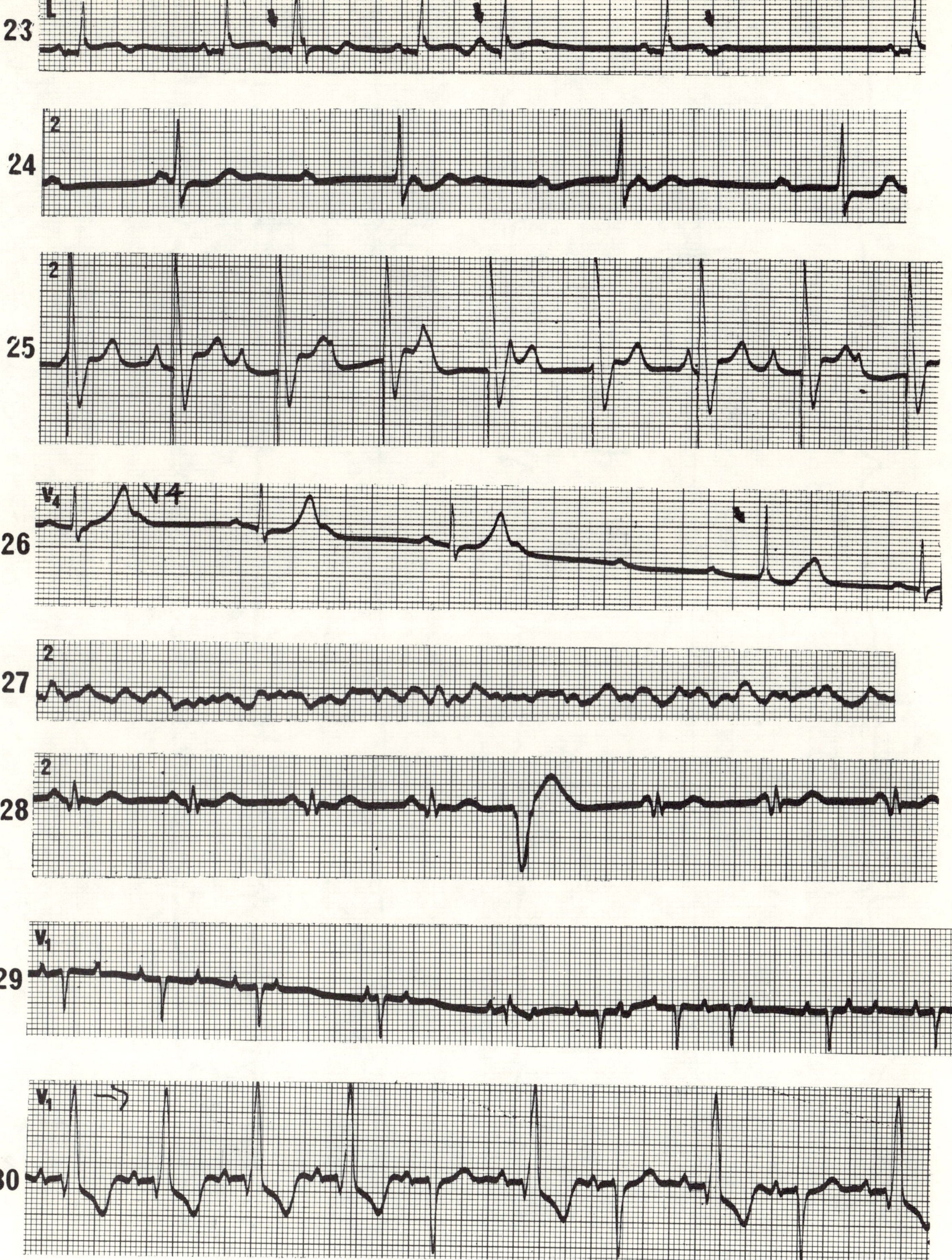

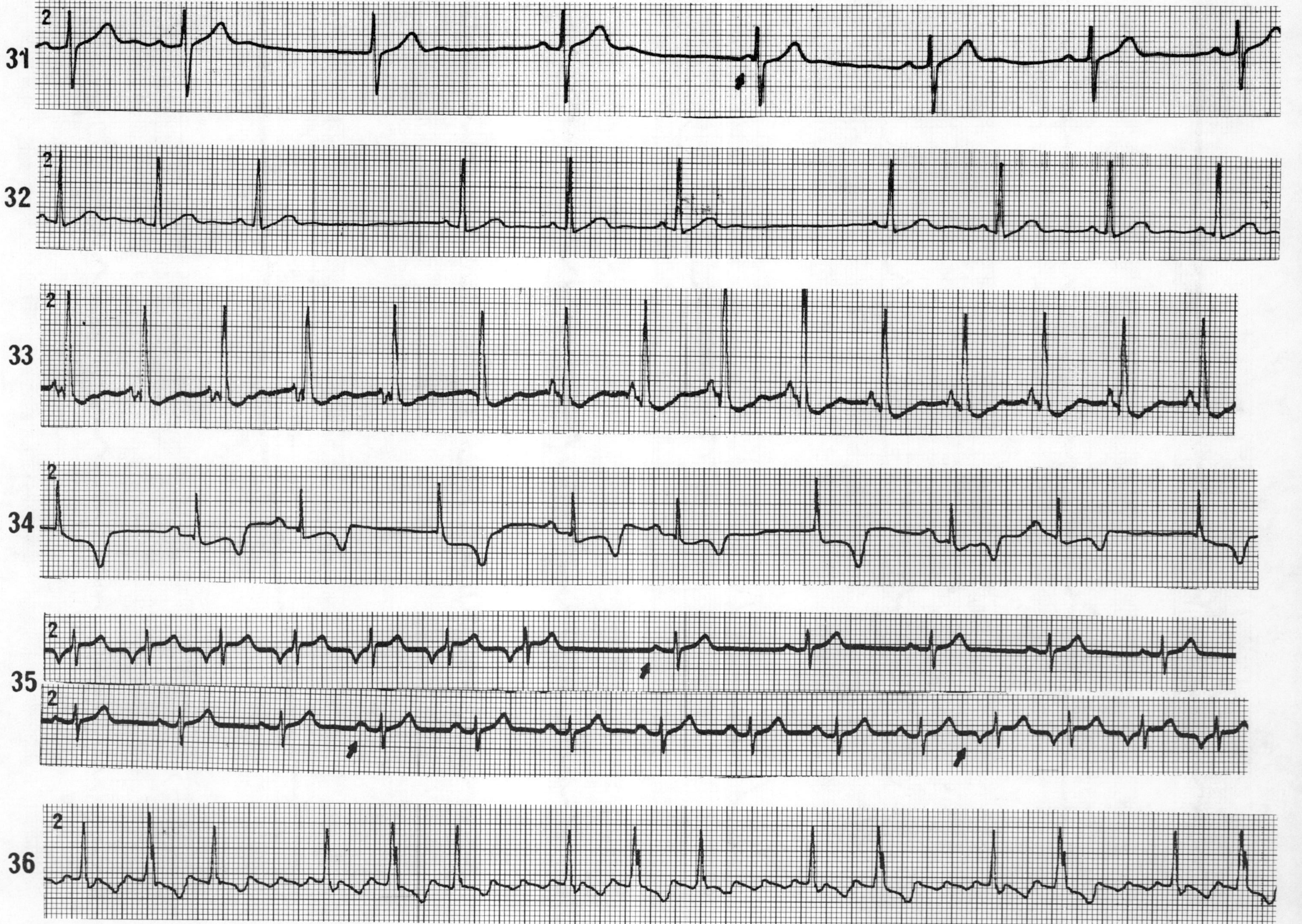

31
2
32
2
33
2
34
2
35
2
2
36
2

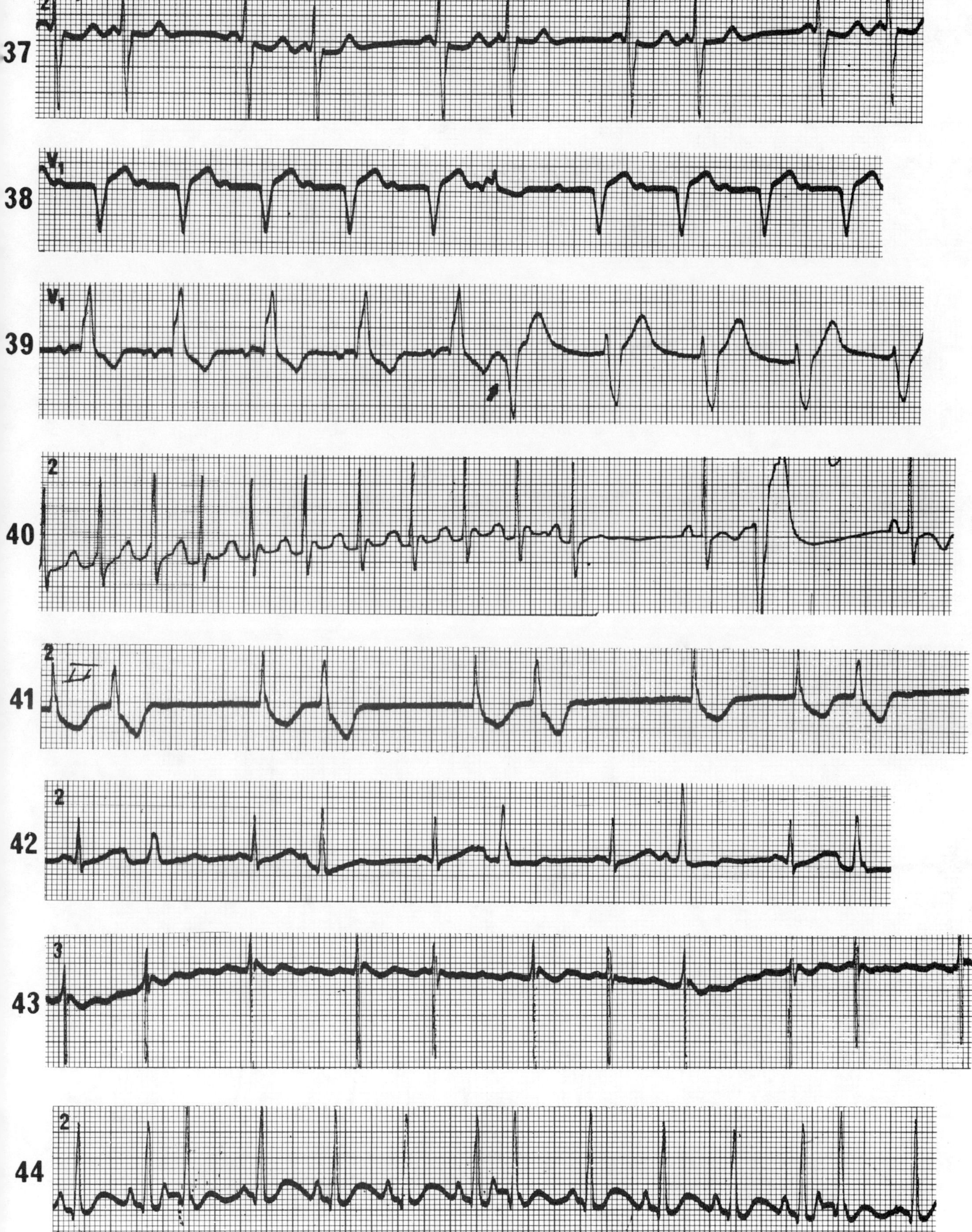

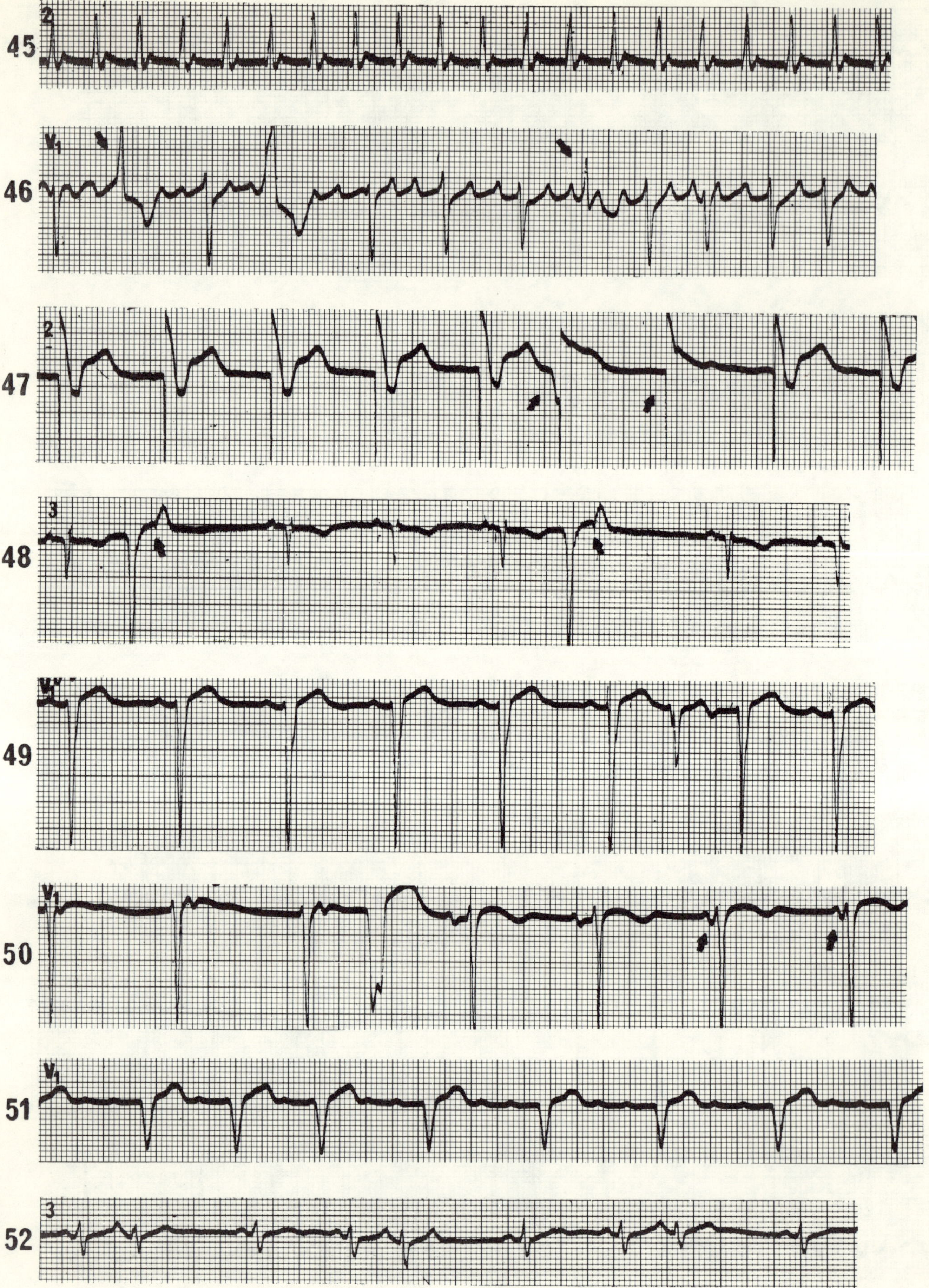

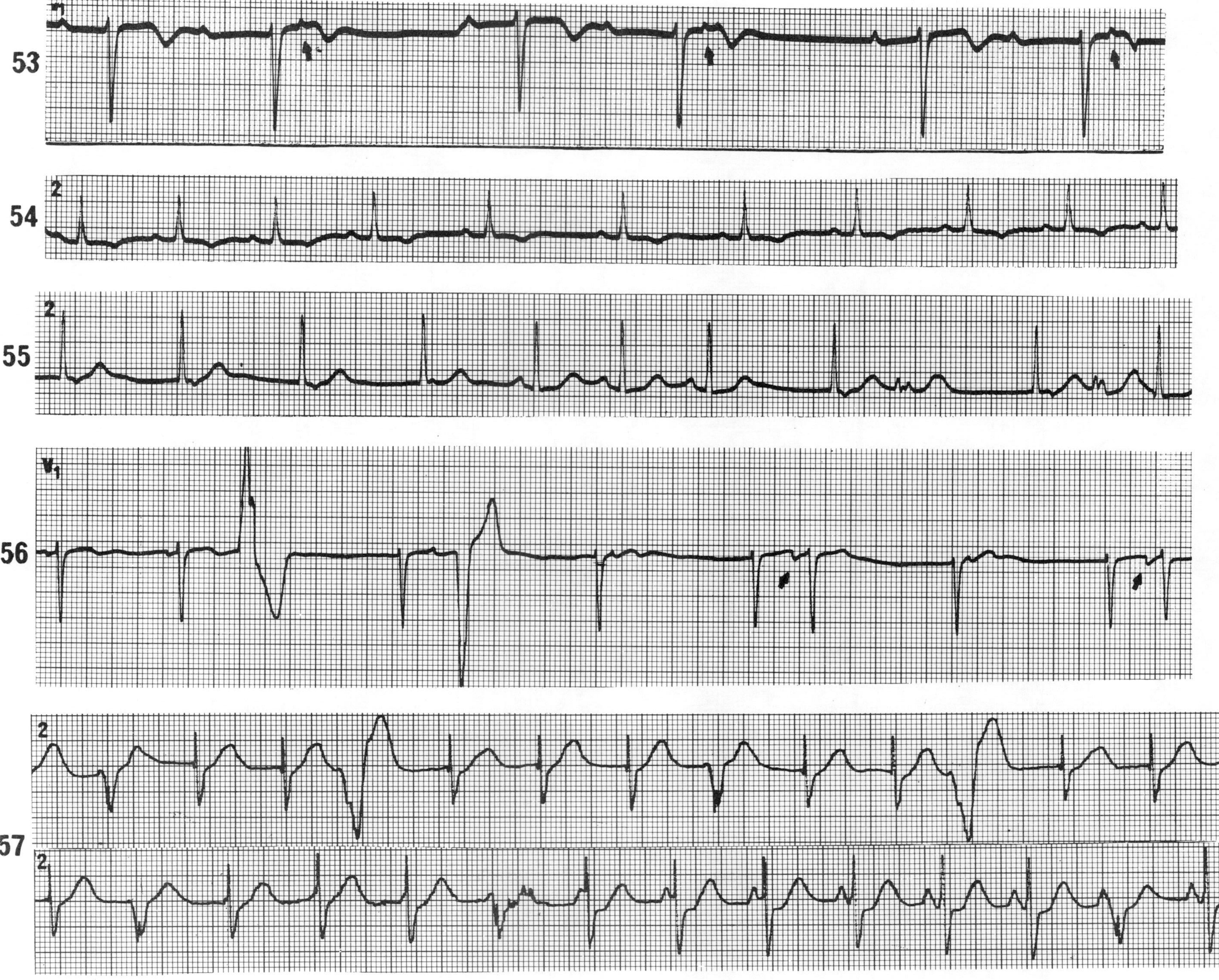

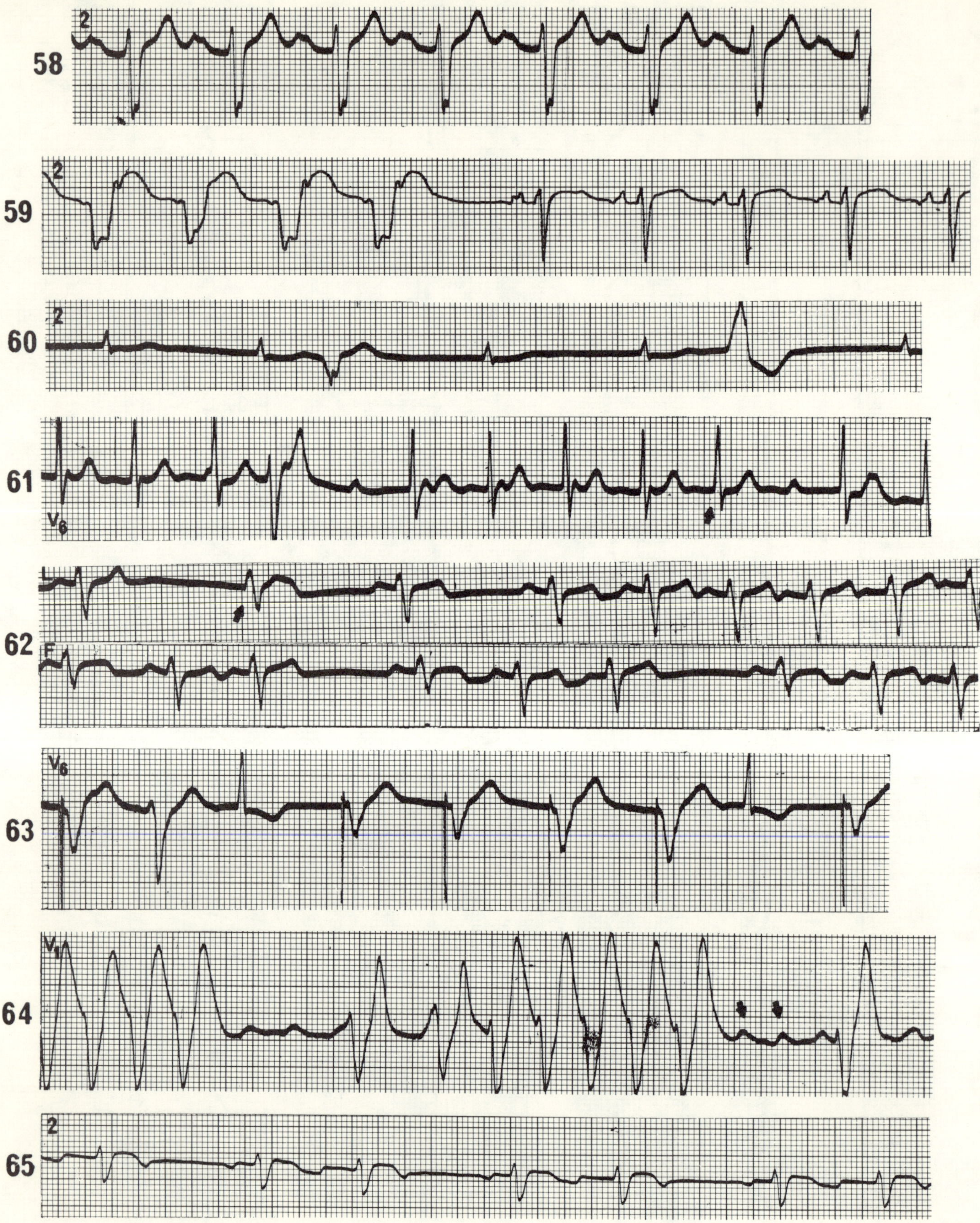

58
59
60
61
62
63
64
65

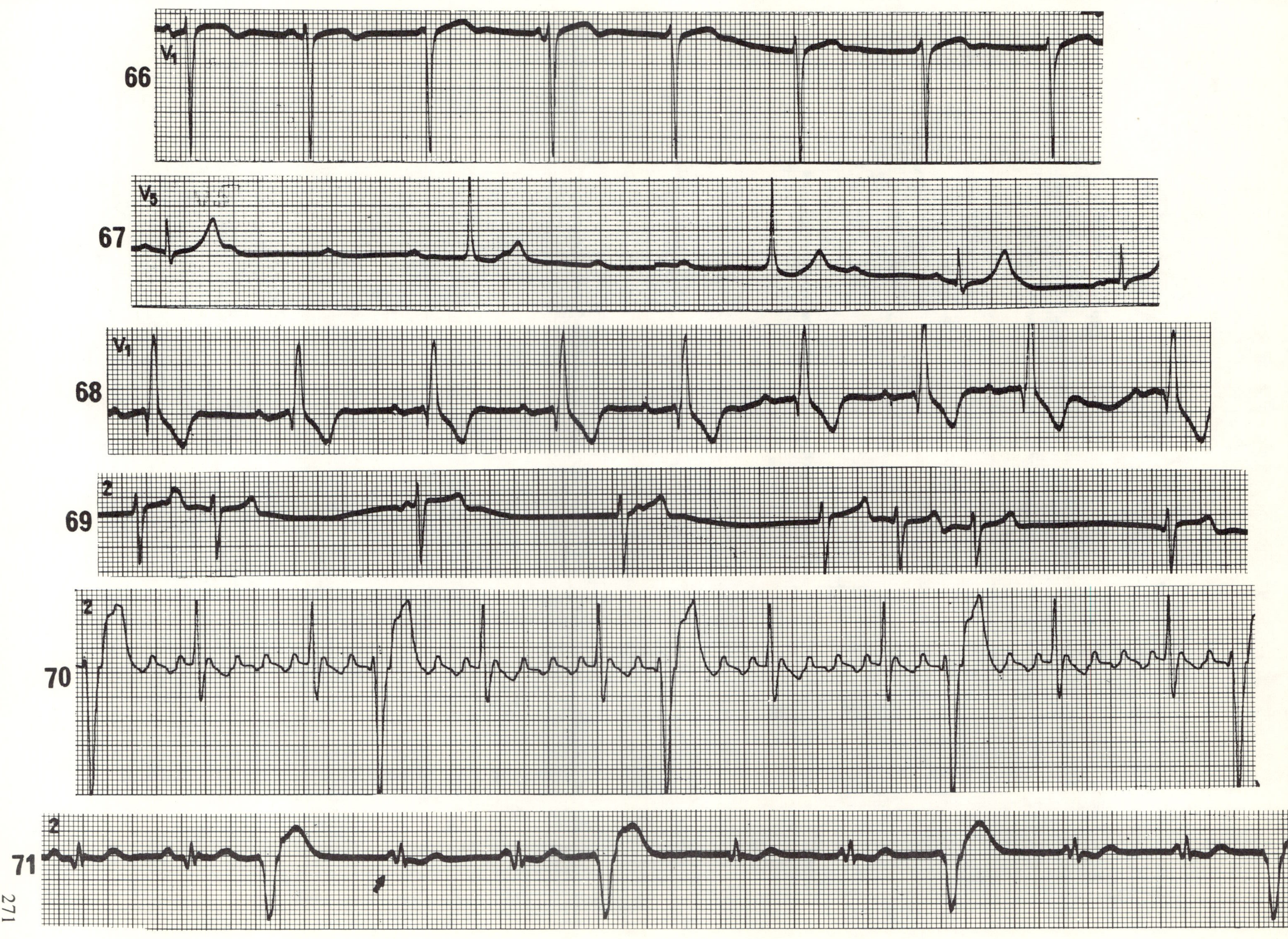
66 V₁
67 V₅
68 V₁
69 2
70 2
71 2

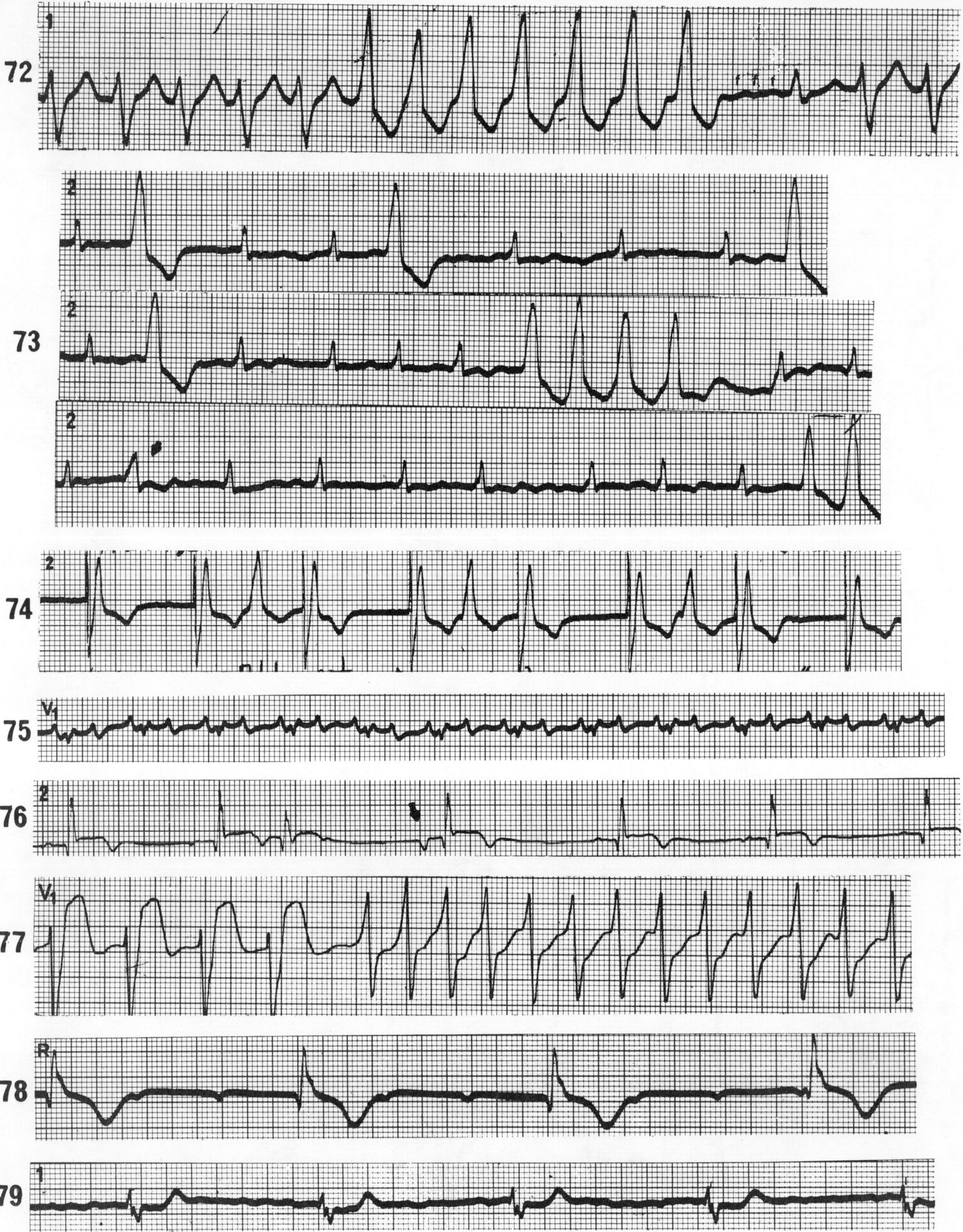

72

73

74

75

76

77

78

79

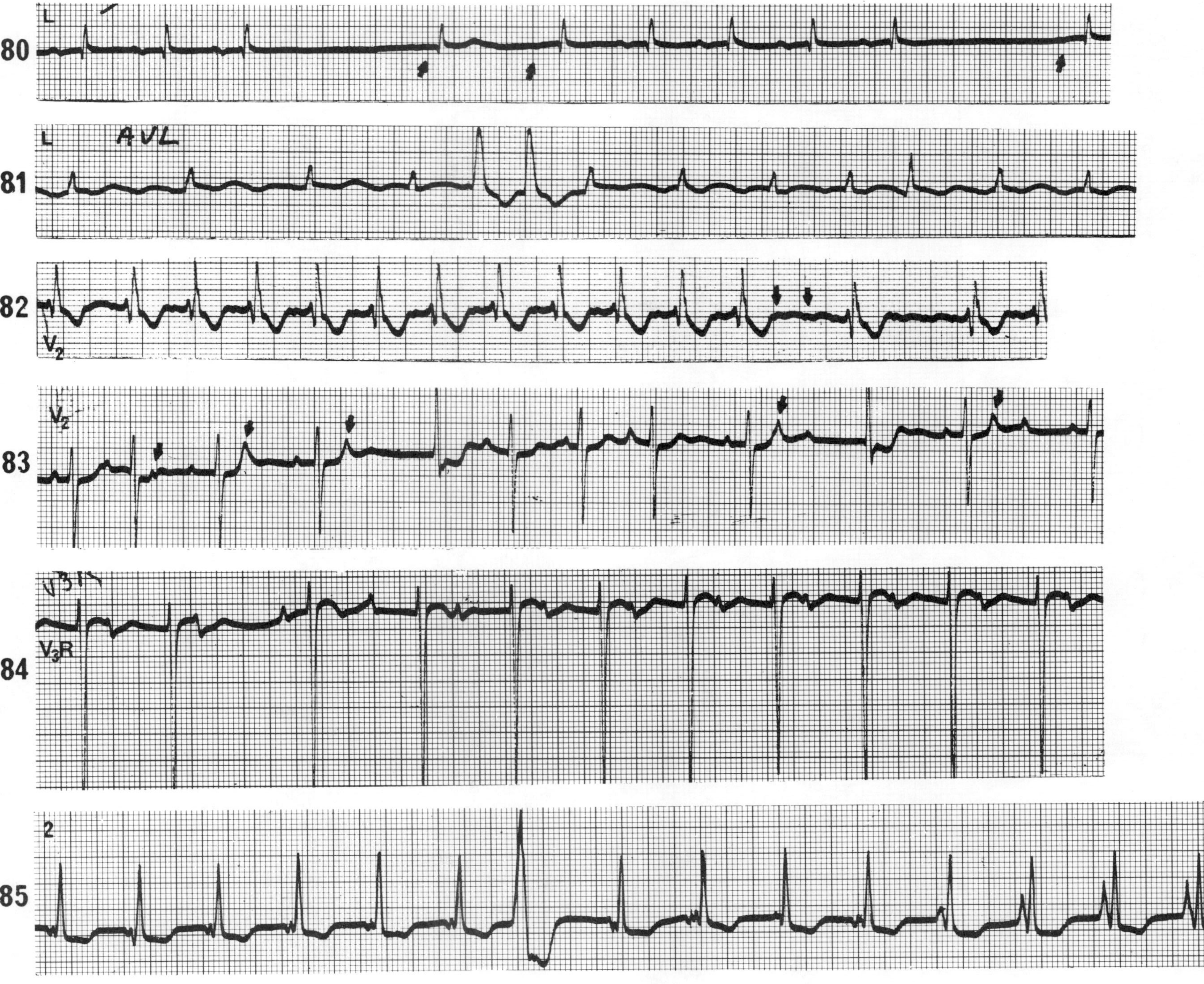

273

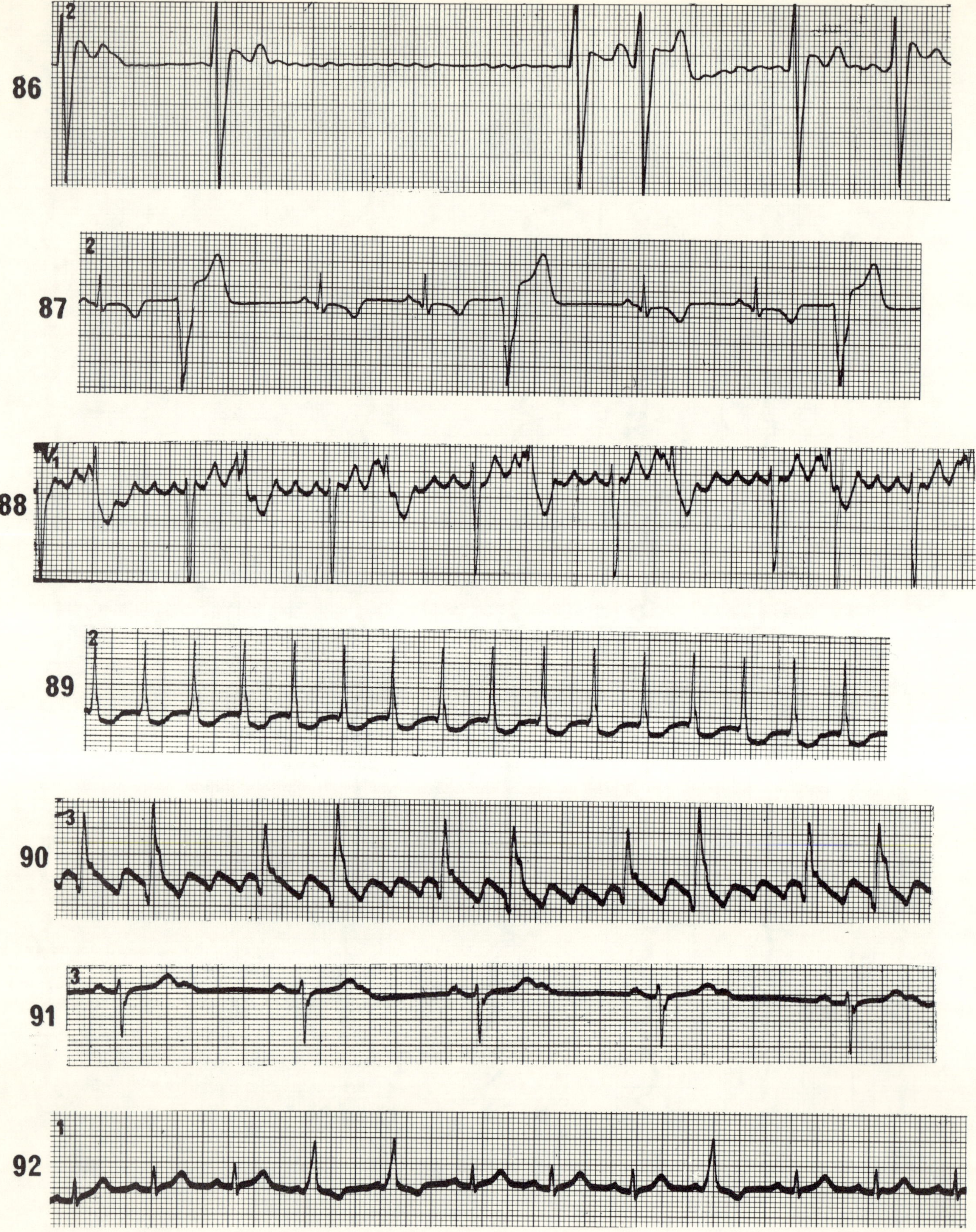

86

87

88

89

90

91

92

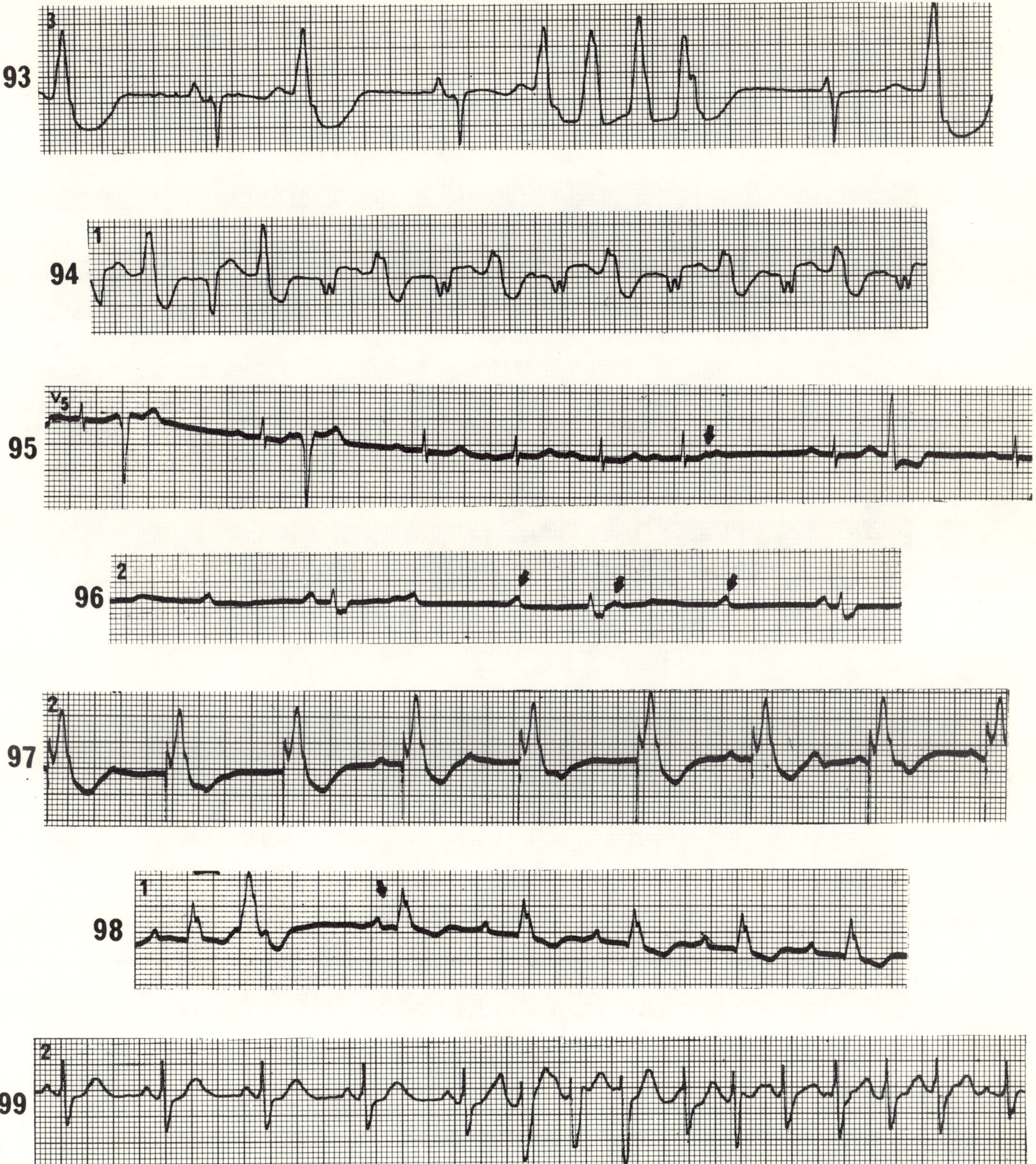

93

94

95

96

97

98

99

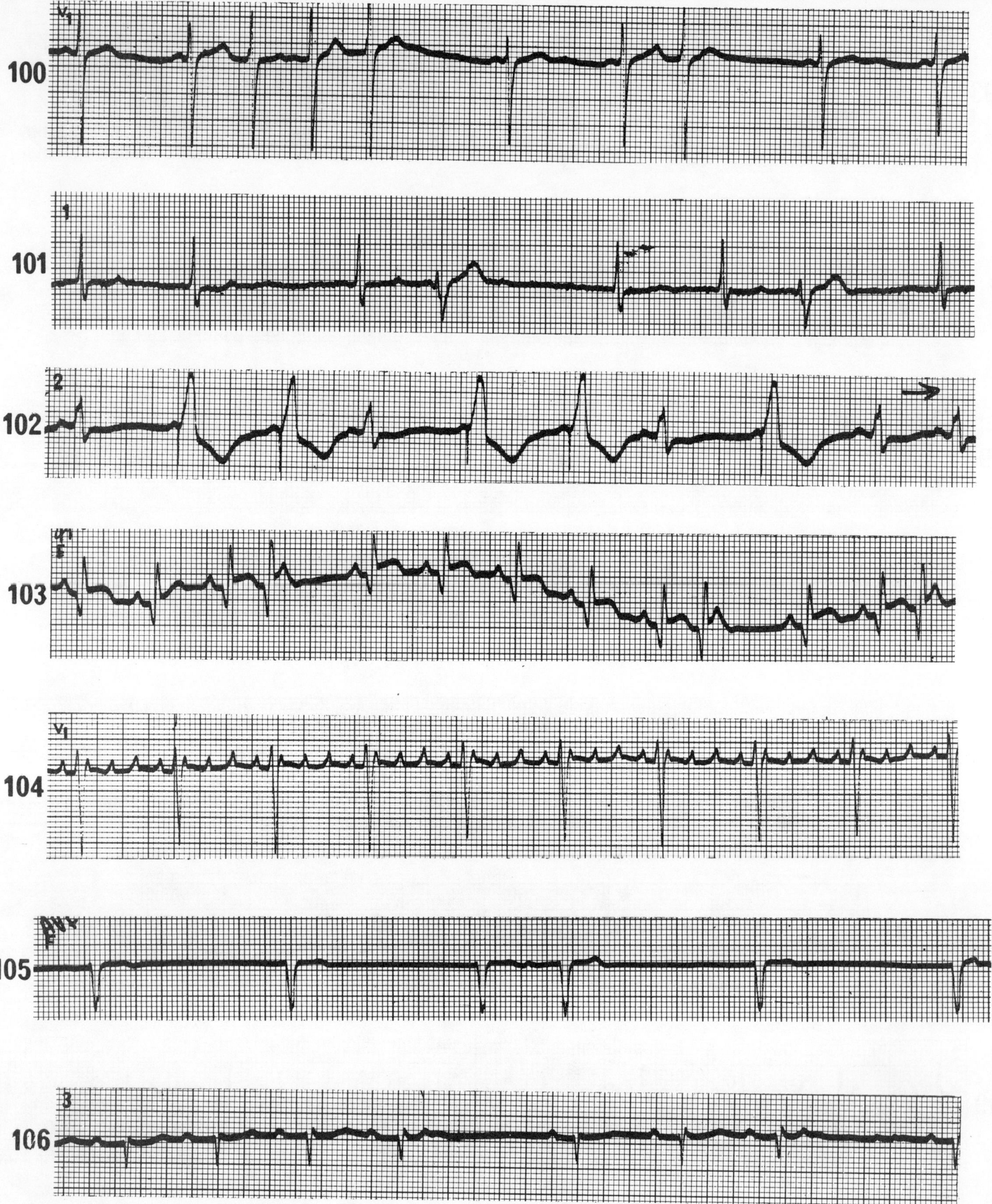

V1
100
1
101
2
102
103
V1
104
aVF
105
3
106

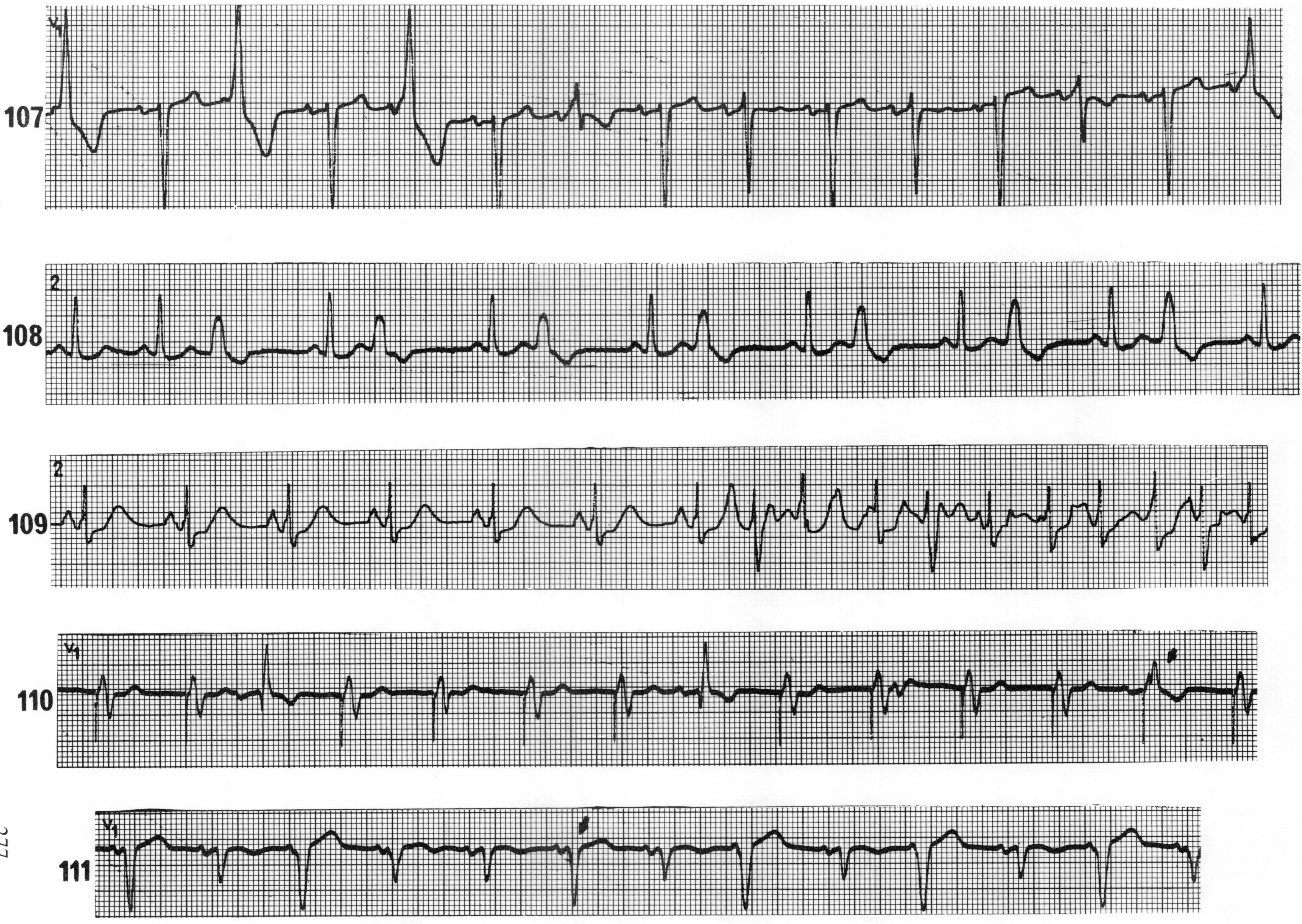

107
108
109
110
111

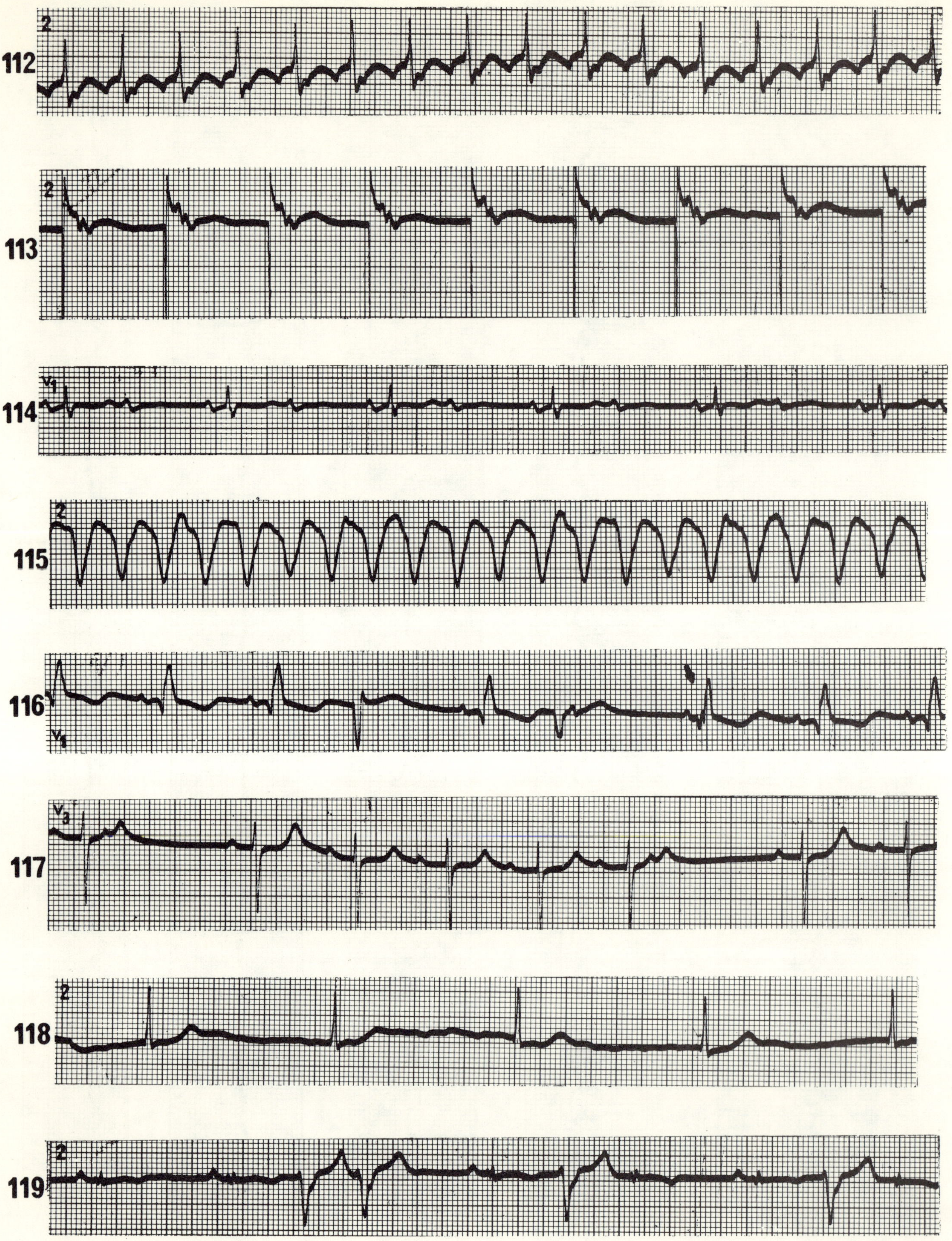

112
2
113
2
114
V₁
115
2
116
V₁
V₃
117
V₃
118
2
119
2

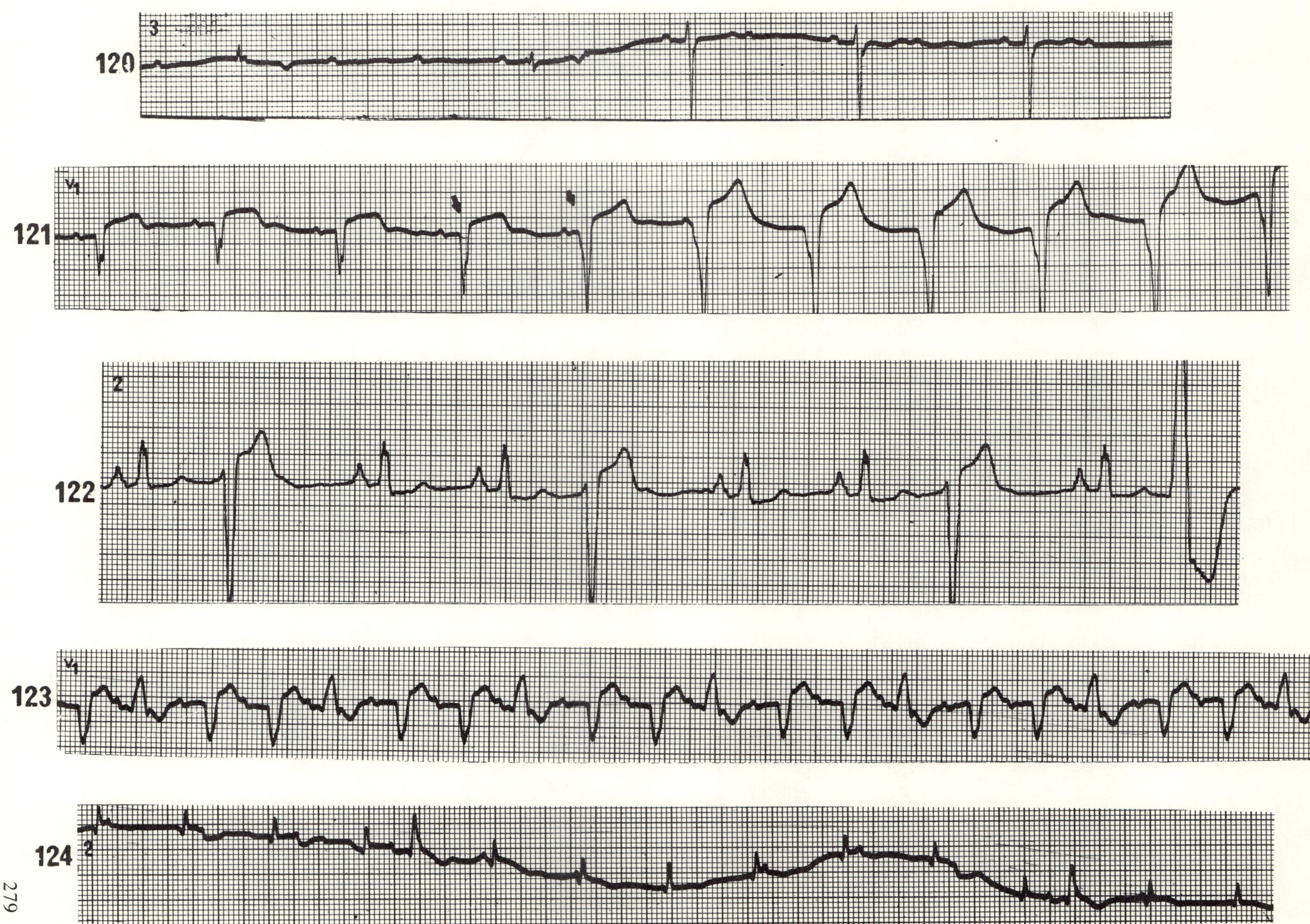

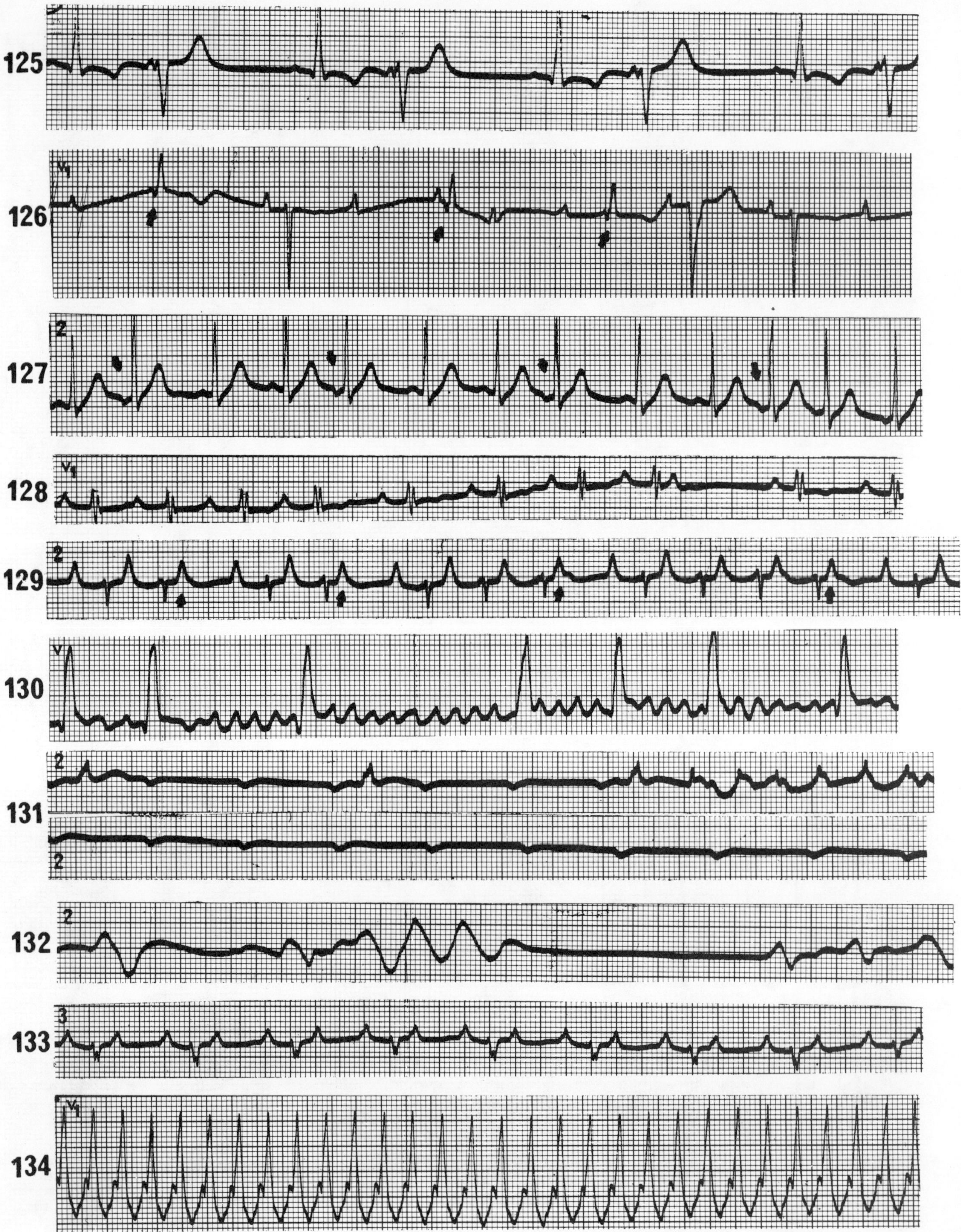

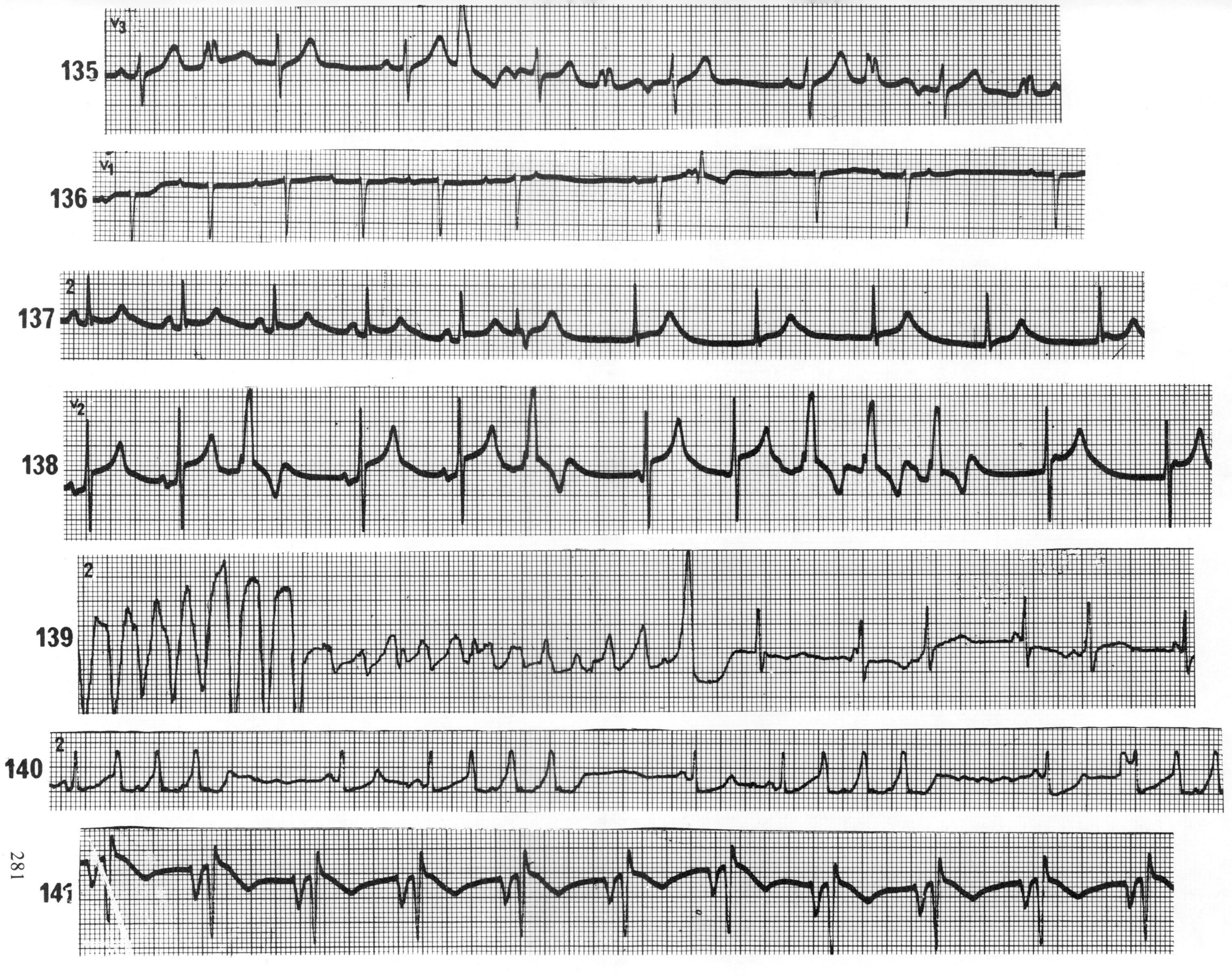
135 V3
136 V1
137 2
138 V2
139 2
140 2
141 V1
281

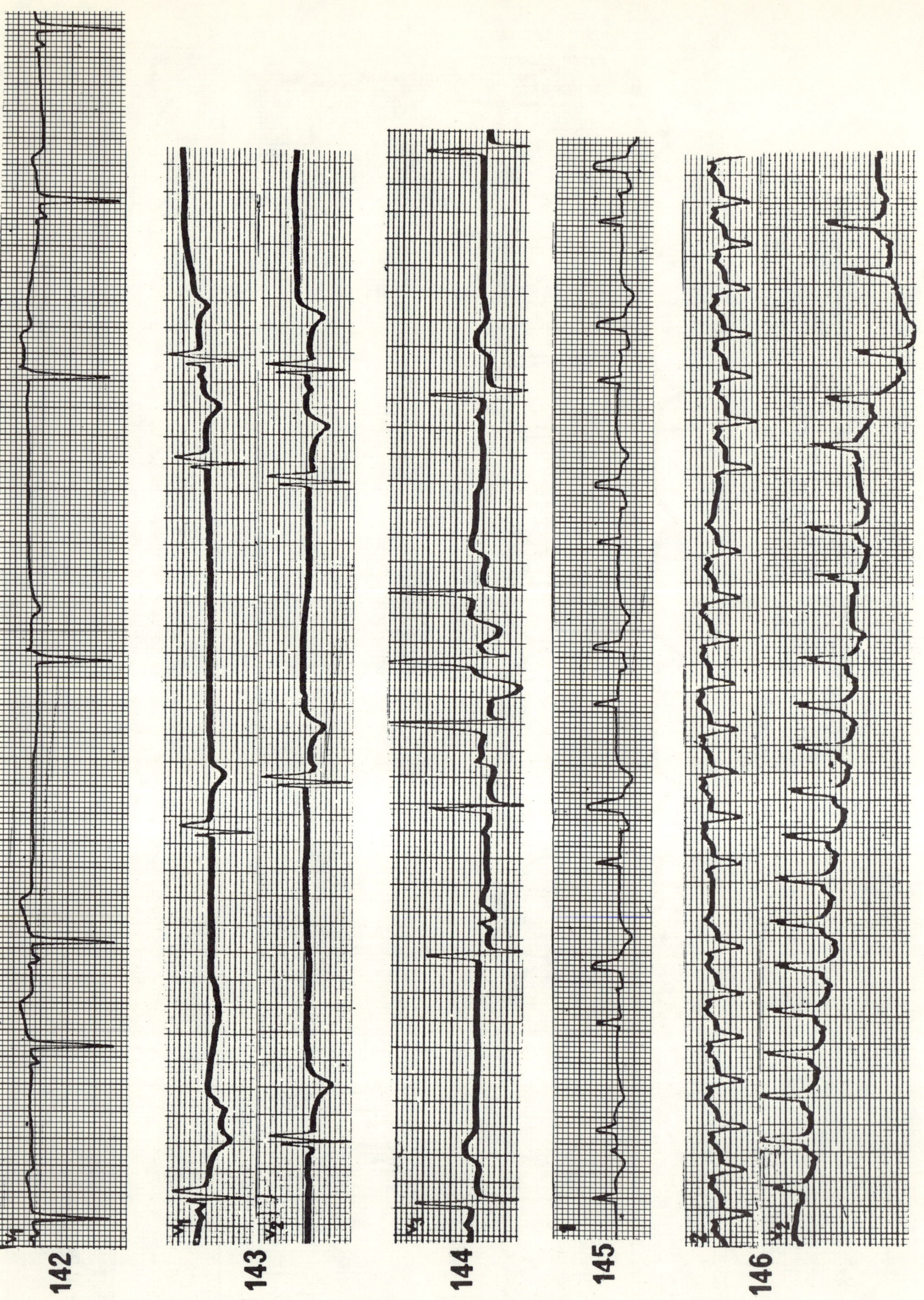

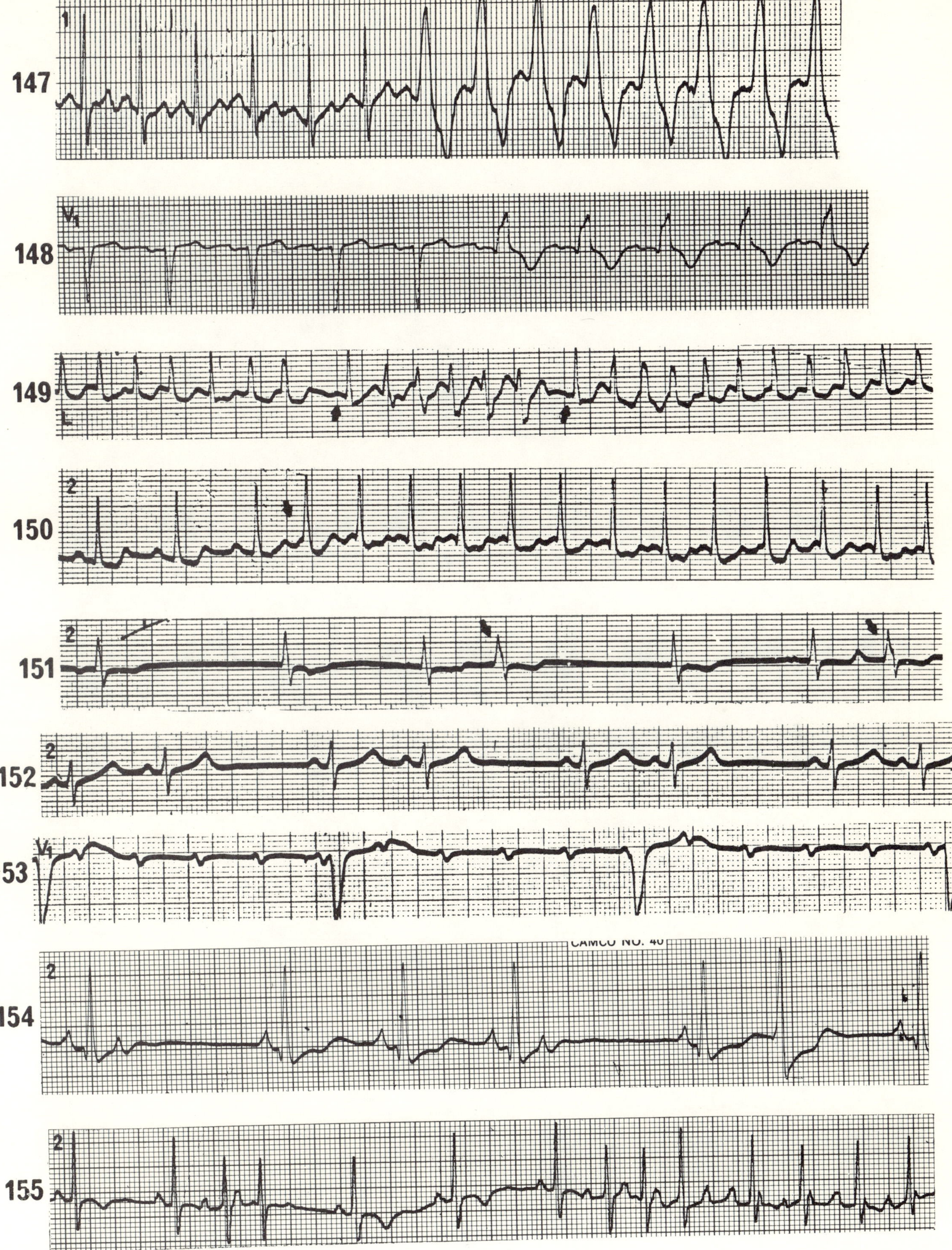

RITHMO-QUIZ INTERPRETATION

1 - FIRST DEGREE A-V BLOCK AND RIGHT BUNDLE BRANCH BLOCK. The P-R interval is prolonged (0.28 sec.) and the QRS complexes are wide and typical of a right bundle branch block. The rhythm is sinus.

2 - SINUS TACHYCARDIA AND SECOND DEGREE A-V BLOCK MOBITZ TYPE II. The second P wave is blocked in the A-V junction. Notice that the sinus rate is 130/minute and that the P-R interval of the sinus beats conducted to the ventricle is 0.20 seconds (first degree A-V block). This indicates a decreased A-V conduction which becomes clearly evident when the P wave is blocked (second degree A-V block).

3 - ATRIAL EXTRASYSTOLES. P¹ waves are buried in the preceding T waves; the QRS complexes are similar to those of sinus beats.

4 - PAROXYSMAL ATRIAL TACHYCARDIA. A brief salvo of PAT with 1:1 A-V conduction may be recognized in the central part of the tracing. The basic rhythm is a sinus tachycardia.

5 - DEMAND PACEMAKER - QRS INHIBITED PACING. The artificial impulses show complete ventricular capture. Two ventricular extrasystoles are followed by two sinus beats conducted to the ventricles. The sinus and extrasystolic potentials inhibits the pacemaker. The standby interval is 760 msec.

6 - SINO-ATRIAL BLOCK AND JUNCTIONAL ESCAPE BEAT. The second beat is followed by a pause determined by the absence of sinus impulses. The pause terminates with the appearance of a junctional escape beat followed by a normal sinus rhythm.

7 - VENTRICULAR TACHYCARDIA. The great majority of QRS complexes are wide and bizarre, typical of a ventricular ectopic focus. The third and seventh complexes are fusion beats while the twelfth QRS is a supraventricular beat with complete ventricular capture.

8 - ATRIAL PAROXYSMAL TACHYCARDIA. At least three brief paroxysms are recognizable; the average rate is 170/minute. The paroxysms cease abruptly and allow for the emergence of a sinus rhythm.

9 - VENTRICULAR TACHYCARDIA. The rate is rapid (270/minute) and slightly irregular and the QRS complexes are wide and bizarre. P waves are not recognizable.

10 - ATRIAL FIBRILLATION. The baseline is undulated. P waves or P¹ waves are not present. The third QRS complex is not a ventricular extrasystole but a supraventricular beat with aberrant ventricular conduction. This terminates a shorter cardiac cycle and has a morphology of a right bundle branch block type.

11 - TRANSITION FROM A SINUS RHYTHM INTO A CORONARY SINUS RHYTHM. The third P wave is an atrial fusion beat (between a sinus and a coronary sinus impulse). Notice that the P wave morphology of the fusion beat is something in between the morphology of the first two sinus P waves and the P¹ wave of a coronary sinus beat. The P¹-R interval is 0.16 seconds.

12 - FIRST DEGREE A-V BLOCK AND BLOCKED ATRIAL EXTRASYSTOLES. The P-R interval of 0.24 seconds indicates a decreased conduction velocity in the A-V junction (first degree A-V block). Two slightly premature atrial extrasystoles (arrows) are not conducted to the ventricles.

13 - ATRIAL TRIGEMINY. An atrial extrasystole follows two sinus beats. The P¹ waves are buried into the descending branch of the preceding T wave.

14 - THIRD DEGREE A-V BLOCK (COMPLETE A-V BLOCK). The atrial rate is 69/min. while the ventricular is 30/min. There is no relation between P waves and the QRS complexes of idio-ventricular origin. A ventriculo-phasic sinus arrhythmia is present and is particularly evident in the last two P waves of the tracing.

15 - INTERPOLATED VENTRICULAR EXTRASYSTOLES. The extrasystoles do not have a fixed coupling. The P-R interval of the following sinus beat is prolonged and indicates a concealed retrograde ventriculo-atrial conduction of the extrasystole. It must be kept in mind that it is difficult to separate this situation with a "return extrasystole". The resultant rhythm is of a trigeminal type.

16 - "HIGH" JUNCTIONAL RHYTHM. The P^1 waves are inverted and the P^1-R interval is 0.10 seconds. The non simultaneous atrial unipolar electrogram of the lower tracing clearly show P^1 waves before each QRS. The rate is 52/min.

17 - ATRIAL TRIGEMINY WITH PROLONGED A-V CONDUCTION. The sinus beats have a borderline P-R interval (0.20 seconds). The slight prematurity of the extrasystolic impulse, occurring every third beat, reveals the latent pathology of the A-V conduction system (P^1-R equals 0.28 sec.).

18 - SINO-ATRIAL BLOCK AND SINO-ATRIAL WENCKEBACH. The rhythm is sinus. Two long pauses are present and they are almost multiple of two sinus cycles (S-A block). The central sequence is a sino-atrial Wenckebach period of 7:6 (notice the progressive shortening of the P-P intervals until an asystolic pause is reached. The P-R intervals of the Wenckebach sequence remain constant. Therefore, the S-A block is preceded by a S-A Wenckebach phenomenon.

19 - VENTRICULAR PARASYSTOLE. The coupling interval of the ectopic beats with the preceding sinus beats is variable. There is a common denominator interectopic interval (the interval between the second and third extrasystole is exactly twice the basic interectopic interval); fusion beats are not present in this case.

20 - SECOND DEGREE A-V BLOCK, MOBITZ TYPE II AND INTERMITTENT VENTRICULAR ABERRATION. The A-V block is constant and of the 2:1 type. The second, fourth and last QRS are normal while the others present a slight abnormality in the intraventricular conduction. The blocked P waves are easily visible. The atrial rate is 95/min. and the ventricular 48/min.

21 - ATRIAL EXTRASYSTOLES. The P waves of the atrial extrasystoles are easily recognized. They seem to emerge in a constant fashion after every four sinus beats (allorhythmia).

22 - ATRIAL FIBRILLATION AND HIGH DEGREE OF A-V BLOCK. The third and fourth QRS are ventricular escape beats for the presence of a high degree of A-V block in the transmission of atrial impulses. The second QRS (arrow) is a fusion beat between a supraventricular and an idio-ventricular impulse. The fine undulation of the baseline is due to atrial fibrillatory waves. The A-V conduction is restored in the last beats. A similar picture can be due to Digitalis toxicity.

23 - ATRIAL EXTRASYSTOLES. They are indicated by the arrows. The coupling interval is variable while the interectopic interval is constant. This suggests an atrial parasystolic focus. The first PAC is conducted with aberration to the ventricles. The second PAC presents an almost normal intraventricular conduction. The last PAC is so premature that it is blocked in the A-V junction. The compensatory pauses are incomplete.

24 - THIRD DEGREE A-V BLOCK AND SUBSIDIARY JUNCTIONAL PACEMAKER. The P waves and QRS complexes are independent. The normal morphology of the QRS's suggest that the subsidiary pacemaker is localized proximally to the bifurcation of the His bundle. A ventriculo-phasic sinus arrhythmia is present.

25 - ARTIFICIAL PACEMAKER. FIXED RATE PACING. Pacemaker impulses are recognizable with a rate of 73/minute and a complete ventricular capture. The atria are depolarized by the S-A node (rate equals 95/min.) and none of the P waves conducts to the ventricles. A third degree A-V block is present.

26 - SECOND AND THIRD DEGREE A-V BLOCK. The first three beats show a second degree A-V block of the 2:1 type. They are followed only by sinus P waves for the presence of a complete A-V block. The pause terminates with the appearance of a junctional escape beat (arrow).

27 - VENTRICULAR FIBRILLATION. The fibrillatory waves have a small amplitude and they are more difficult to be cardioverted.

28 - A-V DISSOCIATION. The first four beats are of sinus origin. They are followed by a ventricular extrasystole and by three beats with P waves overimposed on the QRS. Therefore, an A-V dissociation is present between the sinus node and the escape junctional pacemaker.

29 - CHAOTIC ATRIAL TACHYCARDIA. Numerous, rapid, irregular atrial waves are present. Some of them are conducted to the ventricles with P^1-R intervals of different lengths; others are blocked in the A-V junction. A QRS complex (middle of the tracing) is conducted with ventricular aberration. It must be kept in mind that some P^1 waves may be "echo beats". The resulting ventricular rhythm is irregular and simulate the ventricular response of an atrial fibrillation.

30 - INTERMITTENT RIGHT BUNDLE BRANCH BLOCK. The first four beats are conducted to the ventricles with a complete right bundle branch block. The following beats present an intermittent right bundle branch block (every other QRS). The sinus rate and the P-R intervals are constant in the entire tracing.

31 - JUNCTIONAL ESCAPE BEATS AND A-V DISSOCIATION. The pause following the first two sinus beats (determined by an S-A block or a marked sinus bradycardia) terminates with a junctional escape beat. A sinus beat and another junctional escape beat follow. The QRS of the escape beat (arrow) is overimposed on the sinus P wave and, therefore, during this beat an A-V dissociation is present. A sinus bradycardia follows.

32 - 2:1 S-A BLOCK. Notice the sudden halving of the cardiac rate from 75 to 32 per minute; this is due to a 2:1 S-A block which determines the two pauses within an otherwise regular cardiac cycle.

33 - WANDERING PACEMAKER. The first five beats present P^1 waves and P^1-R intervals of a "high" junctional origin. The pacemaker migrates from the junction to the S-A node (the rate is slightly faster and the morphology of the P waves is of a sinus type).

34 - JUNCTIONAL ESCAPE BEATS. An unusual trigeminal rhythm is present in this tracing. The "triplets" are formed by two sinus beats and a junctional escape beat. The latter is probably induced by the absence of a sinus impulse because of the S-A block.

35 - CORONARY SINUS RHYTHM. The tracings are continuous. They show first a transition of a coronary sinus rhythm into an atrial escape rhythm (first arrow), then into a sinus rhythm (second arrow) and, finally, in a coronary sinus rhythm (third arrow). Notice the three different configurations of the atrial activation waves.

36 - ATRIAL FLUTTER WITH VARIABLE A-V RATIO. A 2:1 block is present in the high areas of the A-V junction while a 4:3 and 3:2 Wenckebach mechanism is operating in the distal part. This determines variable A-V ratios of 4:1 and 3:1. Notice that the second QRS always shows an aberrant ventricular conduction (Ashman phenomenon) and that the ventricular rhythm changes from a trigeminy into a bigeminy.

37 - ATRIAL BIGEMINY. Notice the short P-R interval of the sinus beat (0.12 seconds) and the different morphology of the P^1 wave (coronary sinus rhythm?).

38 - FIRST DEGREE A-V BLOCK. The P-R interval is 0.28 seconds. A ventricular extrasystole is present.

39 - VENTRICULAR TACHYCARDIA. The first five beats are of a sinus origin and present a conduction with complete right bundle branch block. A ventricular extrasystole (arrow) allows the emergence of an idio-ventricular focus. P or P^1 waves are not visible and it is therefore possible that the ectopic beats conducts in a retrograde fashion to the atria.

40 - ATRIAL FLUTTER. The tracing shows a spontaneous cessation of an atrial flutter with a 2:1 A-V ratio, and a prompt restoration of sinus beats. A ventricular extrasystole follows the first sinus beat.

41 - ATRIAL FIBRILLATION AND JUNCTIONAL EXTRASYSTOLES. There is a fixed coupling of the extrasystoles with the preceding beats. The ventricular rhythm is of the bigeminal type. Only the last extrasystole follows two QRS's conducted to the ventricles. An alternative explanation is that the rhythm is of a junctional origin because of a sinus arrest (the rate would be that of the last four QRS's) and the beats with fixed coupling intervals are not extrasystoles but "echo beats" (reciprocal bigeminy).

42 - ATRIAL BIGEMINY. The coupling interval of the P^1 waves is variable and determines the different degrees of aberrant ventricular conduction of the PAC's.

43 - DEMAND PACEMAKER. QRS-SYNCHRONOUS PACING. The basic rhythm is an atrial flutter with a variable A-V conduction. All the QRS's are conducted to the ventricles from the fluttering atria and are sensed by the pacemaker. The pacer delivers an impulse which doesn't capture the ventricles because it falls 20 msec. after the beginning of the spontaneous QRS, and therefore, in the period of ventricular refractoriness.

44 - SINUS TACHYCARDIA AND ATRIAL EXTRASYSTOLES.

45 - SUPRAVENTRICULAR TACHYCARDIA. The small deflections which follow the QRS complexes may be P¹ waves of a "low" junctional tachycardia, or P¹ waves of an atrial tachycardia with a first degree A-V block.

46 - ATRIAL FLUTTER-FIBRILLATION AND VENTRICULAR PARASYSTOLE. Rapid and irregular atrial waves are present and their amplitude is between that of an atrial flutter and fibrillation. The ventricular rate is irregular. The beat indicated by the arrows are fusion beats between the atrial and the parasystolic impulses. (fourth QRS complex)

47 - DEMAND PACEMAKER. QRS-SYNCHRONOUS PACING. The great majority of QRS's are ventricular capture beats by a fixed rate pacemaker. The two arrows indicate a ventricular extrasystole and a supraventricular beat conducted to the ventricles. Both are sensed by the pacemaker which delivers an impulse in the ventricular refractory period (QRS-synchronous pacing).

48 - VENTRICULAR EXTRASYSTOLES WITH RETROGRADE CONDUCTION TO THE ATRIA. The premature beats are followed by evident P¹ waves (arrows). The ventriculo-atrial conduction time is 0.22 seconds.

49 - INTERPOLATED VENTRICULAR EXTRASYSTOLE. The sinus rhythm is not disturbed by the premature beat and the post-extrasystolic beat presents a prolonged P-R interval which indicates a concealed and retrograde penetration of the extrasystolic impulse in the A-V junction.

50 - A-V DISSOCIATION AND JUNCTIONAL RHYTHM. The first three QRS's are junctional and dissociated from the bradycardic sinus P waves. The ventricular extrasystole facilitates the passage of two sinus impulses through the A-V junction (capture beats). The A-V dissociation between the sinus and the junctional pacemakers it follows (the two arrows indicate sinus P waves too close to the QRS's to be conducted to the ventricles).

51 - ATRIAL TACHYCARDIA WITH A VARIABLE A-V BLOCK. The A-V block varies between 3:1 and 2:1.

52 - ATRIAL EXTRASYSTOLES. They have a trigeminal pattern and the second extrasystole shows a slight ventricular aberration.

53 - A-V WENCKEBACH AND INVERSE RECIPROCAL BEATS. The rhythm is sinus and the "couplets" of QRS's are determined by: (a) a sinus impulse conducted to the ventricles with a marked A-V delay (P-R equals 0.30 seconds); (b) a sinus impulse with further prolongation of the A-V conduction (P-R equals 0.52 seconds); (c) an impulse which returns to the atria and is blocked. (the "echo" P¹ waves are indicated by the arrows).

54 - RESPIRATORY SINUS ARRHYTHMIA. Notice the gradual and phasic widening and shortening of cardiac cycles with no variations of the P wave morphology and of the P-R intervals.

55 - "LOW" JUNCTIONAL RHYTHM, SINUS RHYTHM AND RE-ENTRY EXTRASYSTOLES. The first four beats are of a "low" junctional origin (the small deflections following the QRS's are P¹ waves). They are followed by three sinus beats, junctional beats and ventricular extrasystoles. The impulse of the last ventricular extrasystole is reflected in the A-V junction and returns to the ventricles.

56 - SINUS BRADYCARDIA, MULTIFOCAL EXTRASYSTOLES, A-V DISSOCIATION WITH VENTRICULAR CAPTURE BEATS. After the first extrasystole there is an emergence of a junctional escape beat which initiates an A-V dissociation. When sinus waves fall far enough from the preceding QRS's (arrows) they cross the A-V junction and conduct to the ventricles (ventricular capture beats).

57 - "MID" JUNCTIONAL TACHYCARDIA, VENTRICULAR EXTRASYSTOLES AND A-V DISSOCIATION. The upper tracing shows a rhythm of "mid" junctional origin, with a rate of 85 minute, interrupted by several ventricular extrasystoles with variable coupling intervals. The lower tracing shows the transition from a junctional into a sinus rhythm through several beats which show A-V dissociation. Endiastolic ventricular extrasystoles are present.

58 - INTRA-ATRIAL BLOCK, FIRST DEGREE A-V BLOCK AND RIGHT BUNDLE BRANCH BLOCK. The P wave is wide (0.16 seconds) and biphasic. The P-R interval is 0.30 seconds and the QRS duration is 0.12 seconds.

59 - VENTRICULAR TACHYCARDIA WITH RETROGRADE CONDUCTION TO THE ATRIA. P¹ waves follow the QRS's of the ventricular ectopic focus. The tachycardia stops suddenly and is followed by the restoration of a sinus rhythm.

60 - ATRIAL FIBRILLATION AND MULTIFOCAL VENTRICULAR EXTRASYSTOLES.

61 - FIRST DEGREE A-V BLOCK AND WENCKEBACH PHENOMENON. The clue of the arrhythmia is offered by the P wave following the ventricular extrasystole. The sinus wave, which has a markedly prolonged A-V conduction (P-R equals 0.44 seconds) initiates a 6:5 A-V Wenckebach period. The P waves are hidden in the ST segment of the preceding beats and have a very long P-R interval. The arrow indicates a blocked P wave buried in the QRS.

62 - S-A BLOCK AND S-A WENCKEBACH. The first four beats of the upper tracing show pauses due to a 2:1 S-A block (the arrow indicates a junctional escape beat which terminate one of the pauses). The following rhythm presents progressively shorter P-P intervals, until they reach a pause (S-A Wenckebach). The lower tracing presents S-A Wenckebach periods of 4:3.

63 - DEMAND PACEMAKER. QRS-INHIBITED PACING. The pacemaker delivers impulses at a fixed rate of 75/minute and with good ventricular capture. The PVC (second QRS) and the two conducted sinus beats (the third and before last QRS's) do not show an artificial impulse and allow for the identification of the type of pacing.

64 - ATRIAL TACHYCARDIA WITH ABERRANT VENTRICULAR CONDUCTION. The conduction is of a 1:1 type and the QRS complexes are aberrant and simulate salvos of ventricular tachycardia. The longer pauses, with a 3:1 A-V block, allow for a clear visualization of the atrial waves (arrows) and for the understanding of the mechanism of the arrhythmia.

65 - 3:2 A-V WENCKEBACH. The ventricular rhythm is of a bigeminal type and P waves are barely recognizable on the baseline.

66 - A-V DISSOCIATION. A sinus beat with ventricular capture is followed by a dissociation between sinus and junctional impulses (P waves first approach and are finally buried in the QRS complexes).

67 - SECOND DEGREE A-V BLOCK AND INTERMITTENT THIRD DEGREE A-V BLOCK. The first and last complexes show a second degree A-V block, Mobitz type II. Two junctional escape beats appear after a long diastolic pause due to the sudden appearance of a complete A-V block.

68 - S-A WENCKEBACH. Notice the progressive shortening of the P-P interval to the pause preceding the last beat of the tracing. The P-R interval is constant.

69 - RETROGRADE WENCKEBACH, RECIPROCAL BEATS AND RECIPROCAL RHYTHM. The tracing starts with junctional beats showing a delayed conduction to the atria. The impulse returns to the ventricles ("echo beat"). The junctional rhythm restarts with a P¹ wave which at first precedes, then is simultaneous and, finally, follows the QRS complex and determines two salvos of reciprocal beats (reciprocal rhythm).

70 - ATRIAL FLUTTER AND PROBABLE VENTRICULAR PARASYSTOLE. The A-V ratio is of a 4:1 type. The extrasystoles have a constant interectopic interval, they determine an A-V ratio of 6:1 for the concealed V-A conduction of the extrasystolic impulse.

71 - A-V DISSOCIATION AND VENTRICULAR PARASYSTOLE. The PVC's have a variable coupling interval and a constant interectopic interval; this suggests a ventricular parasystolic focus. The A-V dissociation between the sinus node and the A-V junction begins after the first ventricular ectopic beat (arrow).

72 - ATRIAL FIBRILLATION WITH ABERRANT CONDUCTION AND VENTRICULAR TACHYCARDIA. The first five QRS's are irregular and show an aberrant ventricular conduction. A salvo of seven beats of a ventricular tachycardia ceases abruptly and is followed by a brief pause which shows the fibrillatory waves (f). The first conducted beat following the pause has the advantage of a longer repolarization time and is less aberrant.

73 - ATRIAL FIBRILLATION AND VENTRICULAR PARASYSTOLE. The first tracing shows three ectopic ventricular beats, with a variable coupling interval, within the rhythm of an atrial fibrillation. The second tracing shows the real firing rate of the ventricular ectopic focus (ventricular tachycardia). The fusion beat of the third tracing (arrow) confirms the diagnosis of ventricular parasystole. Another pair of ventricular ectopic beats are present.

74 - ARTIFICIAL PACEMAKER - FIXED RATE PACING. The cardiac stimulation has a rate of 72/min. Ventricular extrasystoles are "sandwiched" between two pacemaker beats.

75 - ATRIAL TACHYCARDIA WITH 2:1 A-V BLOCK.

76 - ATRIAL ESCAPE BEATS. The atrial extrasystole (third beat) is followed by a pause and a beat with a sharply different P¹ wave. This is therefore an atrial escape beat.

77 - ATRIAL FIBRILLATION AND VENTRICULAR TACHYCARDIA. An alternative explanation is that of a junctional tachycardia with ventricular aberration.

78 - THIRD DEGREE A-V BLOCK (COMPLETE). The atrial rate is 93/minute while the ventricular rate of 30/minute and is determined by an idio-ventricular pacemaker.

79 - ATRIAL FIBRILLATION AND THIRD DEGREE A-V BLOCK (COMPLETE). The atrial fibrillatory waves are evident (f) and the ventricular rate is slow and regular. The ventricles are, in fact, activated by an idio-ventricular pacemaker for the presence of a complete A-V block.

80 - S-A BLOCK AND ATRIAL ESCAPE BEATS. The first three sinus beats are followed by a long pause, due to an S-A block, which terminates with two atrial escape beats (arrows). A sinus rhythm is then restored; only after four beats the sinus impulses are again blocked in the S-A junction. The following pause is terminated by an atrial escape beat (notice the different morphology between the escape beat P¹ waves and the sinus P wave).

81 - ATRIAL FLUTTER AND VENTRICULAR ABERRATION. The atrial flutter has a variable A-V ratio. The two aberrant beats, in the middle of the tracing, are not ventricular extrasystoles but supraventricular beats with aberrant conduction. They terminate a long-short cycle (Ashman phenomenon). At the end of the tracing another beat with slight ventricular aberration is present (11th QRS).

82 - ATRIAL FLUTTER. The tracing does not offer a good visualization of the F waves of the atrial flutter and would lead one to think of a sinus tachycardia. Two brief moments of a 4:1 A-V block clearly show the F waves and allow for the masurement of the atrial rate (270/min.). The atrial flutter has a basic 2:1 A-V ratio.

83 - CHAOTIC ATRIAL TACHYCARDIA AND JUNCTIONAL ESCAPE BEATS. P¹ waves are present, with different morphologies and different P¹-R interval. An alternative explanation suggests that the P¹ waves, indicated by the arrows, are inverse reciprocal beats (sinus beats which during their trip to the ventricles, reflect and return to the atria). Since the echo beats are markedly premature, they are not conducted to the ventricles. Two junctional escape beats terminate the pause determined by the P¹ waves blocked in the A-V junction.

84 - A-V WENCKEBACH. The first two beats close an A-V Wenckebach sequence (the second P wave is blocked). A new sequence follows, first with a shorter P-R interval and then again with a progressive delay in the A-V conduction.

85 - JUNCTIONAL RHYTHM AND A-V DISSOCIATION. The first six beats show inverted P¹ waves with P¹-R intervals of 0.08 seconds. They indicate a "high" junctional origin of the pacemaker. The ventricular extrasystole determines an A-V dissociation for the appearance of a new atrial pacemaker, (notice the tall and peaked P¹ waves in the last four beats).

86 - ATRIAL FIBRILLATION WITH A HIGH DEGREE OF A-V BLOCK. Atrial fibrillatory waves appear evident during the long asystolic pause determined by the high degree of A-V block.

87 - VENTRICULAR TRIGEMINY. The PVC's have a fixed coupling interval.

88 - ATRIAL FLUTTER-FIBRILLATION AND VENTRICULAR BIGEMINY. In a similar situation the possibility of a ventricular parasystolic focus must also be ruled out.

89 - SUPRAVENTRICULAR TACHYCARDIA.

90 - ATRIAL FLUTTER WITH A-V BLOCK VARYING FROM 4:1 to 2:1 AND PRODUC-TION OF A BIGEMINAL RHYTHM. A Wenckebach mechanism is working and the intra-ventricular conduction of every other QRS of the "couplets" is slightly aberrant.

91 - SECOND DEGREE A-V BLOCK, MOBITZ TYPE II.

92 - INTERMITTENT WOLFF-PARKINSON-WHITE SYNDROME. The "delta" waves (pre-excitatory waves) are easily recognized. They determine a short P-R interval and a wide QRS complex.

93 - VENTRICULAR EXTRASYSTOLES AND VENTRICULAR TACHYCARDIA. The extrasystoles are of the endiastolic type and with a variable coupling interval. A brief salvo of ventricular tachycardia is followed by junctional escape beats showing A-V dissociation.

94 - BIDIRECTIONAL VENTRICULAR TACHYCARDIA. Notice the alternating polarity of the ventricular ectopic beats.

95 - MULTIFOCAL PVC'S AND BLOCKED ATRIAL EXTRASYSTOLE. The blocked PAC is indicated by the arrow.

96 - THIRD DEGREE A-V BLOCK AND VENTRICULO-PHASIC SINUS AR-RHYTHMIA. The arrows indicate the irregular sinus P waves, one of which is "attracted" by the preceding QRS.

97 - ARTIFICIAL PACEMAKER. FIXED RATE PACING. Artificial stimulation at the rate of 66/min. Sinus P waves are not conducted to the ventricles for the presence of a complete A-V block.

98 - FIRST DEGREE A-V BLOCK AND LEFT BUNDLE BRANCH BLOCK. An interesting phenomenon may be observed. The ventricular extrasystole which follows the first sinus beat does not reach the atria in a retrograde fashion (as is demonstrated by the unchanged sinus rhythm). Therefore, a complete compensatory pause would be expected, but this doesn't hap-pen. This is explained by the post-extrasystolic beat which presents a shorter P-R interval and which is either a) a sinus beat with a "facilitated A-V conduction" (while other beats have a first degree A-V block) or b) a junctional escape beat which emerges before the conducted sinus P waves.

99 - ASHMAN'S PHENOMENON. The tracing presents the beginning of a paroxysmal atrial flutter. The first three QRS's of the paroxysm have an aberrant ventricular conduction, and they terminate a "long-short" cardiac cycle.

100 - ATRIAL EXTRASYSTOLE WITH PROLONGED P^1-R INTERVAL. Three atrial ex-trasystoles (third, fourth, fifth QRS) and a single atrial extrasystole (eighth QRS) clearly show a prolonged P^1-R interval when compared to the basic P-R interval.

101 - ATRIAL FIBRILLATION AND VENTRICULAR EXTRASYSTOLES. Two of the beats are premature and have a fixed coupling interval. The configuration of right bundle branch block type may suggest the possibility that the premature beats are junctional extrasystoles with ventricular aberration.

102 - DEMAND PACEMAKER. QRS-INHIBITED PACING. The potentials of the sinus beats conducted to the ventricle inhibit the pacemaker. The pacemaker fires at a fixed rate of 75/minute and is triggered after an escape interval of 800 msec.

103 - JUNCTIONAL EXTRASYSTOLES. The morphology of the extrasystoles is similar to that of sinus beats. They are not preceded by P^1 waves and are followed by sinus P waves which find the A-V junction refractory and which are blocked.

104 - ATRIAL FLUTTER WITH A STABLE 4:1 A-V RATIO.

105 - RETROGRADE WENCKEBACH AND RECIPROCAL BEAT. The first three beats show a P^1 wave which first precedes, then is buried and, finally, follows the QRS. The delay in the conduction to the atria of the third junctional impulse is such to allow for its reflection and re-entry to the ventricles ("echo beat"). The sequence tends to repeat as it can be observed in the last two QRS's.

106 - FIRST DEGREE A-V BLOCK AND BLOCKED PAC'S. The A-V conduction improves slightly in the post-extrasystolic beat.

107 - PARASYSTOLIC VENTRICULAR BIGEMINY. The first three ectopic beats are parasystolic beats with complete ventricular capture. They are followed by fusion beats with different morphology and which alternate with sinus beats. While the coupling interval is variable, the interectopic interval is constant.

108 - VENTRICULAR BIGEMINY. The pause following the first ventricular extrasystole induces the repetition of the extrasystole in the form of bigeminy. This is found quite often in the clinical practice, and particularly in subjects with sinus bradycardia, ("bigeminy rule" of Katz and Pick: "Clinical Electrocardiography: 1. "The Arrhythmias". Lean-Febiger, Philadelphia, 1956).

109 - PAROXYSMAL ATRIAL FIBRILLATION. The atrial extrasystoles which initiate the paroxysm are easily recognized.

110 - DEMAND PACEMAKER. QRS-INHIBITED PACING. The two sinus beats conducted to the ventricles inhibit the artificial stimulation. The arrow indicates a fusion beat between the sinus and the artificial impulse.

111 - VENTRICULAR PARASYSTOLE. The arrow indicates a fusion beat.

112 - ATRIAL FLUTTER WITH A CONSTANT 2:1 A-V RATIO. Some of the F waves are buried into the ST segment.

113 - ARTIFICIAL PACEMAKER. Fixed rate pacing with retrograde atrial activation. P¹ waves follow the ventricular activation complexes.

114 - SECOND DEGREE A-V BLOCK, MOBITZ TYPE II.

115 - VENTRICULAR TACHYCARDIA.

116 - VENTRICULAR EXTRASYSTOLES WITH VARIABLE COUPLING INTERVAL. The beat following the second extrasystole is a junctional escape beat which shows an A-V dissociation. (arrow).

117 - BLOCKED ATRIAL EXTRASYSTOLES.

118 - ATRIAL FIBRILLATION AND COMPLETE A-V BLOCK. Atrial fibrillatory waves are recognizable and the ventricular rate is perfectly regular. The pacemaker which controls the ventricles is located in the junction.

119 - VENTRICULAR EXTRASYSTOLES WITH REPETITIVE BEHAVIOR.

120 - INTERMITTENT THIRD DEGREE A-V BLOCK. The first two QRS complexes, with a rate of 25/min., are independent from the sinus P waves for the presence of a complete A-V block. The A-V conduction is partially re-established in the following beats (rate equals 44/min.), and the A-V block is transformed into a second degree A-V block Mobitz type II.

121 - VENTRICULAR TACHYCARDIA. The arrows indicate fusion beats at the beginning of the ventricular tachycardia. The rate of the ventricular ectopic focus is not elevated (66/min.) but it is enough to suppress the sinus rate. Sinus P waves remain undisturbed and appear like small deflections on the ST segment of the ectopic beat.

122 - VENTRICULAR TRIGEMINY AND MULTIFOCAL VENTRICULAR EXTRASYSTOLES.

123 - FIRST DEGREE A-V BLOCK AND ENDIASTOLIC VENTRICULAR EXTRASYSTOLES. The extrasystoles follow sinus P waves and suggest the presence of a parasystolic focus.

124 - A-V DISSOCIATION AND VENTRICULAR CAPTURE BEATS. Two sinus impulses cross the A-V junction and capture the ventricles (they fall 224 msec. after the junctional QRS).

125 - VENTRICULAR BIGEMINY. The ventricular extrasystoles have a fixed coupling interval.

126 - CHAOTIC ATRIAL TACHYCARDIA. Of the numerous and irregular atrial waves, only three are conducted to the ventricles. The other QRS complexes (arrows) are ventricular escape beats which follow the blocked P¹ waves.

127 - JUNCTIONAL TRIGEMINY. Two sinus beats are followed by a "high" junctional extrasystole. The premature beat indicated by the last arrow initiate a "high" junctional rhythm.

128 - FIRST DEGREE A-V BLOCK AND BLOCKED ATRIAL EXTRASYSTOLES. Notice that the P-R interval of the blocked extrasystole is shorter than other P-R intervals.

129 - A-V WENCKEBACH. Several types of Wenckebach are present (3:2, 4:3, 5:4). The blocked P waves are indicated by the arrows. The beat which is the shortest P-R interval and which initiates the Wenckebach sequence shows a first degree A-V block (P-R interval equals 0.28 sec.).

130 - ATRIAL FLUTTER-FIBRILLATION.

131 - SECOND DEGREE A-V BLOCK, VENTRICULAR TACHYCARDIA, ASYSTOLE. The atrial rate is 85/min. The first three QRS's are conducted to the ventricles with a 3:1 A-V block. They are followed by a salvo of ventricular tachycardia and by a ventricular asystole (second tracing) while the atrial rate remains unchanged and all the P waves are blocked in the A-V junction.

132 - CHAOTIC CARDIAC ACTIVITY. AGONAL TRACING.

133 - ATRIAL TACHYCARDIA WITH A 2:1 A-V CONDUCTION. The P^1 wave which conducts to the ventricles has a P^1-R interval of 0.24 sec.

134 - ATRIAL TACHYCARDIA WITH A 1:1 A-V CONDUCTION AND VENTRICULAR ABERRATION. The tracing simulates a ventricular tachycardia.

135 - MULTIFOCAL AND INTERPOLATED EXTRASYSTOLES WITH CONCEALED V-A CONDUCTION. Notice the prolongation of the P-R interval of the sinus beats which follow the extrasystoles. This indicates a concealed penetration of the extrasystolic impulse within the A-V junction.

136 - FIRST DEGREE A-V BLOCK AND ATRIAL EXTRASYSTOLES. Two P^1 waves are blocked while one conducts to the ventricles with a right bundle branch block aberration.

137 - JUNCTIONAL ESCAPE RHYTHM. An atrial extrasystole with aberrant conduction is followed by an escape "mid" junctional rhythm.

138 - ATRIAL EXTRASYSTOLES WITH ABERRANT VENTRICULAR CONDUCTION, A-V DISSOCIATION AND JUNCTIONAL RHYTHM. It can be easily noticed how the PAC's with ventricular aberration simulate ventricular extrasystoles (P^1 waves are, however, recognizable before each QRS with a right bundle branch block). The second extrasystole determines an A-V dissociation between the sinus node and the A-V junction. A salvo of three extrasystoles is followed by a slower "mid" junctional rhythm.

139 - SPONTANEOUS CESSATION OF TACHYCARDIA AND VENTRICULAR FIBRILLATION. Some junctional beats and atrial extrasystoles follow the cessation of the ventricular arrhythmia.

140 - SALVO OF VENTRICULAR TACHYCARDIA. "Three or more extrasystoles form a ventricular tachycardia." The ventricular ectopic beats are followed by small deflections which represent retrograde atrial activation.

141 - ATRIAL UNIPOLAR ELECTROGRAM. NORMAL SINUS RHYTHM.

142 - JUNCTIONAL ESCAPE BEATS. The third beat is an atrial extrasystole and it is followed, after an asystolic interval of two seconds, by two junctional escape beats and by the restoration of a bradycardic sinus rhythm.

143 - JUNCTIONAL RHYTHM WITH RETROGRADE WENCKEBACH AND RECIPROCAL BEATS. The two tracings show the P^1 waves of a junctional focus which first precede, then are buried and, finally, follow the QRS allowing for the reflection of the impulse and ventricular capture ("echo beats").

144 - INVERSE RECIPROCAL RHYTHM. The second QRS is of a "low" junctional origin and with a delayed conduction to the atria (R-P^1 equals 0.26 seconds). The three beats with aberrant conduction in the middle of the tracing originate from the preceding sinus beats with impulses reflecting to the atria and the ventricles. They originate a brief sequence of an inverse reciprocal rhythm. The aberration is due to the "Ashman phenomenon".

145 - RECIPROCAL BIGEMINY OR A-V DISSOCIATION WITH VENTRICULAR CAP-TURE BIGEMINY? The diagnostic dilemma cannot be solved with such a short tracing and both possibilities are valid. In reciprocal bigeminy the pacemaker is situated in the A-V junction and the impulse travels with delay to the atria. This permits the "reflection" and the re-entry of the impulse to the ventricles ("echo beats"). In A-V dissociation with ventricular capture bigeminy, a sinus and a junctional pacemakers are simultaneously present and dissociated. Since the rates are very close the dissociation is isorhythmic. The dissociated sinus P waves fall far enough from the junctional QRS and capture the ventricles.

146 - ATRIAL TACHYCARDIA WITH A-V WENCKEBACH PHENOMENON. Notice the "group beating" of the upper tracing (L2). The better visualization in L2 of the P¹ waves and the P¹-R intervals allows for a precise identification of the mechanism of the arrhythmia.

147 - INTERMITTENT LEFT BUNDLE BRANCH BLOCK. There is a slight increase in the cardiac rate from 140/min. to 150/min. (critical cardiac rate) and this is sufficient to determine a block in the conduction of the left bundle. The aberrantly conducted beat simulate a ventricular tachycardia.

148 - INTERMITTENT RIGHT BUNDLE BRANCH BLOCK. The intraventricular conduction disturbance appears without any modification of the sinus rate. The P-P intervals and the P-R intervals remain constant throughout the tracing.

149 - PAROXYSMAL ATRIAL TACHYCARDIA AND ASHMAN PHENOMENON. The beats indicated by the arrows are of sinus origin and with a normal ventricular conduction. They are followed by a paroxysmal atrial tachycardia with aberrant ventricular conduction.

150 - PAROXYSMAL ATRIAL TACHYCARDIA WITH 2:1 A-V BLOCK. The first three beats are of sinus origin. The atrial extrasystole indicated by the arrow initiates a paroxysm of PAT.

151 - JUNCTIONAL RHYTHM AND RECIPROCAL BEATS. The "echo beats" are indicated by the arrows. The junctional impulses show a progressive delay in the conduction to the atria (retrograde Wenckebach phenomenon).

152 - BIGEMINAL RHYTHM AND S-A WENCKEBACH. The beats are grouped in couplets. The P waves and the P-R intervals are constant and equal. The pause is determined by a sinus impulse blocked in the S-A junction and which does not appear on the tracing (third impulse of 3:2 S-A Wenckebach). This type of rhythm may be mistaken for atrial bigeminy.

153 - ATRIAL TACHYCARDIA AND THIRD DEGREE A-V BLOCK. The atrial rate is 130/min. The ventricular rate is 28/min. The P¹ waves are totally independent from the idio-ventricular QRS's.

154 - BLOCKED ATRIAL EXTRASYSTOLES. Two blocked PAC's are easily recognized with P¹ waves buried into the ST segment of the preceding beats and followed by a ventricular ex-trasystole.

155 - PAROXYSMAL ATRIAL FLUTTER. Two atrial extrasystoles heralds the appearance of a flutter. Note that an identical sequence of PAC's initiates the paroxysm. The first three beats of the flutter present a 1:1 A-V conduction and an A-V Wenckebach mechanism.

REFERENCES

BOOKS

Hoffman, B. F., and Cranefield P. F.: « *Electrophysiology of the Heart* », McGraw-Hill, New York, 1960.

Katz, L. N., and Pick, A.: « *Clinical Electrocardiography: I. The Arrhythmias,* » Lea and Febiger, Philadelphia, 1956.

Bellet, S.: « *Clinical Disorders of the Heart Beat,* » 2d ed., Lea and Febiger, Philadelphia, 1963.

Dreifus, L. S., Likoff, W., and Moyer J.H.: « *Mechanisms and Therapy of Cardiac Arrhythmias,* » Grune and Stratton, New York and London, 1966.

Prinzmetal, M., Corday, E., Brill, I.C., Oblath, R.W., and Kruger, H.E.: « *The Auricular Arrhythmias,* » Charles C. Thomas, Pubblisher, Springfield, Ill., 1952.

Scherf, D., and Cohen, J.: « *The Atrioventricular Node and Selected Cardiac Arrhythmias,* » Grune and Stratton, Inc., New Yorkk, 1964.

Greenwood, R.J., and Finkelstein, D.: « *Sinoatrial Heart Block,* » Charles C. Thomas, Publisher, Springfield, Ill., 1964.

Siddons, H., and Sowton, E.: « *Cardiac Pacemakers* », Charles C. Thomas, Illinois, 1967.

Hurst J.W. and Logue R.B.: « *The Heart* », New York, McGraw-Hill Co., 1970.

Thalen, H.J.Th., Van Den Berg, J.W., Homan Van Der Heide, J.N., and Nieveen, J.: « *The Artificial Cardiac Pacemaker* », Netherlands, Charles C. Thomas, 1969.

Marshall, R.J., and Shepherd, J.T.: « *Cardiac Function In Health and Disease* », Philadelphia, W.B. Saunders Co., 1968.

Zimmerman, H.A., Bersano, E., and Dicosky, C.: «*The Auricular Electrocardiogram* », Illinois, Charles C. Thomas, 1968.

Lindsay, A.E., and Budkin, A.: « *The Cardiac Arrhythmias* », Chicago, Year Book Medical Publishers, Inc., 1969.

Burch, G.E., and Winsor, T.: « *A Primer of Electrocardiography* », P᠎ ᠎delphia, Lea and Febiger, 1966.

De Carvalho, A.P., De Mello, W.C., and Hoffman, B.F.: « *The Specialized Tissues of the Heart* », Amsterdam, Elsevier Publishing Co., 1961.

Chou, T., and Helm, R.A.: « *Clinical Vectorcardiography* », New York, Grune and Stratton, 1967.

Zimmerman, H.A.: « *Intravascular Catherization* », Illinois, Charles C. Thomas, 1966.

PAPERS

Arrhythmias secondary to abnormal impulse formation

Hoffman, B. F., and Cranefield, P. F.: *The Physiological Basis of Cardiac Arrhythmias, Am. J. Med., 37:670, 1964.*

Pick, A., Langendorf, R., and Katz, L. N.: *Depression of Cardiac Pacemakers by Premature Impulses, Am. Heart J., 41:49, 1951.*

Mounsey, P.: Intensive Coronary Care: *Arrthythmias after Acute Myocardial Infarction, Am. J. Cardiol., 20:475, 1967.*

Scherf, D.: *The Mechanism and Treatment of Extrasystoles, Progr. Cardiovas. Dis., 2:370, 1960.*

Stock, E., Goblee, A., and Sloman, G.: *Assessment of Arrhythmias in Myocardial Infarction, Brit. M. J., 1:719, 1967.*

Kistin, A., and Landowne, M.: *Retrograde Conduction from Premature Ventriculare Contractions, a Common Occurrence in the Human Heart, Circulation, 3:738, 1951.*

Surawicz, B., and MacDonald, M.G.: *Ventriculare Ectopic Beats and Fixed and Variable Coupling: Incidence, Clinical Significance and Factors Influencing the Coupling Interval, Am. J. Cardiol., 13:198, 1964.*

Meltzer, L. E., and Kitchell, J.B.: *The Incidence of Arrhythmias Associated with Acute Myocardial Infarction, Progr. Cardiovas. Dis., 9:50, 1966.*

Soloff, L.A.: *Ventricular Premature Beats Diagnostic of Myocardial Disease, Am. J. M. Sc., 242:315, 1961.*

Smirk, F.H., and Palmer, D.G.: *A Myocardial Syndrome, with Particular Reference to the Occurrence of Sudden Death and of Premature Systoles Interrupting Antecedent T Waves, Am. J. Cardiol., 6:620, 1960.*

Sandler, I.A., and Marriott, H.J.L.: *The Differential Morphology of Anomalous Ventricular Complexes of RBBB-type in Lead V1: Ventricular Ectopy versus Aberration, Circulation, 31:551, 1965.*

Bisteni, A., Medrano, G.A., and Sodi-Pallares, D.: *Ventricular Premature Beats in the Diagnosis of Myocardial Infarction, Brit. Heart J., 23:521, 1961.*

Langendorf, R., Pick, A., and Winternitz, M.: *Mechanism of Intermittent Ventricular Bigeminy: I. Appearance of Ectopic Beats Dependent upon Length of the Ventricular Cycle, the « Rule of Bigeminy, » Circulation, 11:422, 1955.*

Benchimol, A., Lasry, J.E., and Carvalho, F. R.: *The Ventricular Premature Contraction: Its Place in the Diagnosis of Ischemic Heart Disease, Am. Heart J., 65:334, 1963.*

Lown, B., Wyatt, N.F., and Levine, H.D.: *Paroxysmal Atrial Tachycardia with Block, Circulation, 21:129, 1960.*

Shine, K.I., Kastor, J.A. and Yurchak, P.M.: *Multifocal Atrial Tachycardia: Clinical and Electocardiographic Features in Thirty-two Cases, Circulation, 36 (suppl. II): 236, 1967.*

Lown, B., Marcus, F., and Levine, H.D.: *Digitalis and Atrial Tachycardia with Block: A Year's Experience, New England J. Med., 260:301, 1959.*

Marriott, H.J.L.: *Nodal Mechanisms with Dependent Activation of Atria and Ventricles, in L.S. Dreifus, and W. Likoff (eds.), « Mechanisms and Therapy of Cardiac Arrhythmias, » Grune and Stratton, Inc., New Yorkk, 1966, pp. 412-418.*

Bellet, S.: *Diagnostic Features and Management of Supraventricular Arrhythmias, Progr. Cardiovas. Dis., 8:483, 1966.*

Lown, B. and Levine, H.D.: *P. Atrial Arrhytmias, Digitalis and Potassium. New York, Landsberger Medical Books, Inc., 1958.*

Lown, B., Marcus, F. and Levine H.D.: *Digitalis and atrial tachycardia with block. A year's experience. N. Eng. J. Med. 260:301, 1959.*

Lown, B., Wyatt, N.F. and Levine, H.D.: *Clinical progress. Paroxysmal atrial tachycardia with block. Circulation 21:129, 1960.*

Jewitt, D.E., Balcon, R., Raftery, E.B., and Oram, S.: *Incidence and Management of Supraventricular Arrhythmias after Acute Myocardial Infarction, Lancet, 2:734, 1967.*

Goble, A.J., Sloman, G., and Robinson, J.S.: *Mortality Reduction in a Coronary Gare Unit, Brit. M. J., 1:1005, 1966.*

J.W. Linhart and G.A. Pupillo: *Supraventricular tachycardias: treatment by electrical pacing of the right atrium and ventricle (presentato per pubblicazione).*

Fosmoe, R.J., Averill, K.H., and Lamb, L.E.: *Electro-cardiographic Findings in 67,375 Asymptomatic Subjects: II. Supraventricular Arrhythmias, Am. J. Cardiol., 6:84, 1960.*

Morgan, W.L., and Breneman, G. M.: *Atrial Tachycardia with Block Treated with Digitalis, Circulation, 25:787, 1962.*

Kissane, R. W., Brooks, R., and Clark, T.E.: *Relation of Supraventricular Paraoxysmal Tachycardia to Heart Disease and the Basal Metabolic Rate, Circulation, 1:950, 1950.*

Freirmuth, L. J., and Jick, S.: *Paroxysmal Atrial Tachycardia with Atrioventricular Block, Am. J. Cardiol., 1:584, 1958.*

Irons, G.V., and Orgain, E.S.: *Digitalis-induced Arrhythmias and Their Management, Profr. Cardiovas. Dis., 8:539, 1966.*

Scherf, D., Romano, F.J., and Terranova, R.: *Experimental Studies on Auricular Flutter and Fibrillation, Am. Heart J., 36:241, 1948.*

Delman, A.J., and Stein, E.: *Atrial Flutter Secondary to Digitalis Toxicity, Circulation, 29:593, 1964.*

Halmos, P.B.: *Direct Current Conversion of Atrial Fibrillation, Brit. Heart J., 28:302, 1966.*

Culler, M.R., Boone, J.A. and Gazes, P.C.: *Fibrillatory Wave Size as a Clue to Etiological Diagnosis, Am. Heart J., 66:435, 1963.*

Gouaux, J.L., and Ashman, R.: *Auricular Fibrillation with Aberration Simulating Ventricular Paroxysmal Tachycardia, Am. Heart J., 34:366, 1947.*

Thurmann, M., and Janney, J.G.: *The Diagnostic Importance of Fibrillatory Wave Size, Circulation, 25: 991, 1962.*

Rosselot, E., Haque M., and Vyden J.K., and al.: *Paradoxically Narrow Ectopic Beats, The New Physician, February, 1969.*

Haft, J.I., Lau, S.H., and Stein, E., and al.: *Atrial Fibrillation Produced by Atrial Stimulation, Circulation, 37:70, 1968.*

Vyden, J.K., Allen, H.N., and Gale, L.A., and al.: *Spontaneous Reversal of Ventricular Fibrillation, The New Physician, April, 1969.*

Delman, A.J., Robinson, G., and Stein, E., and al.: *Precise Determination of Cardiac Arrhythmias During Open Heart Surgery by Monitoring of Myocardial Electrograms, Am. J. Cardiol., 21:714, 1968.*

Kastor, J.A., and Yurchak, P.M.: *Recognition of Digitalis Intoxication in the Presence of Atrial Fibrillation, Annals of Internal Medicine, 67:1045, 1967.*

Hoffman, B.F. and Singer, D.H.: *Effects of Digitalis on Electrical Activity of Cardiac Fibers, Progr. Cardiovas. Dis., 7:226, 1964.*

Stibitz, G.R., and Rytank, D.A.: *On the Path of the Excitation Wave in Atrial Flutter, Circulation, 37:75, 1968.*

Cohen, H.E., Kahn, M., and Donoso, E.: *Treatment of Supraventricular Tachycardias with Catheter and Permanent Pacemakers, Am. J. Cardiol., 20:735, 1967.*

Enescu, V., Boszormenyi, E., and Utsu, F., and al.: *A-V Nodal Rhythm and Wandering Pacemaker During Anesthesia, The New Physician, January, 1966.*

Enescu, V., Boszormenyi, E., and Utsu, F., and al.: *Atrial Premature Beats, Paroxysmal Atrial Flutter, and Fibrillation, The New Physician, March, 1966.*

Haque, M., Protopapas, T., and Vyden, J.K., and al.: *High, Mid and Low Nodal Rhythm, The New Physician, January, 1968.*

Langendorf, R., Pick, A., and Katz, L.N.: *Ventricular Response in Atrial Fibrillation, Circulation, 32:69, 1965.*

Pick, A.: *Arrhythmias and Potassium in Man, Am. Heart J., 72:295, 1966.*

Hurst, J.W., and Myerburg, R.J.: Cardiac Arrhythmias: Evolving Concepts (II), Mod. Con. of Cardiovascular Disease, 37:79, 1968.

Hurst, J.W.: *Arrhythmias in Context, Hospital Practice, July, 1967.*

Imperial, E.S., Carballo, R. and Zimmerman, H.A.: *Disturbances of Rate, Rhythm and Conduction in Acute Myocardial Infarction, Am. J. Cardiol., 5:24, 1960.*

Ambrust, C.A., and Levine, S.A.: *Paroxysmal Ventricular Tachycardia: A Study of One Hundred and Seven Cases, Circulation, 1:28, 1950.*

Cohn, L.J., Donoso, E., and Friedberg, C.K.: *Ventricular Tachycardia, Prog. Cardiovas, Dis., 9:29, 1966.*

Lesch, M., Lewis, E., Humphries, J.O., and Ross, R.S.: *Paroxysmal Ventricular Tachycardia in the Absence of Organic Heart Disease: Report of a Case and Review of the Literature, Ann. Int. Med., 66:950, 1967.*

Gianelly, R., Griffin, J.R., and Harrison, D.C.: *Propranolol in the Treatment and Prevention of Cardiac Arrhythmias, Ann. Int. Med., 66:667, 1967.*

Schrire, V. and Vogelpoel, L.: *The Clinical and Electrocardiographic Differentiation of Supraventricular and Ventricular Tachycardias with Regular Rhythm, Am. Heart J., 49:162, 1955.*

Dressler, W., and Roesler, H.: *The Occurrence in Paroxysmal Ventricular Tachycardia of Ventricular Complexes Transitional in Shape to Sinoauricular Beats, Am. Heart J., 44:485, 1952.*

Kistin, A.D.: *Retrograde Conduction to the Atria in Ventricular Tachycardia, Circulation, 24:236, 1961.*

Stock, J.P.P.: *Repetitive Paroxysmal Ventricular Tachycardia, Brit. Heart J., 24:297, 1962.*

De Sanctis, R.: *Electrical Conversion of Ventricular Tachycardia, J.A.M.A., 191:632, 1965.*

Castellanos, A.: *The Genesis of Bidirectional Tachycardia, Am. Heart J., 61:733, 1961.*

Gianelly, R., von der Groeben, J.O., Spivack, A.P., and Harrison, D.C.: *Effect of Lidocaine on Ventricular Arrhythmias in Patients with Coronary Heart Disease, New England J. Med., 277:1215, 1967.*

Cohen, L.S., Buccino, R.A., Morrow, A.G., and Braunwald, E.: *Recurrent Ventricular Tachycardia and Fibrillation Treated with a Combination of Beta-adrenergic Blockade and Electrical Pacing, Ann. Int. Med., 66:945, 1967.*

Pick, A., and Langendorf, R.: *Differentiation of Supraventricular and Ventricular Tachycardias, Progr. Cardiovas. Dis., 2:391, 1960.*

Arrhythmias secondary to abnormal impulse conduction

Lister, J.W., Stein, E., Kosowsky, B.D., Lau, S.H., and Domato, A.N.: *Atrioventricular Conduction in Man: Effect of Rate, Exercise, Isoproterenol and Atropine on the P-R Interval, Am. J. Cardiol., 16:516, 1965.*

Penton, G.B., Miller, H., and Levine, S.A.: *Some Clinical Features of Complete Heart Block, Circulation, 13:801, 1956.*

Zoob, M., and Smith, K.S.: *The Aetiology of Complete Heart-block, Brit. M. J., 2:1149, 1963.*

Lev, M.: *The Pathology of Complete Atrioventricular Block, Progr. Cardiovas. Dis., 6:317, 1964.*

Lemberg, L., Castellanos, A., and Berkovits, B.V.: *Pacemaking on Demand in AV Block, J.A.M.A., 191:12, 1965.*

Scherf, D., Cohen, J., and Orphanos, R.: *Retrograde Activation of Atria in Atrioventricular Block, Am. J. Cardiol.*, 13:219, 1964.

Jackson, A.E., and Bashour, F.A.: *Cardiac Arrhythmias in Acute Myocardial Infarction: I. Complete Heart Block and Its Natural History, Dis. Chest,* 51:31, 1967.

Lown, B.: *in «Cardiac Pacing and Cardioversion,» Charles Press, Philadelphia, 1967, p. 7.*
Harris, A., and Bluestone, R.: Treatment of Slow

Scott, M.E., Geddes, J.S., Patterson, G.C., Adgey, A.A.J., and Pantridge, J.F.: *The Management of Complete Heart Block Complicating Acute Myocardial Infarction, Lancet,* 2:1382, 1967.

Arrhythmias secondary to abnormal impulse formation and conduction

Marriott, H.J.L., Schubart, A.F., and Bradley, S. M.: *A-V Dissociation: A Re-appraisal, Am. J. Cardiol.*, 2:586, 1958.

Marriott, H.J.L., and Menendez, M.M.: *A-V Dissociation Revisited, Progr. Cardiovas, Dis.,* 8:522, 1966.

Castellanos, A., Azan, L., and Calvino, J.M.: *Dissociation with Interference between Pacemakers Located within the A-V Conducting System, Am. Heart J.,* 56:562, 1958.

Pick, A.: Dissociation: *A Proposal for a Comprehensive Classification and Consistent Terminology, Am. Heart J.,* 66:147, 1963.
Miller, R., and Sharrett, R. H.: Interference Dissociation, *Circulation,* 16:803, 1957.

Marriott, H.J.L.: *Atrioventricular Synchronization and Accrochage, Circulation,* 14:38, 1956.

Hwang, W., and Langendorf, R.: *Auriculoventricular Nodal Escape in the Presence of Auricular Fibrillation, Circulation,* 1:930, 1950.

Moe, G.K., and Mendez, C.: *The Physiologic Basis of Reciprocal Rhythm, Progr. Cardiovas. Dis.,* 8:461, 1966.

Bix, H.H.: *Various Mechanisms in Reciprocal Rhythm, Am. Hearth J.,* 41:448, 1951.

Marriott, H.P.L.: *Personal Communication, 1970.*

Moe, G.K., Preston, J.B., and Burlington, H.: *Physiologic evidence for a dual A-V transmission system. Circulation Research* 4:357, 1956.

Hoffman, B. F., Moore, E.N., Stuckey, J., and Cranefield, P.F.: *Functional properties of the atrioventricular conduction system. Circulation Research* 13: 308, 1963.

Cohen, S.I., Lau, S.H., Haft, J.I., and Damato, A.N.: *Experimental production of aberrant ventricular conduction in man. Circulation* 36:673, 1967.
Heart Rates Following Acute Myocardial Infarction, Brit. Heart J., 28:631, 1966.

Scherf, D., and Bornemann, C.: *Parasystole with a Rapid Ventricular Center, Am. Heart J.,* 62:320, 1961.
Schamroth, L.: *Ventricular Parasystole with Slow Manifest Ectopic Discharge, Brit. Heart J.,* 24:731, 1962.

Scherf, D., Bornemann, C., and Yildiz, M.: *A-V Nodal Parasystole, Am. Heart J.,* 60:179, 1960.

Scherf, D., Yildiz, M., and De Armas, D.: *Atrial Parasystole, Am. Heart J.,* 57:507, 1959.

Scherf, D., and Boyd, L.J.: *Three Unusual Cases of Parasystole, Am. Heart J.,* 39:650, 1950.

Corday, E., and Vyden, J.K.: *Resuscitation after Myocardial Infarction: A Clinical Appraisal, J.A.M.A.,* 200:781, 1967.

Javier, R.P., Narula, O.S., Samet, P.: *Atrial Tachysystole (Flutter?) with Apparent Exit Block, Circulation,* 40:179, 1969.

Pick, A.: *Electrocardiographic features of exit block. In Mechanisms and Therapy of Cardiac Arrhythmias: Fourteenth Hahnemann Symposium, edited by L. S. Dreifus and W. Likoff. New York, Grune and Stratton, Inc., 1966, p. 469.*

Hiss, R.G. and Lamb, L.E.: *Electrocardiographic findings in 122,043 individuals. Circulation* 25:947, 1962.

Wolff, L.: *Anomalous atrio-ventricular excitation (Wolff-Parkinson-White syndrome). Circulation* 19:14, 1959.

Sears, G.A. and Manning, G.W.: *The Wolff-Parkinson-White pattern in routine electrocardiography. Canad. Med. Ass. J.* 87:1213, 19622.

Langendorf, R., Lev. M. and Pick, A.: *Auricular fibrillation with anomalous A-V excitation (WPW syndrome) imitating ventricular paroxysmal tachycardia. A case report with clinical and autopsy findings and critical review of the literature. Acta Cardiol.* 7:241, 1952.

MISCELLANEOUS

S.S. Barold, G.A. Pupillo, J.J. Gaidula and J. W. Linhart: *Chest wall stimulation in tre evaluation of patients with implanted ventricular inhibited demand pacemakers. British Heart Journal* 33:783, 1970.

A.J. Trevino, B.M. Beller, R.C. Talley, J.W. Linhart, and G.A. Pupillo: *Chest wall stimulation: a method of demand QRS blocking pacemaker suppression in the study of arrhythmias. American Heart Journal* 81: 20, 1971.

J.W. Linhart, and G.A. Pupillo: *Left ventricular enddiastolic pressure elevation in angina pectoris with normal left ventricular function. American Heart Journal (accettato per pubblicazione).*

Rosenbaum, M., and Lepeschkin, E.: *The Effect of Ventricular Systole on Auricular Rhythm in Auriculoventricular Block, Circulation,* 11: 240, 1955.

Nathan, D.A., Samet, P., Center, S. and Wu, C.Y.: *Long-term correction of complete heart block. Clinical and physiologic studies of a new tlpe of implantable synchronous pacer. Prog. Cardiov. Dis.* 6:538, 1964.

Chardack, W.M., Gage, A.A., and Greatbatch, W.: *A transistorized, self-contained implantable pacemaker for the long-term correction of complete heart block. Surgery* 48:643, 1960.

Sowton, E.: *Ventricular-triggered pacemakers: Clinical experience, Brit. Heart J.* 30:363, 1968.

Nathan, D.A., Center, S., Wu, C.Y., and Keller, W.: *An implantable, synchronous pacemaker for the longterm correction of complete heart block, Circulation* 27:682, 1963.

Chardack, W.M., Gage, A.A., and Greatbatch, W.: *Correction of complete heart block by a self-contained and subcutaneously implanted pacemaker. J. Thoracic and Cardiovas. Surg.* 42:814, 1961.

Brown, W.H.: *A study of the esophageal lead in clinical electrocardiography. Amer. Heart J.* 12:1, 1936.

Hellerstein, H.K., Prichard. W.H. and Lewis, R.L.: *Recording of intracavitary potentials through a single lumen saline filled catheter. Pro. Soc. Exp. Biol. Med.* 71:58, 1949.

Fohman, L.R. and Williams, H.M.: *Percutaneous right heart catheterization using polyethylene tubing. Amer. J. Cardiol.* 4:373-378, 1959.

Vogel, H.H.K., Tabari, K., Averill, K.H. and Blount, S.F., Jr.: *A simple method for identifying P. waves in complex arrhythmias. Amer. Heart J. 67:158-167, 1964.*

Kistin A.D. and Bruce, J.C.: *Simultaneous esophageal and standard electrocardiographic leads for the study of cardiac arrhythmias. Amer. Heart J. 53:65, 1957.*

Copeland, G.D., Tullis, I.F. and Brody, D.A.: *Clinical evaluation of a new esophageal electrode, with particular reference to the bipolar esophageal electrocardiogram. Amer. Heart J. 57:862, 874, 1959.*

Manuel, C. J., Avanz, C.L. and Castellanos, A., Jr.: *Valor de las derivaciones esofàgicas en las arritmias complejas. Rev. Cubana Cardiol. 16:293, 1955.*

Scherlag, B.J., Lau, S.H., Helfant, R.H., Berkowitz, W.D., Stein, E., and Damato, A.N.: *Catheter technique for recording His bundle activity in man. Circulation 39:13, 1969.*

Damato, A.N., Lau, S.H., Berkowitz, W.D., Rosen, K.M., and Lisi, K.R.: *Recording of specialized conducting fibers (A-V nodal, His bundle, and right bundle branch) in man using an electrode catheter technic. Circulation 39:435, 1969.*

Gold, H., and Corday, E.: *Vasopressor Therapy in the Cardiac Arrhythmias, New England J. Med., 260: 1151, 1959.*

Moss, A.J., and Aledort, L.M.: *Use of Edrophonium (Tensilon) in the Evaluation of Supraventricular Tachycardias, Am. J. Cardiol., 17:58, 1966.*

Lown, B., Perlroth, M. G., Kaidbey, S., Abe, T. and Harken, D.E.: *«Cardioversion» of atrial fibrillation: A report on the treatment of 65 episodes in 50 patients. New Eng. J. Med. 269:325, 1963.*

Lown, B.: *«Cardioversion» of arrhythmias. Mod. Conc. Cardiov. Dis. 33:863-873, 1964.*

Morris, J.J., Kong, Y., North, W.C. and McIntosh, H.D.: *Experience with «cardioversion» of atrial fibrillation and flutter. Amre. J. Cardiol. 14:94, 1964.*

Lown, B., Amarasingham, R. and Neuman, J.: *New method for terminating cardiac arrhythmias. Use of synchronized capacitor discharge. J.A.M.A. 182:548, 1962.*

Rodensky, P.L. and Wasserman, F.: *Esophageal electrocardiography. Selected clinical applications. Amer. Heart J. 64:444, 1962.*

Gilbert, R., Eich, R.H., Smulyan, H., Keighley, J. and Auchincloss, J.H., Jr.: *Effect on circulation of conversion of atrial fibrillation to sinus rhythm. Circulation 227:1079, 1963.*

Broch, O.J. and Muller, O.: *Hemodynamic studies during auricular fibrillation and after restoration of sinus rhythm. Brit. Heart J. 19:222, 1957.*

Sarnoff, S.J. and Mitchell, J.H.: *The regulation of the performance of the Heart. Amer. J. Med. Med. 30:747, 1961.*

Braunwald, E., Frye, R.L., Aygen, M.M. and Gilbert, J.W., Jr.: *Studies on Starling's Law of the heart. III. Observations in patients with mitral stenosis and atrial fibrillation on the relationships between left veitricular end diastolic segment, length, filling pressure, and the characteristics of ventricular contraction J. Clin. Invest. 39:1874, 1960.*

Ferrer, M.I. and Harvey, R.M.: *The value of converting atrial fibrillation to normal sinus rhythm. Amer. Heart J. 68:725, 1964.*

Samet, P., Bernstein, W. and Levine, S.: *Significance of the atrial contribution to ventricular filling. Amer. J. Cardiol. 15:195, 1965.*

Sarnoff, S.J., Gilmore, J.P. and Mitchell, J.H.: *Influence of atrial contraction and relaxation on closure of mitral valve. Circ. Res. 11:26, 1962.*

Skinner, N. S., Jr., Mitchell, J.H. and Wallace, A.G.: *Hemodynamic effect of altering the placement of atrial systole. Clin. Res. 10:180, 1962.*

Mitchell, J.H., Gilmore, J.P. and Sarnoff, S.J.: *The transport function of the atrium. Factors influencing the relation between mean left atrial pressure and left ventricular end diastolic pressure. Amer. J. Cardiol. 9:237, 1962.*

Ferrer, M.I. and Harvey, R.: *Some hemodynamic aspects of cardiac arrhythmias in man. Amer. Heart J. 68:153-165, 1964.*

Nakano, J.: *Effects of atrial and ventricular tachycardias on the cardiovascular dynamics. Amer. J. Physiol. 206:547-552, 1964.*

Wégria, R., Frank, C.W., Wang, H.H. and Lammerant, J.: *The effect of atrial and ventricular tachycardia on cardiac output, coronary blood flow and mean atrial blood pressure. Circ. Res. 6:624-632, 1958.*

Bevegard, S.: *Observations on the effect of varying ventricular rates on the circulation at rest and during exercise in two patients with an artificial pacemaker. Acta Med. Scand. 172-615, 1962.*